D1239237

CLINICAL PODOGERIATRICS

CLINICAL PODOGERIATRICS

ARTHUR E. HELFAND, D.P.M.
Editor

Professor and Chairman, Department of Community Health
Pennsylvania College of Podiatric Medicine
Philadelphia, Pennsylvania
Chief, Department of Podiatry and Director of Podiatric Education
James C. Guiffré Medical Center
Philadelphia, Pennsylvania
Adjunct Professor of Medicine, Jefferson Medical College
Thomas Jefferson University and Thomas Jefferson University Hospital
Philadelphia, Pennsylvania
Member, Technical Committee on Health Services, 1981
White House Conference on Aging

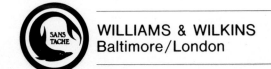

WILLIAMS & WILKINS
Baltimore/London

Copyright ©, 1981
Williams & Wilkins
428 East Preston Street
Baltimore, MD 21202, U.S.A.

Made in the United States of America

Library of Congress Cataloging in Publication Data

Main entry under title:

Clinical podogeriatrics.

   Bibliography: p.
   Includes index.
   1. Podiatry. 2. Geriatrics. I. Helfand, Arthur E.
RD563.C64   618.97′7585   80-21582
ISBN 0-683-03951-2

Composed and printed at the
Waverly Press, Inc.
Mt. Royal and Guilford Aves.
Baltimore, MD 21202, U.S.A.

Dedication

To the people I love

My wife, Myra,
My children, Jennifer Bess and Lewis Aaron
My parents, Nathan and Esther Helfand

Foreword

My initial contact with Dr. Helfand was while he was a student at Temple University. He demonstrated a keen interest in clinical knowledge and research and, following his residencies at our hospital, he joined our staff. He assisted in the development of our podiatry clinic and residency program and demonstrated an interest in the foot problems of our elderly population. Between 1962 and 1965, Dr. Helfand directed the first clinical research project to be funded by the Federal Government, in cooperation with the Philadelphia Department of Public Health. The project, called "Keep Them Walking," produced much data which clearly identified the foot health and care needs of the elderly.

His efforts were recognized early as he served as a consultant for "Feet First" and completed the initial chapter on foot problems for the elderly in a major manual developed by the Gerontological Society, again sponsored by the Public Health Service. He served as a Founder of the Pennsylvania College of Podiatric Medicine, was an initial faculty appointee and served as its first Clinical Director to establish the College's clinical teaching program. His direction of a subsequent longitudinal study of the elderly at the South Mountain Restoration Center in cooperation with the Pennsylvania Department of Public Welfare again demonstrated the special foot care needs of the elderly.

His contributions to the literature have been significant with major segments devoted to the elderly and diabetic patient. His didactic and clinical approach has always maintained an educational and public health base in an effort to deliver a quality service within reasonable cost boundaries.

Dr. Helfand established the first podiatric services at Thomas Jefferson University Hospital and brought his efforts to the professional schools in the disciplines of podiatry, pharmacy, medicine, nursing and public health.

Calling on his background and experience, Dr. Helfand has enlisted the knowledge of a multidisciplinary group of guest authors from most of the health fields dealing with the care of the elderly. Their end result has been the evolution of a text that provides a realistic and compassionate approach to the principles of foot care for the elderly which is most practical.

The need to maintain an ambulatory population is most significant when applied to the elderly. The social implications of immobility are segregation and institutionalization. Perhaps the phrase that has been used so many times, i.e., Keep Them Walking, still needs to be heard in louder tones by those who establish health care programs for the elderly. Foot care is many times not included, thus eliminating not only a comprehensive approach to care but a vital multidisciplinary element.

We are most pleased that our Hospital has had a part to play in the development of this text and to note that its editor and many guest authors practice together. The close family that we have at our institution is well reflected in this text which we know will benefit many health care providers and the patients they serve.

We congratulate those who have undertaken this major work and look forward to improved health care for our elderly.

JAMES C. GIUFFRÉ, M.D.
Executive and Medical Director
Chairman, Division of Surgery
James C. Giuffré Medical Center
Philadelphia, Pennsylvania

Preface

Podogeriatrics can be defined, in the broadest clinical sense, as that segment of health service which concerns itself with the human foot and aging. One should recognize that our ultimate responsibility lies in the care of the elderly and that the foot is but just one part of that total and comprehensive approach. We must always remember that the head bone is connected to the foot bone and that a multidisciplinary approach is needed particularly when we consider the aged.

Why should we really care about the elderly anyway? True, there are more old people today and there will be even more tomorrow. But are their complaints and concerns real or do we as practitioners merely provide a service to keep people calm in their declining years? In order to answer this question, we must ask, "Who are the elderly?" Are they just a group of people who are alone, neglected, poor, sick, frightened and about to die anyway? Is walking and the ability to move about so important? Why not consider social segregation and institutionalization to avoid all problems? Are they people who really need help from us? Do they realize that their life is behind them or what life is really about? Have they lost their freedom? And what about their inner resources? Are they our parents and older relatives? Perhaps if we look into a mirror and recognize that with God's given life, we are the elderly, the path for all of us in the health and social professions becomes quite clear. If we are to make sure that what we now recognize as inadequate care for the elderly does not happen again . . . to us . . . our road for dedication, research, education and care becomes quite evident.

In developing this text on foot problems related to aging, it was not our intent to provide a research text or to develop an encyclopedia on all of the foot problems that can occur in aging patients. Our goal was to deal with a practical presentation of those problems which are most common and those situations which most need consideration. Our guest authors have come from many fields but we have all shared practice experiences together in the same institutions and programs. We all have seen the changes that take place with aging and, in particular, those changes which effect the human foot as part of a whole person.

The health care delivery system provides many constraints on the delivery of needed and quality foot care services to the elderly. We need to remember that most elderly patients do not understand our systems and are many times so frightened, that they only seek care when problems are severe, hospitalization is mandatory and the outcome of care is guarded. Many times, the "old race horse" once stopped, never seems to move again, thus creating wards of society.

We hope and trust that this effort will stimulate not only the health care providers to deliver a quality service, but will motivate research and insure adequate educational programs to insure that our health professionals understand the total process of aging and are compassionate in their responses to the needs of the elderly. That we shall do something is quite evident . . . the unanswered question is *when*?

ARTHUR E. HELFAND, D.P.M.

Acknowledgment

On July 20, 1980, Seward P. Nyman, D.P.M. passed away. He served as Executive Director of the American Podiatry Association during my personal involvement with the Association. His ability to see a far vista for the field of podiatric involvement in aging led me down a path which helped create this text, and his support for many projects in aging brought each of us to recognize that our involvement in the field of gerontology was critical. Dr. Nyman was my mentor. His passing will leave a void for many but with the knowledge that the world is much better because he was here.

ARTHUR E. HELFAND, D.P.M.

Contributors

Morris Barrett, M.P.H.
Assistant Professor of Community Health, Pennsylvania College of Podiatric Medicine, Philadelphia, Pennsylvania; Program Administrator, PASS Program, Philadelphia, Pennsylvania

Joseph Bruno, P.T.
Director, Department of Physical Therapy, James C. Giuffré Medical Center, Philadelphia, Pennsylvania; Clinical Professor, Department of Community Health, Pennsylvania College of Podiatric Medicine, Philadelphia, Pennsylvania

Stanley N. Cohen, M.D.
Clinical Associate Professor of Medicine, Thomas Jefferson University, Jefferson Medical College, Philadelphia, Pennsylvania; Associate Professor of Medicine, Pennsylvania College of Podiatric Medicine, Philadelphia, Pennsylvania; Attending, Department of Medicine, Thomas Jefferson University Hospital, Philadelphia, Pennsylvania

Jay H. Davidson, M.D.
Clinical Associate Professor of Medicine, The Hahnemann Medical College, Philadelphia, Pennsylvania; Director, Division of Medicine and Chief, Department of Gastroenterology, James C. Giuffré Medical Center, Philadelphia, Pennsylvania; Attending Staff, Albert Einstein Medical Center, Northern Division, Philadelphia, Pennsylvania

Ernestine Estes, M.S.W.
Assistant Professor of Community Health, Pennsylvania College of Podiatric Medicine, Philadelphia, Pennsylvania; Associate Executive Director, West Philadelphia Mental Health Consortium, Philadelphia, Pennsylvania

James C. Giuffré, M.D.
Executive and Medical Director, Chairman, Division of Surgery, James C. Giuffré Medical Center, Philadelphia, Pennsylvania; Professor Emeritus of Surgery, Pennsylvania College of Podiatric Medicine, Philadelphia, Pennsylvania; Clinical Professor of Surgery, The Hahnemann Medical College and Hospital, Philadelphia, Pennsylvania

Arthur E. Helfand, D.P.M.
Professor and Chairman, Department of Community Health, Pennsylvania College of Podiatric Medicine, Philadelphia, Pennsylvania; Chief, Department of Podiatry and Director of Podiatric Education, James C. Giuffré Medical Center, Philadelphia, Pennsylvania; Adjunct Professor of Medicine, Department of Medicine, Jefferson Medical College and Podiatrist, Thomas Jefferson University Hospital, Department of Orthopedic Surgery, Philadelphia, Pennsylvania; Consultant, Philadelphia Veterans Administration Medical Center, Philadelphia, Pennsylvania; Consultant, Podiatry, Philadelphia Department of Public Health, Philadelphia, Pennsylvania; Consultant, Wills Eye Hospital, Podiatry, Philadelphia, Pennsylvania; Consultant, Podiatry, Veterans Administration Central Office, Washington, D.C.; Member, Technical Committee on Health Services, 1981 White House Conference on Aging, Washington, D.C.; Visiting Associate Professor of Orthopedic Surgery and Rehabilitation, The Hahnemann Medical College, Philadelphia, Pennsylvania

Neil J. Kanner, D.P.M.
Associate Professor of Community Health, Pennsylvania College of Podiatric Medicine,

Philadelphia, Pennsylvania; Consultant, Philadelphia Veterans Administration Medical Center, Philadelphia, Pennsylvania; Consultant, Diabetes Information Center, Garfield G. Duncan Research Foundation and Diabetes Clinic, Pennsylvania Hospital, Philadelphia, Pennsylvania; Staff, James C. Giuffré Medical Center, Philadelphia, Pennsylvania; Staff, Parkview Hospital, Philadelphia, Pennsylvania

Frank A. Mattei, M.D.
Chief, Department of Orthopedic Surgery and Assistant Medical Director, James C. Giuffré Medical Center, Philadelphia, Pennsylvania; Clinical Associate Professor of Orthopedic Surgery and Rehabilitation, Hahnemann Medical College, Philadelphia, Pennsylvania; Chief, Department of Orthopedic Surgery, St. Agnes Hospital, Philadelphia, Pennsylvania; Attending, Department of Orthopedic Surgery, Methodist Hospital, Philadelphia, Pennsylvania

Edward L. Tarara, D.P.M.
Chief, Podiatry Section, Mayo Clinic, Rochester, Minnesota (Retired)

Vincent N. Tisa, D.P.M.
Associate Professor of Community Health, Pennsylvania College of Podiatric Medicine, Philadelphia, Pennsylvania; Clinical Assistant Professor of Orthopedic Surgery and Rehabilitation, The Hahnemann Medical College and Hospital, Philadelphia, Pennsylvania; Consultant, Philadelphia Veterans Administration Medical Center, Philadelphia, Pennsylvania; Staff, James C. Giuffré Medical Center, Philadelphia, Pennsylvania; Staff, Methodist Hospital, Philadelphia, Pennsylvania; Staff, Garden State Community Hospital, Marlton, New Jersey

Bruce I. Weiner, Pharm.D., D.P.M.
Assistant Professor of Community Health, Pennsylvania College of Podiatric Medicine, Philadelphia, Pennsylvania; Chief, Podiatry, Section of Orthopedic Surgery, Department of Surgery, Philadelphia Veterans Administration Medical Center, Philadelphia, Pennsylvania; Staff, James C. Giuffré Medical Center, Philadelphia, Pennsylvania

Contents

List of Figures

chapter 1

Primary Foot Care for the Elderly

Arthur E. Helfand, D.P.M.

During the course of a lifetime, the human foot undergoes a great deal of trauma, use, misuse and neglect. The very stress of involvement in today's society; the usual degenerations associated with aging such as systemic diseases and focal impairment; and the environmental factors associated with walking make painful feet a common cause of discomfort in the elderly. The ability to move about, render self-care and remain an active and productive member of society is lost when foot problems deter these activities. If we remember that motivation is the key to health care of the aged and that keeping patients walking is the catalyst for that motivation, the need for podiatric programs in all health delivery systems becomes self-evident.

To the aged, the poor, and patients laboring under physical or mental impairment, the inability to move about means social segregation, a loss of efficiency, declining health and resultant personality and emotional changes. In effect, our elderly patients have three strikes against them in the health area. In baseball, three strikes and you are out, and in a very real sense, the aged are out too. Out of health, out of time, out of usefulness, out of enjoyment—out of everything, except life—and that, too, is running out. Foot problems produce immobility, and this deprives our elderly of their self-respect and increases the social poverty that they now face. To be old, poor and sick automatically requires the need for rehabilitation in the total sense, and that converts some of the negatives to positives. Practitioners cannot attempt to make

everything right again; this would be an unrealistic goal. But we can keep people walking and help our elderly establish goals that identify their fullest capacity to cope with life in the situations in which they find themselves. Perhaps we can help the elderly achieve the dignity of age, for this may be all that is left of life.

There are many factors that contribute to the development of foot problems in the elderly, including the following:

1. The degree of walking.
2. The duration of hospitalization or institutionalization.
3. Previous types of podiatric care and management.
4. The environment.
5. Emotional adjustments.
6. Current medications and therapeutic programs.
7. Associated systemic and localized disease processes.
8. Past foot conditions and/or pedal manifestations of disease.

In identifying common foot problems in the elderly, we must look at people who happen to have a foot complaint or impairment and consider podiatric care as part of comprehensive health care, recognizing the interdisciplinary approach needed to develop a proper projection.

In general, our aged patient is usually taking more than one drug at any given time and may have unusual sensitivities to drugs in general. He usually is very susceptible to local infection due to the anatomic location of the foot itself. The atrophy associated with degenerative neuromusculoskeletal disease and the avascular status and neuropathic changes associated with diabetes and arteriosclerosis further complicate patient management.

In addition, the geriatric individual is frequently confused and may have a lower threshold of emotional stress. His ambulatory status is often limited by his general physical deterioration, his environment and the social poverty that most of our elderly are faced with. Our elderly patient usually has one or more chronic systemic diseases and is more prone to injure his lower extremities. Thus, a minor problem in the young is a major problem in the old, requiring early diagnosis, appropriate therapy and care, continued management and proper health education to prevent exacerbations of preexisting conditions.

To add to these complicating factors, the aged are more prone to immobility, impairment, disability, hospitalization and surgery following even minor foot infections. They have tissue that does not heal well and are generally a greater risk than the average population.

The skin is among the first structures to demonstrate changes. The earliest sign is usually a loss of hair due to a diminishing vascular supply and the gradual appearance of brownish pigmentations. Anhidrosis, dry skin and fissures usually follow these early changes.

Dryness, in turn, may lead to pruritus. Other pertinent areas for consideration include contact dermatitis, tinea pedis and localized pyodermas. Because of the usual coexistence of fixed deformities, some form of peripheral vascular disease and the possible presence of diabetes, any infective process can lead to ulceration, necrosis and the need for hospitalization.

During the geriatric years, one can usually demonstrate all of the onychial dystrophies and diseases in even a small population sample. Thickened toenails as either onychauxis or onychogryphosis are part of the geriatric picture. By comparing the onychial structures on the hands and feet of the same patient, it is easy to demonstrate the effects of repeated microtrauma, vascular impairment to the digits and the end result of our environment. In many cases, the normal flat status of the nail is lost and curvature takes place. Hyperkera-

totic lesions form in the nail folds and pain and discomfort become apparent.

Neglect or mistreatment usually results in infection, requiring much greater concern than the management needed to prevent those complications. Onychomycosis or tinea unguium is also more common in the geriatric patient. This disease also tends to thicken the toenails. There is no question that repeated microtrauma from the toe box of a shoe and the warm, moist environment of the shoe itself contribute to the etiology of this condition. In these cases, for example, the nail becomes loosened from the bed. With thickening and enlargement, the possibility of traumatic nail avulsion by the patient becomes a reality. Should this occur, secondary bacterial infection is assured. The same concern must be voiced about the early recognition and prompt treatment of onychia and paronychia, before bone involvement requires amputation.

Various hyperkeratotic lesions, such as tyloma and the multiple varieties of heloma, are of concern to the elderly patient. The associated fixed deformities, arthritic changes and a loss of muscle mass further complicate walking.

The biomechanical or pathomechanical changes which occur in the musculoskeletal system serve as the prime etiologic factor for their development. It should be noted that the presence of hyperkeratosis is a natural protective mechanism and a symptom of pressure and is always secondary to some other lesion or condition. Management requires a realistic approach to the patient's complaint and the etiologic factors involved. Some of the pathologies include the following: pes planus and pes valgo planus, plantar imbalance, fascitis, myofascitis, tendonitis, myositis, hallux valgus (bunion), digitus flexus (hammer toe), phalangeal rotational deformities, phalangeal hyperostosis, differential metatarsal patterns, neuritis, atrophy, calcaneal spurs and hallux limitus. There is usually a decrease in work tolerance, and a marked limitation of motion can easily be demonstrated.

Many systemic diseases produce serious foot complications. Osteoarthritis or degenerative joint disease is a major factor in limiting walking. Fixed deformities and inflammatory reactions to repeated microtrauma produce pain, stiffness and swelling. In most cases, fascitis, calcaneal erosions and spur formation, periostitis and tendonitis are the primary demonstrable clinical entities in the elderly.

Existing pathomechanical deformities of the feet increase pain and limit motion and the ambulatory ability of the patient. Another significant factor to consider is inadequate foot care at earlier ages.

The primary form of traumatic arthritis is usually present in the elderly as hallux limitus and hallux rigidus. These conditions require continued management to maintain walking, as the first segment is needed for the kick-off phase of gait.

Other forms of arthritis (i.e., neurotrophic, infectious, gouty and rheumatoid) usually produce clinical manifestations and changes that are degenerative in nature. Gross asymptomatic changes are seen in the neurotrophic form, while gout produces acute and intense pain. The continued use of diuretics for hypertension can produce a gout-like syndrome in the elderly. Gout may be ruled out in any case involving significant pain and swelling. The end result of rheumatoid arthritis is deformity and atrophy. Contractures and rigidity gradually change the gait pattern in the elderly and make the patient more susceptible to falls.

Diabetes mellitus is a significant foot morbidity state in the geriatric patient. Many times a foot lesion will be the initial cause of a patient seeking care. The pedal manifestations involve multiple systems and are associated with a variety of symptoms and signs, such as paresthesias, sensory impairment, motor weakness, reflex loss, neurotrophic arthropathy, muscle atrophy, dermopathy, absent pedal pulses and the clinical findings of peripheral vascular impairment. The dread neurotrophic or diabetic ulceration is directly related to microangiopathy and neuropathy. Infection, necrosis and terminal gangrene are common unless early diagnosis and total management can be achieved. For example, ulcerations can be precipitated by continuous pressure and local vascular impairment. Counterpressure by hyperkeratotic lesions and continued microtrauma and continued friction with thrusting and shearing of the plantar structures almost always result in ulceration. Coexistent pathomechanical prob-

lems, fixed contractures and deformities add to the total consideration of this clinical entity.

Peripheral arterial insufficiency is present in the elderly patient in varying degrees. Overt indications of decreased arterial supply in the feet include muscle fatigue, cramps, claudications, pain, coldness, pallor, paresthesias, burning, atrophy of soft tissues, trophic dermal changes such as dryness and loss of hair, absent pedal and related pulses, and abnormalities in the various vascular function tests.

Many times calcification can be demonstrated during an x-ray examination. Pain attributed to pathomechanical causes in the feet may be ischemic in character and due to a lack of oxygenated blood to the part.

Edema, related either to cardiorenal disease or dependency, may be the first real sign of peripheral arterial complications.

Pedal ulcerations in the aged, associated with arterial insufficiency, are extremely slow to heal and many times are complicated by diabetes mellitus. The loss of collateral circulation and the possibility of occlusion from vasospasm provide an ever-present liability to the patient. A conservative approach should be instituted in the management of these complications.

Many diseases of the neurologic system can also affect the foot and walking. The postcerebral vascular accident patient can have his entire rehabilitative state delayed by a local painful foot condition or lesion. Prolonged hyperkeratotic lesions frequently do not disappear with prolonged bed rest, as epidermal hyperplasia still creates keratosis.

The problems of delivering podiatric services to the aged are the same as those faced by other services in the delivery system. However, comprehensive health care programs and systems must include podiatric service as part of their primary approach. Agencies and governmental programs must provide for an early and direct clinical entry of the patient who is to receive podiatric care. Podiatrists must be included as part of the primary medical care team and must be involved in the outreach, education and social aspects of geriatric care.

Podiatric services must also be part of the primary care team's programs to provide for continued management and interdisciplinary care programs. Appropriate support must also include administrative policies, reimbursement, staff training, records (utilization and review), laboratory, x-rays, pharmaceutical, health education and social services. Communities themselves must become involved in health care and foot care if our elderly are to remain noninstitutionalized members of society.

It would be difficult for me to visualize a comprehensive community hospital or an extended care or nursing home facility without podiatric services. Perhaps the true key to the future is involvement of all health and related personnel in planning appropriate care programs and services, including health education and prevention.

Most podiatric services are covered by Medicare under the same provisions as other providers of medical care. The exclusions present for any provider eliminate many of the procedures that can be employed to pre-

vent costly complications. However, at the present time, Medicare provides the most coverage of any governmental or private carrier program. It should also be noted that the exclusions listed for foot care do not apply to any other part of the human body. We trust that the anatomic segregation will soon diminish.

The key to identifying foot problems lies in the ability of the practitioner to recognize the problem, look for abnormalities, and listen to the complaints of the patient. Finally, let me identify some goals that can be easily established for podiatric programs for the elderly:

1. Improve healing.
2. Reduce pain.
3. Maintain and increase range of motion.
4. Maintain and improve muscle effort.
5. Encourage walking.
6. Prevent complications, and
7. Keep them walking.

chapter 2

The Podiatric Examination of the Elderly Patient

Arthur E. Helfand, D.P.M.

Examining aging patients who happen to have foot complaints involves a multidisciplinary approach to the examination process. In order to evaluate the aging patient properly, we must really first perceive some of the activities that are related to elderly individuals seeking care and provide some assurance that dignity will be maintained in the delivery of that care.

We need to recognize that all people have reasons or motivations for doing the things that they do or choose not to do. Perhaps it might be stated that motivation is the key to health care of the aged and that maintaining some degree of ambulation is one of the catalysts for that motivation. We need to begin to think of elderly people who happen to have foot problems and not permit our evaluation of the aging patient to include only the foot. For to deal with an end organ only and not deal with the patient inhibits an appropriate diagnosis and an appropriate approach to a therapeutic program.

In evaluating the aging patient we must recognize that we must satisfy the needs of the elderly and must place emphasis on what they are able to do rather than on what they have lost. We need not only focus on what the elderly patient can do but must encourage the elderly to do for themselves and actively participate in what they are able to accomplish. We need to acknowledge the intrinsic work of the individual, his right to membership in society, his right to be individualized, his right to be appreciated, and his right to

be needed. We must recognize that the elderly must retain their ability to be responsible citizens in the community. Even if that community is a long-term care facility, maintaining responsibility gives the elderly a reason to live and move about.

We in podiatry recognize that the foot is not the total problem of the elderly patient. But it is a link in the chain that deals with the total health of the patient. It is one of the catalysts that permit the elderly to remain ambulatory, to identify their fullest capacity for life and to cope with whatever situation they find themselves in.

In evaluating the elderly patient's foot problems, we need to bear in mind that we should establish attainable goals for the elderly based on their physical disabilities, functional losses, medical problems, and psychological and social interactions, and break down barriers so that the patient can obtain quality health care.

If we are to evaluate the elderly and their foot problems, we should really look at the primary factors that create these problems in the aged. These include the degree of ambulation, the duration of institutionalization or hospitalization, the previous types of care and management, the environment, their emotional adjustment to limitation, their current medications and therapeutic programs, all of their related and associated medical disorders, their past podiatric or foot problems and the primary pedal manifestations of systemic disease.

It is essential to obtain an appropriate data base in the evaluation of the elderly patient (Table 2.1 and the screening form Table 2.2). This should include the name and date of the examination, the patient's date of birth, known height and weight, previous occupation, marital status, and his current living status in society. There should also be an appropriate review of family history as it may be known.

The next area of primary consideration should be the chief complaint of the patient. This should be the main symptom or symptoms, as stated in the patient's own words, which precipitated his seeking an evaluation and/or care. It would be appropriate to record such data in the patient's own terms and to attempt to place a time frame on the development of the primary symptoms. It is also helpful to look into the economic, social and psychologic factors that may be related to the current complaint of the patient. It might be well to review the patients symptoms from various points of view so that there is some clarity on the part of the elderly as to his or her concerns.

There should be a detailed account of other present conditions and illnesses as a result of the patient's review. It should include the duration, location, severity, other treatment programs and general symptoms involved, with all related podiatric and medical findings. The review of the present illnesses should also include a categorical review of the events leading up to all existing illnesses and new symptoms or conditions which have occurred during the course of any treatment program. It might be well to obtain the patient's own interpretation of his health status, both generally and in relation to his foot health. It is essential to determine the quality of pain and to compare that quality of pain with the patient's tolerance to pain and a comparison with other painful episodes. The evaluation should include the patient's medical and surgical history, including such areas of review as infections, operations, fractures, injuries, and drug sensitivities that are related to lower extremity involvement. It is also important to ascertain any evidence of asthma and/or allergies. In addition, some concern should be placed on the total well being of the patient, his capacity for activity and his general energy status. We need to review the patient's experience with fatigue

in relation to recreation or activity, types of fatigue, and the relationship of fatigue to worry itself. Some inquiry should be made as to the patient's sleep pattern with specific references to any dependence upon drugs or alcohol to help induce sleep. Our review should also include any current weight changes and their relationship to food intake. Evidence of fever, chills or night sweats accompanied by changes in the perspiration activity of the patient as a whole should be noted. The patient's tolerance to heat and cold should be part of his medical history. A concern for patient pallor or anemia must also be accompanied by a concern for experiences of bleeding or bruising tendency. In the review of infection, it is important to ascertain both the type and frequency of known infections, the severity and duration of such experiences and the previous modes of treatment and their effectiveness. The medical history of the elderly patient should also attempt to ascertain the degree of nervousness of the patient. Complaints such as tension, anxiety, general feelings and ability to concentrate, known phobias or myths of the patient, special fears, or general worriment, may not only relate to the onset of the problem but will definitely have a strong relationship to the effects of any treatment program. The reaction of patients to existing medication is essential, not only in relation to the disease under treatment, but to signs of the patient's ability to respond.

The next major element in the evaluation of the elderly patient should be a systems review and should include the concerns of the patient in relation to head problems such as headache, eyes, ear changes, nose or sinus problems, relationships of eating and soreness in the oral cavity. Any changes that occur in the neck should also be noted, such as swellings, goiter, pain resistance, frequent sore throats and/or voice changes.

Any symptoms that relate to the respiratory system should be noted, such as pain or cough, wheezing or difficult breathing, blood spitting, a previous history of pneumonia or bronchitis, and the relationship to smoking.

The cardiovascular system should be reviewed with the patient to determine if he is currently under care or presenting any symptoms which may be related to the cardiovascular system. Such symptoms as shortness of breath, cyanosis, pain or discomfort in the

Table 2.1.

Podiatric Evaluation Form

Chart No.

Name

Age _____ Sex: ☐ M ☐ F;　　Race: ☐ W ☐ NW

☐ S ☐ M ☐ W ☐ D ☐ Sep.　　Weight _____ pounds; Height _____ inches.

Chief Complaint:

Present Condition and Illness: Duration, location, severity, treatment, general symptoms

Systems Review: Significant findings of medical evaluation

Past Medical and Surgical History: Infections, operations, fractures, injuries, and drug sensitivities related to lower extremity involvement. Asthma and/or allergies.

Past Podiatric History:

Occupational History: Exposures, military, geographic locations, present occupation, % weight bearing,
flooring

Social History: Use of tea, coffee, alcohol, tobacco, sleeping habits, sedatives and hypnotics, narcotics
and other drugs, hobbies, interests, + reaction of patient to condition or illness.

Subjective Symptoms:

Hyperkeratotic and Other Related Dermatologic Lesions:
Onychial evaluations and impressions:

Peripheral Vascular Evaluation: Pulses, color, temperature, trophic changes, edema, varicosities, night
cramps, claudication, fatigue, burning, etc.:

Function Tests:
1. Skin temperature
2. Venous filling and plantar ischemia
3. Ophthalmoscopic
4. Oscillometric　　　　　　　Blood Pressure_____

	Left	Right
Thigh	_____	_____
Leg	_____	_____
Foot	_____	_____

Orthopedic and Orthodigital Evaluation: Foot type, gait, postural deformities, palpation, range of motion, angulations, etc.

Radiographic findings relating:

Neurologic Evaluation: Gait, reflexes (patellar, Achilles, superficial plantar), ankle clonus, vibratory
sense, other and impressions:

Drug History: Antihypertensives, antidiabetics, cortisone, sedatives, topicals, antibiotics, allergies, etc.

Summary of Findings:

Impressions:

Special Notations:

Projected Treatment Plan:

Table 2.2.
Pennsylvania College of Podiatric Medicine Screening Form

 PENNSYLVANIA COLLEGE OF PODIATRIC MEDICINE

SCREENING FORM   Case No._____

Patient's Name_____

Address_____

_____

Phone Number_____ Date Examined_____

Age_____ Sex M ___ F_____ Race W_____ NW_____

Weight_____ In pounds   Height_____in inches

Name & Address of Other Health Facilities_____

_____

_____

_____

_____

Foot Complaints by Patient

Swelling of Feet	_____	Painful Toe Nails	_____
Painful Feet	_____	Infections	_____
Corns	_____	Cold Feet	_____
Calluses	_____	Other	_____
Bunions	_____	None	_____

PAST HISTORY

Heart Disease	_____	Circulatory Disease	_____
High Blood Pressure	_____	Allergy	_____
Diabetes	_____	Other	_____
Arthritis	_____	None	_____

SOCIAL STATUS

M_____S _____ W_____ D_____ Sept. _____

Occupation_____

_____

DERMATOLOGIC EVALUATION

Hyperkeratosis	_____	Dry Skin	_____
Onychauxis	_____	Tinea Pedis	_____
Infection (Bacterial)	_____	Other	_____
Ulceration	_____	Verruca	_____
Onychomycosis	_____	None	_____

FOOT ORTHOPEDIC EVALUATION

Hallux Valgus	_____	Hallux Rigidus	_____
Anterior Imbalance	_____	Morton's Syndrome	_____
Digiti Flexus	_____	Bursitis	_____
Pes Planus	_____	Other	_____
Pes Valgoplanus	_____	None	_____

A

8

VASCULAR EVALUATION

    Coldness   _____   Claudication   _____

    Trophic Changes   _____   Varicosities   _____

    Dorsalis Pedis Absent (L or R) _____   Other   _____

    Posterior Tibial Absent (L or R) _____   None   _____

    Night Cramps   _____

NEUROLOGIC EVALUATION (Check if Absent or Abnormal)

    Achilles   _____   Superficial Plantar _____

    Vibratory   _____   Other   _____

TYPE OF STOCKING

    Nylon   _____   Other   _____

    Cotton   _____   None   _____

    Wool   _____

TYPE OF GARTER

    Circular   _____

    Other   _____

    None   _____

Footwear Satisfactory   Yes_____ No_____

Foot Hygiene Satisfactory   Yes_____ No_____

IMPRESSIONS

    Primary_____

    Secondary_____

    Other_____

For Care, To_____

_____

_____

_____

Recommendations_____

_____

_____

_____

_____

_____

_____

Examiner_____

B

CL–110 R67A

chest, the effects of posture on digestion, palpitations, histories of murmurs or rheumatic disease, blood pressure history, and edema of the extremities should be noted. The vascular system should be reviewed as to previous episodes of claudication, coldness, cyanosis, color changes, ulcers of skin changes. Any vasospastic manifestations should be noted, including varicose veins and a history of phlebitis.

The gastrointestinal system, urinary system, and genital changes should also be noted for the record if identified by the patient.

The general musculoskeletal system should be reviewed. Symptoms such as joint pain, stiffness, or swelling should be clearly illicited from the patient. Any history of injuries and their sequelae, or other related inflammatory changes, should be noted. The degree of disability or deformity produced by any musculoskeletal change should be noted so that some attempt can be made to ascertain an appropriate prognosis related to any foot problem. Any evidence of back pain or stiffness should also be recorded. If there is a history of any fracture, special attention should be paid to the healing time, any special problems, or a relationship to bone pain.

Any changes which the patient has noted in the skin, hair or nails should be noted. A history of previous skin diseases or allergies should be recorded. Chronic lesions of any type on the part of the patient should be noted. If there have been any changes in any moles or nevi anywhere in the body, these also should be noted. A past history of fungal infections and changes due to exposure to sunlight in the elderly are essential in the planning of a therapeutic program for the aged.

There should be a review of the central and peripheral nervous systems to include such factors as intellect, memory, judgment and patient self-control. Any speech disturbance should be considered an important factor in the review of the elderly patient. Motor functions such as weakness, clumsiness, spasticity or involuntary movements should be noted. Sensory functions such as parathesias, hyperthesias, abnormal pain sensations in the skin or any impairment with the perception of pain should be recorded. Autonomic functions such as color changes or postural dizziness should also be considered as part of the review of the elderly patient.

It is also important to be aware that the psychological activities of the patient are also related to his foot problems and his ability to ambulate. Any tension on the part of the patient or nervous fatigue may also relate to his ambulatory status. Some patients feel embarrassed about the looks of their feet or a lack of confidence in their ability to ambulate normally; these feelings of inadequacy will also affect the total outcome of the patient's response to any treatment. Difficulties in expressing emotions or feeling lonely, or living alone, will also relate to the total manifestation of any foot problem and its therapeutic regime. Patients may have fears in relation to their foot problems or their ability to ambulate. These need to be considered in relation to any total treatment program. There should be an appropriate podiatric history on the part of the patient as it relates to the specific management of foot problems he has had over the years. This might also include a personal and family history of similar types of foot problems. It is also essential to obtain some review of the patient's occupational activity, including any exposure to military activity, specific geographic locations of occupation or activity, the percent of weight bearing during areas of activity or occupation, and the type of flooring the individual has generally been exposed to. The social history of the patient should also include patient's use of tea, coffee, alcohol, tobacco or other drugs. Hobbies and interests of the patient should also be recorded, and it is essential to determine the patient's own reaction to his or her condition or illness.

The physical examination of be patient who is being reviewed for a foot problem includes several basic areas. The initial area is the skin. The presence of hyperkeratotic or other related dermatologic lesions should be clearly identified. The onychial examination should not only focus on the patients primary concern but deal with all of the nail problems, including a comparison of nail health on the foot with nail health on the hand. The skin should be noted for general texture, temperature, color, moisture, elasticity, the presence of subcutaneous tissue, and the atrophic qualities of the skin itself. Signs of scratching or scaling should be noted along with pigmentation. Any scarring should be noted. Any infection or neoplastic change should be identified and should clearly be delineated as to whether it is local or general.

The peripheral vascular evaluation of the aging patient should include the dorsalis pedis pulse, posterior tibia pulse, popliteal pulse and, if needed, the femoral pulse. The patient's temperature should be noted, and trophic changes should be recorded such as atrophy and changes in hair growth as well as skin pallor. Edema and varicosities should be clearly identified. The patient's complaint of night cramps and claudication should also relate to his symptoms of fatigue and burning. Evidence of vascular insufficiencies to the toenails, the presence of blebs, ulcerations, or gangrene—including its type, onset and level of infection—should be noted as part of the peripheral vascular evaluation of the patient. Blood pressure should be recorded as part of the peripheral vascular and general systemic evaluation of the elderly patient. Special studies, including such functional tests as skin temperature, venous filling time, ischemia, Doppler flow studies, ophthalmoscopic evaluations, oscillimetric evaluation, and plethysmographic evaluation, should be included in assessing the peripheral vascular status of the elderly patient, when such studies are indicated on the basis of symptoms and other physical findings.

The foot orthopedic evaluation of the elderly patient should include appropriate biomechanical measurements where indicated. There should be some indication of the foot type and gait of the patient in relation to postural deformities, palpation for osseous deformities, a review of range of motion, and changes in the normal angulation of the patient. There should be a review of the digital structure and function of the patient to include contractural deformities of the digits as well as the relationship of the toes to the metatarsal shafts. Where bunion deformity is clear, an appropriate notation should be made as to the type and degree of activity of the hallux abducto valgus deformity. Where there is a bunionette or varus deformity of the fifth digit on the fifth metatarsal, this should also be appropriately reported. It would be appropriate to review radiographically the foot of the elderly patient where pain is present. Special notation should be paid to the degree of osteoporosis, other areas of demineralization, old findings of osteomyelitis, neoplastic changes in bone, and the

degree of arthritic changes that are related to the small or large joints of the foot. There should be a clear review of the relationship of foot function to the ankle and its relationship to gait. It is important to recognize that the foot orthopedic evaluation of the elderly patient must relate to existing deformity with the patient's ability to adjust his ambulatory activity to that deformity. Although the abnormalities may be present, it is many times quite feasible for the elderly to provide an appropriate adjustment to meet their functional needs. When considering definitive therapy for foot orthopedic problems, one must be cognizant of the fact that changes in a functionally adapted position result in a new educational process for ambulation and may require a long period of adjustment. Footwear should be evaluated as to whether it is consistent with patient needs.

The neurologic evaluation of the elderly patient should include such aspects as the patient's mental status and his behavioral activities. Motor function should be reviewed to include some element of muscle evaluation, particularly the muscle groups in the lower extremities. Gait should be evaluated along with the primary reflexes involved in the foot itself such as the patella reflex, Achilles reflex and superficial plantar reflex. Evidence of ankle deformity should be recorded. The vibratory sense should be evaluated for the foot and other areas of the lower extremities to ascertain the degree of pallesthesia. Pain, touch and temperature should be evaluated. Discomfort on muscle compression or tendon compression should be recorded. Proprioception should also include position sense in relation to passive and active movement. Tactile sensation is necessary in the elderly patient, particularly in those patient's with diabetes or peripheral vascular disease. Signs of nerve root irritation should be clearly delineated. Motor functions should include the evaluation of involuntary movement, localized wasting of muscles in any area, muscle power in relation to movement, muscle tone and coordination.

An appropriate drug history of the elderly patient is essential in relation to the management of foot problems. It should include a clear delineation of drugs that are being used as antihypertensives, drugs to control diabetes mellitus, cortisone, sedatives, any topical medications, all antibiotics and their reactions in the patient, and drugs used for the management of allergy.

The summary of findings should be a resume of the patient's primary complaints and the issues that are to be dealt with therapeutically. A listing of the differential diagnoses should include the main diagnostic possibilities. A provisional working diagnosis, or clinical impression, should be formed prior to the onset of any treatment. The prognosis should be clearly delineated and should relate to areas of management as opposed to cure. It is essential in planning any treatment program that the family and related health care practitioners be included in notification of treatment so that there can be a clear coordination of all elements of the health care system in managing the patient. The plan of treatment should be drawn up and should include the specific elements for initial care as well as those elements to be considered in future care. Other additional laboratory or investigatory activities should be discussed with the patient.

Perhaps one of the most important elements in an appropriate evaluation of the geriatric patient and his foot problems, is a frank discussion of realistic aims with the patient, his family, and those related to and responsible for his or her health care. Foot problems in the aged are usually chronic in nature and require periodic review, care and management, similar to other chronic conditions.

chapter 3

Nail Changes Associated with Aging

Arthur E. Helfand, D.P.M.

Nail disorders in the elderly are common. They may be the end result of severe trauma or repeated microtrauma. They may be associated with disease and may present many and varied abnormalities. Nail changes can occur in relation to infections, dietary deficiencies, drug reactions, circulatory disease, diabetes mellitus and degenerative changes associated with aging. They may demonstrate structural abnormalities and, many times, the toenails may demonstrate the first sign of an insidiously developing systemic disorder. The nails of the feet are more significantly affected in aging because of the forces of activity and the environmental factors associated with ambulation and footwear.

In managing changes associated with the aging toenail, one must include the tissues surrounding them and supporting the nail as well as those involving the nail plate itself. Many of the conditions identified are of generic interest only, but they may give rise to a considerable degree of discomfort and pain. The growth of the nail occurs by virtue of an adequate vascular supply and proper nutrition. Classically, nail lesions are identified according to the trophic changes that occur. They include atrophy, hypertrophy and dystrophy. An additional delineation relates to factors surrounding the nail plate, such as infection. Differentiation must be made of those conditions that are congenital or acquired.

The acquired type of atrophy of the toenail is quite common. It generally results from a disturbance of nutrition, infection or injury to the nail. The nail may appear disorganized or totally or partially avulsed. There is generally regrowth, but the original texture of the nail tends to be lost. Alterations may occur in the shape and thickness of the nail.

Atrophy also occurs after the first attack or series of attacks or disturbances in peripheral circulation. These may be commonly demonstrated in the patient with occlusive arterial disease or in a diabetic patient with microvascular disease. These changes tend to be permanent and the nail becomes shriveled and opaque. The nail bed tends to become fibrosed and thickened with onycholysis present; a collection of subungual keratoses and debris is common. There is usually no pain, and treatment generally includes cautious debridement of excess nail to maintain as normal an appearance as possible. Similar changes can occur from senile degeneration of the nail plate or as a result of an early gangrenous condition. Such changes demonstrate the need for foot health education to minimize trauma to the area.

Congenital absence of a nail is known as anonychia. The condition is rare but may be associated with some of the congenital dermatologic diseases. The prime consideration is a historical review of an absent nail. It is extremely important, however, to identify the elderly patient with severe diabetes mellitus of longstanding who may also demonstrate periodic absence of one or more nails through the process of autoavulsion. Patients with a history of small, but otherwise normal, nails are known to have micronychia. Patients with historically large nails are known to have macronychia. These are congenital in origin but tend to increase in size in later life. They may be associated with clubbing of the fingers, and may also be present in some endocrine disorders.

Hypertrophic changes in the nail are common in the elderly. They are generally the end product of excessive activity of the matrix, either through systemic or traumatic disease. Changes which take place in the matrix are permanent. It should be noted that if avulsion of the nail takes place either surgically or naturally, the nail which regrows will be of equal if not greater thickness. In all hypertrophy, the matrix increases in size and thus the nail plate grows with an equivalent thickness. With increased activity in the matrix, cells are produced more rapidly and the hypertrophy increases. Because of the structural changes, the nail cells are produced more rapidly and have a greater cohesive force. Therefore, there is not only an increase in bulk, but there is an increase in hardness of the nail plate itself. There are two primary varieties of hypertrophic nails. They include onychauxis, where the nail plate is enlarged, and onychogryphosis, where the nail plate becomes grossly deformed.

The most common etiologic factor for the formation of onychauxis in the elderly patient is associated with repeated microtrauma. It may be related to a violent injury to the nail matrix, but in this case, a historical review would usually demonstrate a clear knowledge of the incident by the patient and the possibility of an associated fracture of the distal phalanx. When all the nails are affected, the condition generally can be associated with a systemic disorder, which interrupts the normal vascular supply to the nail plate, nail bed and matrix. An example of this would be in patients with obliterative arterial disease and patients with longstanding diabetes mellitus. Pain is generally not a major factor. However, as the hypertrophy continues to develop, even the pressure of bedding can give rise to discomfort in the elderly patient. The nails lose their normal luster and become somewhat opaque. There is usually a collection of subungual debris accompanied by some hyperkeratosis present in the nail bed and lateral nail folds as the nail becomes thicker.

Onychogryphosis is usually associated with a disorder of the matrix and the nail bed. There generally is an increase in the subun-

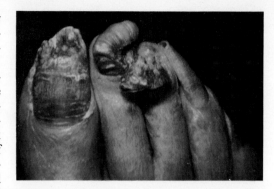

Fig. 3.1 Multiple onychogryphotic toenails, with marked deformity, clinical mycosis, subungual keratosis and subungual hemorrhage.

gual hyperkeratotic tissue, which forms an obstruction to the forward growth of the nail plate. The nail attempts to surmount this barrier and tends to become deformed in the process.

The contour of the nail changes due to the influence of the hyperkeratotic barrier. Where injury affects one side of the matrix only or to a greater degree than the other, there tends to be a sideways growth of the nail plate. The shape of the nail has given rise to the common names of "ram's horn" nail, and "club" nail. Due to much neglect on the part of the elderly, the nail plate itself may increase its deformity and as a result of footwear pressure may demonstrate as a complete semicircle. It is not uncommon to find a neglected nail meeting the underside of the digit. The deformity itself is not generally painful, other than the pressure placed upon footwear. However, the roughness and bulk do increase the tendency for hyperkeratotic tissue and the thickened transverse ridges which may occur generally cause a concentration of pressure which can be painful. In most cases, however, it is not the pain which makes the patient seek treatment, but rather the ugly appearance of the nail itself. Patients with occlusive arterial disease and those with diabetes mellitus need to be particularly concerned about this condition, as external pressure upon the nail plate may produce localized tissue ischemia, giving rise to subungual ulceration, infection and gangrene.

The management of onychauxis and onychogryphosis must not only include professional care, but also patient education. In many instances, there is total neglect on the part of the patient, either from the inability to seek care, be aware that there is a deformity or recognize the potential complications that exist from this pathology. As the nail grows with hypertrophy and deformity, a certain degree of nuisance value is apparent in many patients and/or institutional staffs. The nail itself becomes offensive to look at and the increase in bulk may create an impingement factor on the adjacent digits.

The etiologic factors related to onychauxis and those of onychogryphosis are related to changes that can occur as a result of mild persistent trauma or systemic diseases such as peripheral stasis, peripheral neuritis, syphilis, leprosy and hemiplegia. The hypertrophy of the nail bed related to these conditions also is associated with the presence of onychomycosis, psoriasis of the nails, and other dermatoses. A congenital condition known as pachyonychia causes an extreme thickening of the nails. The nails are generally more solid than those associated with onychauxis or onychogryphosis. There is usually an association of this condition with extreme hyperkeratosis of both the palms and soles of the feet.

The treatment of onychauxis, onychogryphosis and related conditions in the elderly patient generally involves debridement on a periodic basis. Although debridement will not change the future growth of the nail due to the already existing damage to the nail matrix, treatment of this deformity is essential, to provide both a preventive measure for pressure ulcerations and to permit proper ambulation. Treatment is by no means routine. Patients with severe vascular insufficiency or neurologic disease and those with diabetes mellitus represent a significant potential for severe foot problems as a result of these conditions, as they tend to be predisposing factors to pressure necrosis, ulcerations and gangrene. The frequency of debridement of these conditions is totally dependent upon the individual patient. It should be determined during patient management and should be related to the overall systemic disease complications involving the patient. In addition to debridement, the local application of a mild keratolytic agent will assist in eliminating some of the subungual debris and hyperkeratosis beneath the nail plate. An example of such a preparation

would include Keralyt Gel used judiciously in a nonocclusive manner and 20% urea cream used on a regular basis.

Due to the hyperkeratotic tendency involved with the thickening of nail plates, some patients may develop a condition known as pterygium. The patient presents with an abnormal thickening of the eponychium or the posterior nail fold. There is a tendency for the cuticle to spread over the nail plate and this condition is many times associated with vasospastic conditions in addition to hyperkeratosis. Treatment generally consists of adequate debridement of the hyperkeratotic tissue and the use of an emollient for some degree of softening to the area. Onychorrhexis is an exacerbation of the longitudinal ridging that adheres the nail to the nail bed. There may be some longitudinal splitting associated with this condition. It generally is related to dermatoses and nail infections, and may be related to many systemic diseases, senility, injury or induced by a chemical agent. In the diabetic patient where there is a significant degree of small vessel disease, such changes in the nail may be associated with a diabetic onychopathy. Where the nail is hypertrophic in addition to the degree of striation change, there may appear to be a laminated effect to the nail which increases the hypertrophic tendency. Treatment generally involves observation and where there is a degree of hypertrophy, appropriate debridement is required on a periodic basis.

Severe trauma to the nail plate may result in a subungual hematoma. The nail may present with a bruise in the nail bed and a

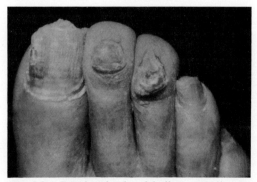

Fig. 3.2 Onychorrhexis of hallux toenail, onychauxis, Beau's line of fourth toenail, subungual keratosis, pterygium and clinical mycosis.

clear evidence of hemorrhage beneath the nail. The patient in the acute phase may well be in severe pain. One of the associated problems in the elderly with this condition is that, due to disease and diminished sensory responses, the patient may be, in fact, in no pain and be unable to effectively view his feet for one reason or another. Where subungual hemorrhage is a result of trauma, radiographic evaluation of the toe involved should be completed to rule out the presence of a fracture of the distal phalanx or other phalanges of the involved digit. The treatment varies depending upon the time the patient is seen. If the patient is seen immediately after trauma and is in severe pain, it is generally necessary to drill a small hole in the nail plate to permit the escape of liquid blood. Once this is completed the pain is usually diminished unless there is an associated fracture.

When the patient is seen later in the disease, and the blood has in fact coagulated, drilling a hole in the nail is generally unnecessary. Gross traumatic effects generally include an ecchymotic appearance of the nail plate with the potential for shedding of the nail. This generally takes place in the form of onychomadesis, which is a freeing of the nail from the posterior nail wall. If the nail becomes loosened from the nail bed, it may be debrided to the point of attachment with little or no pain.

Subungual hemorrhage may also be present with the diabetic patient. The tendency of patients with small vessel disease associated with diabetes mellitus to develop retinal hemorrhages, and problems in the kidney, should also be viewed as a potential for subungual hemorrhage, which is another related area in the diabetic onychopathy syndrome and

bears watching to insure that the initial hemorrhage beneath the nail does not represent the presence of an early focus of gangrene and necrosis.

Inflammatory changes which take place about the posterior nail wall or nail bed which do not present with pus formation at the time of evaluation, are termed an onychia. The inflammatory change of the nail wall and the nail matrix may cause a deformity of the nail plate if continued on an extended basis. It is related to the presence of trauma, infections, and other systemic diseases such as diabetes mellitus and peripheral vascular disease. The condition generally responds to tepid saline or povidone-iodine soaks for short periods of

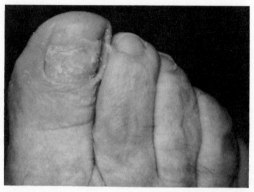

Fig. 3.4 Follow-up of Figure 3.3. Excision of loosened portion of hallux toenail demonstrating new nail. Note pitting of new nail, clinically present in psoriasis.

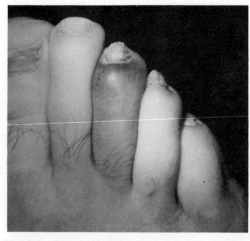

Fig. 3.5 Onychia of third toenail with marked early deformity. Etiologic factor was trauma induced by self-care for onychomycotic third toenail.

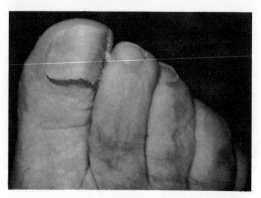

Fig. 3.3 Onychomadesis of hallux toenail.

time. Generally speaking, 15-minute compresses three times a day should bring the condition under control without the presence of infection. Where the trauma is related to shoe pressure, changes should be made to prevent a recurrence of this condition. Where the inflammation is related to systemic disease such as diabetes mellitus or peripheral vascular disease, the patient should be reviewed in guarded condition in relation to the integrity of the digit and one must always recognize the potential for organization of the inflammatory process and the presence of necrosis and gangrene.

Paronychia is a diffuse infection of the tissue adjacent to the nail and occurs with trauma, injury due to chemical agents or bacterial and/or fungal infections. In the aged individual, this problem is severe, as it represents a potential for necrosis and gangrene due to the generalized inadequate vascular supply to the digits themselves. The toe generally is markedly inflamed and redness and swelling do produce pain. Drainage may be present if the patient is seen in the secondary stages of involvement. Treatment generally consists of drainage, appropriate antibiotics, a culture and sensitivity test, and a continuation of patient follow-up to minimize the potentials for gangrenous changes in a generally avascular area for most geriatric patients. The effective process may be quite severe and may necessitate hospitalization if the patient is unable to provide for adequate home care. In the later stages of the infection, lymphangitis and lymphadenitis may be present. Tepid saline and/or povidone-iodine compresses generally also provide an effective means to assist in the establishment of drainage. The condition is associated many times with a diabetic patient and when this occurs it is known as diabetic paronychia. Radiographs should be taken early in the management of this condition to establish a base line of normal bone to clearly identify the potential for osteomyelitis. When this condition leads to chronic osteomyelitis, rigorous antibiotic therapy and bed rest are essential in the total management of this condition. Because of the fact that many elderly patients have severe vascular impairment of the digits, the potential for gangrene should be considered in the management of an acute paronychia.

Subungual and periungual abscesses may be the result of trauma and/or an abnormal pressure activity. Where present, appropriate debridement and drainage are essential. A culture and sensitivity test should be taken and appropriate antibiotics instituted early in the management phase. Radiographs should be completed to develop a data base in relation to normal bone continuity of the patient to minimize the effects or ascertain early any evidence of osteomyelitis. When a subungual abscess is diagnosed, a segment of the nail plate may need to be removed. If the nail plate is well attached to the bed, appropriate regional block anesthesia generally can be employed if the vascular status of the patient is adequate to allow for partial avulsion of the nail plate.

Onychomycosis represents a fungal infection of the toenail. It is frequent in occurrence. It generally causes a severe disturbance in nail growth when the matrix becomes involved and it locally destroys the affected nail. If not managed, it usually provides a source of infection or reinfection to the surrounding skin tending to create a chronic longstanding tinea pedis. The abnormalities of the nail structure may be severe with no treatment and may even prove incapacitating

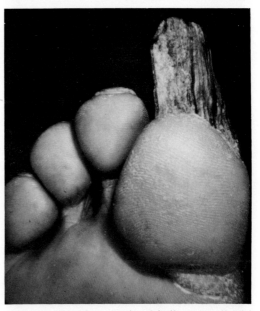

Fig. 3.6 Onychomycosis of hallux toenail with marked hypertrophy and subungual keratosis and debris.

when associated with trauma. The nails generally become thickened if the matrix is involved and present as a mycotic onychauxis. They may also become severely deformed and present as a mycotic onychogryphosis. There is usually some degree of onycholysis or loosening of the nail from the nail bed at the free edge with an associated build up of subungual keratosis and subungual debris. The organisms generally causing the various forms of onychomycosis are varied, but *Trichophyton, Epidermophyton*, or monilial infections, are the most common.

The clinical characteristics of the nails are diverse, varying from a moderate amount of scaling in the lateral nail folds, to complete nail destruction. We usually find a scaling at the free edges of the nail and surrounding tissue. The nail may present with associated other skin manifestations. Usually if a single nail plate is involved, there is a subsequent progression of the disease until many of the nail plates are affected. The nails tend to become hypertrophic and opaque in appearance and the distal portion of the nail may become granular or powdery. There is a characteristic musty odor associated with onychomycosis. The condition may be diagnosed clinically and later confirmed by microscopic examinations and culture. However, the characteristic appearance of the nail plate warrants management to present future complications. The more severe the condition, the greater the destruction of the nail plate. Where the toenails are deformed for other reasons, such as trauma, or as a result of other systemic diseases, onychomycosis increases the deformity and provides an increased liabilty to these diabetic patients. When onychomycosis is accompanied by a bacterial or monilial infection, appropriate antibiotics and/or antimonilial therapy should be utilized prior to the treatment of other types of fungal infections. There is a clinical association between excessive moisture and repeated microtrauma as an etiologic factor in the development of onychomycosis. In addition, in the elderly, where there is generalized lack of vascular supply, therapy becomes difficult and the condition becomes one of management, as with any chronic disease. Shoe trauma as a result of deformity of the nail being continually exposed to a low toe box of the shoe, and excessive perspiration and dark-

ness create an environmental atmosphere that increases the vulnerability of elderly patients to the development of onychomycosis.

The treatment of onychomycosis varies. In the elderly patient systemic antifungal agents generally have proven to be of less value in the long run than in younger patients or in the management of fungal infections of the skin and nails of the hand. Although there have been reported remissions with systemic antifungal agents there tends to be some recurrence once this approach is eliminated. The lack of vascular supply to the nail bed itself may be one of the prime reasons that this approach has been less satisfactory in a general consideration. In addition, inasmuch as many of the elderly patients are already taking many systemic medications, the addition of yet another drug which can produce some lowering of the white count may not be the most appropriate approach in the long range management of onychomycosis. Treatment must include periodic debridement and the removal of the onycholysed segments of the nail plate. The use of a topical fungicide in the management of this condition also has value to help control and limit the infection. However, our experience has demonstrated that one drop of haloprogin applied twice a day does provide some control of the subungual debris, odor and granular appearance of the nail plate. When the matrix of the nail is involved, and the nail becomes deformed, it is unlikely to assume that a cure will occur. However, because the condition can give rise to other associated complications such as chronic tinea, chronic ulcerations and pressure necrosis, debridement and management should be utilized. Twenty to forty percent urea can also be used to soften the nail plate and provide a chemical avulsion of the nail plate, thus providing a better means for the application of topical medication. Depending upon the vascular supply of the patient, surgical avulsion of the nail plate in a geriatric patient may be feasible. However, inasmuch as the most elderly patients do not have an adequate vascular supply, debridement on a periodic basis seems to be the best approach for management. Where the deformity is marked and we are dealing essentially with a young, healthy geriatric patient, a total removal of the nail plate and excision with phenolization of the matrix area does provide a means to eradicate the nail on a permanent basis and thus prevent deformity and pressure in future years when the vascular supply is inadequate. One of the most important factors to consider in the management of tinea unguium or mycotic toenails in the elderly patient is that the condition should be managed as any other chronic disease.

Onychocryptosis is defined as an ingrown toenail. It is present when a segment of the nail plate penetrates the skin, usually producing a periungual abscess and infective process. In the elderly patient who attempts some degree of home care, the inability to see or bend properly generally results in inadequate care provided by the patient with a segment of nail remaining. As the nail grows forward, there is penetration of the nail into the soft tissue where the vascular supply is inadequate. If the patient is diabetic, the result is a secondary infection and abscess formation which generally produce a cellulitis; and with inadequate vascular supply the potential for gangrene and amputation is real. Where the nail is involuted or incurvated there is a tendency for a semicircular character as one views the nail from the distal segment. With this abnormal curvature, there tends to be excessive pressure on the lateral nail folds and nail bed as a result of shoe trauma.

Initial management of the early infected ingrown toenail would include incision and drainage of the periungual abscess and a

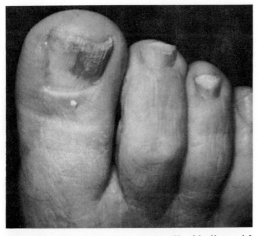

Fig. 3.7 Infected ingrown toenail of hallux with periungual granulation tissue. Subungual hemorrhage is also noted involving the lateral segment of the hallux toenail.

partial excision of the extending portion of the nail plate. Many times local anesthesia is not required for this procedure and it can be effectively done with minimal instrumentational trauma. However, where pain is present, local regional block anesthesia can be employed to excise the offending portion of nail plate. Postoperative management should include the use of a culture and sensitivity test to determine the appropriate antibiotic, appropriate systemic antibiotics, tepid saline, or povidone-iodine compresses, and mild nonnarcotic analgesics for pain. Where the patient has an overlying systemic disease that causes inadequate vascular supply to the area, such as the small vessel disease associated with diabetes mellitus, or peripheral vascular disease such as arteriosclerosis obliterans, this condition should be viewed as a potential for amputation and needs to be managed in a similar manner. Hospitalization may be required even at this early stage of the condition. When the incurvated nail tends to be the prime problem, generally the excision of the small segment of nail plate and the subsequent use of an emollient on a periodic basis would generally maintain control of the problem. Where the nail pressure on the nail folds has become excessive onychophosis or callous nail groove will result and as long as there is continued pressure the hyperkeratosis tends to form. In these cases periodic excision of a segment of the nail plate and continued use of an emollient is an effective means of management and control.

When the infected ingrown toenail is permitted to persist for long periods of time, due to patient inability to distinguish pain or the inability of the patient to recognize that there is a problem, periungual ulcerative granulation tissue generally forms and will organize in a matter of time. This condition generally requires surgical intervention to excise both the periungual ulcerative granulation tissue and the offending portion of nail plate.

Where the deformity of the nail is persistent and provides a continuing degree of discomfort, either through the incurvated activity and the development of repeated onychophosis, or the persistent true ingrown toenail with resultant granulation tissue, ulceration and paronychia, appropriate consideration should be given to either partial or total removal of the nail plate with the adjacent matrix structure. This may be done through either surgical dissection or phenolization. However, concern must be given to the vascular supply of the patient. It is important to recognize in the early geriatric patient that when the potential for this problem exists, surgical revision of the nail plate should be attempted as early as possible to prevent future infective processes and the future potential for gangrene and the loss of an extremity. It should also be noted that the granulation tissue, once organized, does become epithelialized and may produce a granuloma pyogenicum type of lesion. As long as the granulation tissue is present, there will always be a focus of infection in the nail plate area. Topical antibiotics may be used to complement the use of tepid saline and/or povidone-iodine compresses. However, it should be noted that these have limited value, and where the infection is well organized, for the most part, systemic antibiotics should be appropriate. Where surgical intervention may be inappropriate for the management of granulation tissue, topical astringents and their caustics may be used. These include aluminum chloride, ferric subsulfate solution and/or a mild solution of silver nitrate. These can be applied by the patient following judicious instruction.

Pinpoint pressure either reported by the patient or demonstrated through clinical examination of the nail plate may be associated with subungual exostosis. A radiographic examination of the distal phalanx and the lateral projection is used to demonstrate the enlargement or abnormality of the superior distal portion of the distal phalanx. The spur, exostosis and/or hypertrophic area of the bone may present abnormal pressure on the nail bed, accompanied by counterpressure of the nail plate in relation to footwear. This condition in the elderly patient represents a complex treatment approach. Where the vascular supply is adequate, the primary consideration should be to surgically remove the enlarged segment of bone, thereby providing relief of pain for the patient. Where this is not feasible due to the vascular insufficiency of the patient, consideration should be given to periodic thinning of the nail plate and the removal of all pressure from the offending phalanx. This would include the cutting out

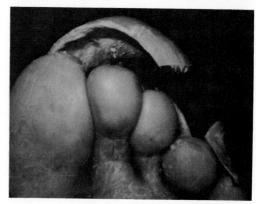

Fig. 3.9 Onychogryphosis with subungual keratosis and clinical onychomycosis.

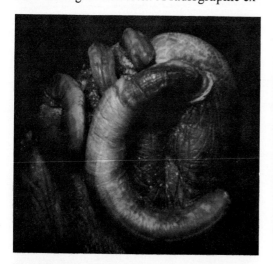

Fig. 3.8 Onychogryphosis of all toenails or ram's horn toenails with clinical mycosis, demonstrating marked neglect on the part of the patient.

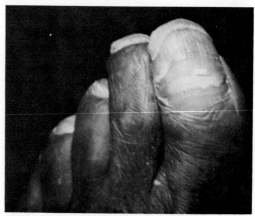

Fig. 3.10 Resolution of onychomycotic hallux toenail, idiopathic resolution as a side effect to chemotherapy for malignancy.

of a toe box of the shoe and the potential use of tube foam to provide adequate relief from pressure.

Associated with this condition is the feasibility to develop a subungual heloma or keratotic lesion in the nail plate. The condition is almost identical in pain to the subungual exostosis and may be present with or without any present abnormality. Management consists of debridement and/or partial removal of the nail plate and the excision of the heloma. Where the pressure is a prime factor, some alteration in footwear is generally required to minimize the occurrence of this particular condition. Subungual heloma must be differentiated from subungual melanoma which, for the most part, is rare but at present is life-threatening. Melanotic areas generally appear darker and may present with a less circumscribed area of discoloration.

A glomus tumor is an abnormal anastomosis in the vascular nail bed. It is generally acutely painful and is not relieved by any conservative measures such as thinning of the nail plate or the use of a protective device for the distal portion of the toe. Pain is acute and generally incapacitating. The appropriate approach is to surgically avulse the appropriate segment of the nail and to excise the tumorous growth.

Onychophosis is the presence of hyperkeratosis or callous formation in the lateral nail grooves. The condition is primarily associated with repeated microtrauma, deformity of the nails, onychauxis, onychogryphosis, onychomycosis, and a xerotic appearance of the lateral nail fold. With nail deformity such as incurvation of nails, the pressure of the nail produces a hyperkeratotic reaction which presents more tissue than can be effectively compensated for by the nail groove. Management involves several principles, which include the use of an emollient to minimize the presence of hyperkeratosis, excision of pressure areas, and surgical revision of the lateral sections of nail and matrix to eliminate pressure from the area. Generally speaking, a low percentage (10%) of salicylic acid used as a nail packing will facilitate the local excision of the hyperkeratotic tissues.

There are several other nail dystrophies that should be noted, as they tend to appear in a geriatric patient. They include Beau's line, which is a transverse ridge marking a repeated disturbance of nail growth. It may occur in relation to trauma or in relation to some systemic disease. It may be seen following an acute myocardial infarction and has been demonstrated in patients undergoing chemotherapy for neoplastic diseases. A diffusion of the lunula may be present on one or more nails. It is dystrophic in character and generally does not have a significant clinical significance other than to be observed. No treatment is generally required for this condition. Onychoschizia is a friable or brittle nail with splitting occurring at the free end or distal portion of the nail plate. It is

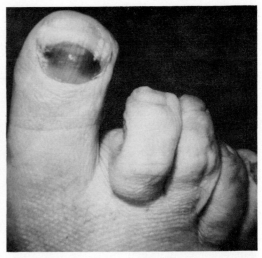

Fig. 3.12 Subungual hemorrhage associated with diabetes mellitus. Onychorrhexis and spotty mycosis are also noted in the hallux toenail. Note should also be made of the digital contractures.

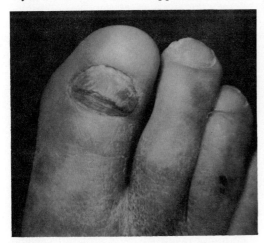

Fig. 3.11 Onychauxis of hallux toenail. Note trophic changes involving the second toe.

usually related to a dietary deficiency and may occur in trauma or in those patients with chemical contact. This condition may also be present in the later stages of syphilis. For the most part, treatment is generally managed where the origin is nutritional in character by an appropriate diet and the use of gelatin systemically. Hapalonychia is a softening of the nails which tend to split easily. It may be associated with the use of strong chemicals, endocrine disturbances, malnutrition, syphilis and chronic arthritis. Treatment again involves the appropriate management of the systemic disease and the improvement of nutrition and the use of gelatin. Hippocratic nails, sometimes called spoon or drumstick nails, if present, usually are associated with chronic respiratory or circulatory disorders. Leukonychia is the presence of white spots or striations in the nail plate. It is generally the result of nutritional deficiency trauma or may be related to some systemic disease. Generally speaking, no treatment is required, other than to provide some continuing observation of the nail plate and improve nutrition. Onychomadesis is generally classified as a shedding of the nails from the posterior nail segment. The etiologic factors include dermatoses such as exfoliative dermatitis, psoriasis, and eczema, and nail infections or severe systemic diseases. Autoavulsion associated with onychomadesis can occur in the diabetic patient, without reason, and this is perhaps its most common occurrence in the geriatric patient. Treatment includes the prevention of infection by the use of appropriate antibiotic therapy as required.

In most cases of psoriasis involving the feet, the nails are also generally affected. In some cases the only manifestation of psoriasis may in fact be the nails themselves or often may occur before there are changes in the skin surrounding the nails. In the early cases of psoriasis of the nails, the nail plates undergo a fine scaling and there is a loss of luster with the nails assuming a whitish opaque appearance. The nail plate may be affected uniformily or the destruction may begin at the distal portion and proceed proximally. In the later stages of the disease, the nail becomes detached from the free edge (onycholysis) and the nail becomes elevated during this process with deformity and fragmentation occurring. A hyperkeratotic friable mass, generally yellow in color, usually accumulates between the nail plate and the nail bed. The growth pattern of the nail may change and marked shortening may occur. The nail may ulcerate and the resultant nail bed may become coated with subungual debris. Multiple Beau's lines result from the interruption of the normal growth process at the matrix so that the nail becomes crossed by many transverse ridges. In many cases onychia punctatia may occur which consists of punctated erosions or fine pitting of the nail plate. The nail appears to have been picked with a needle at various points. The nail plate itself may undergo hypertrophy, thus increasing the elevation of the nail plate. In advanced chronic cases, the nail may become yellow or brownish to black. The nail tends to be scaly and has a worm-eaten appearance. The Beau's lines continue and the nail becomes raised from the bed with subungual hypertrophy present. Partial destruction of the nail plate may take place along the lateral nail folds and the irregularity may resemble some attempt at surgical debridement. In some cases the nails are completely lost from the posterior nail wall (onychomadesis). This condition needs to be differentiated from onychomycosis with the differential diagnosis aided by microscopic evaluation of the scrapings with KOH and an attempt to obtain a positive culture.

Treatment of psoriasis of the nails is generally lengthy and for the most part unsatisfactory. Debridement on a continuing basis is appropriate and an attempt to minimize the hyperkeratosis is extremely important. The patient may be instructed in how to mechanically debride the horny substances on a daily basis at home. Effort should be made to soften the nail as much as possible and a 20–40% urea concentration may be effectively used to provide for a chemical avulsion of the nail plate. Topical steroids may prove to be of some use but, generally speaking, in the aged patient periodic debridement appears to be the most effective means of managing the condition.

Nail changes can occur as the result of many skin diseases. They include such conditions as Darier's disease, acrodermatitis, epidermolysis bullosa, and eczema. They result from minor disturbances in growth to generalized destruction of the nail itself. Scaling, clubbing, splitting may occur. Onycholysis or onychomadesis may also be present. It is extremely important in the geriatric patient to recognize that nail diseases associated with dermatological processes for the most part occur late in the disease and require management of the primary dermatologic disease in order to provide any control of the nail process itself.

Changes do occur as a result of endocrine disorders. In hypothyroidism the nails tend to grow slower, onycholysis is present and a spoon nail appearance tends to develop. In hyperthyroidism, atrophy of the nails is common, onycholysis may be present and there is a significant degree of longitudinal ridging. Atrophy is a frequent occurrence in most endocrine disorders. Onychogryphosis may also be present with endocrine dysfunctions. It should be noted that the nails of the diabetic patient do demonstrate some significant characteristics and they include some degree of thickness, onycholysis, some ungual hemorrhage, possible shedding and exacerbation in the ridging of the nails. Where hypertrophy is a factor associated with diabetes mellitus the diabetic onychopathy does require debridement on a periodic basis to prevent a buildup of counterpressure and ulceration.

In both vasospastic and organic peripheral vascular disease the nails undergo many changes. The severity of the changes is totally related to the underlying state of the vascular disorder. In continued vasospasm, pterygium is a primary factor. It is particularly associated with Raynaud's disease and scleroderma. In organic arterial disease, severe ischemia causes a distortion in the nail plate. Linear growth is slowed and for the most part the nail becomes thickened, rough and dark in color. If the blood supply is free there generally is a sharp line of demarcation between the old and new growth. A reversal of the organic nail changes may well be the best indicator of the evaluation of therapy for chronic circulatory diseases. Diffusion of the lunulae may be the end result of ischemia and is one method of identifying chronic vascular disease in the elderly patient. Where chronic subungual infection accompanies the vascular insufficiency, osteomyelitis of the terminal phalanges is not uncommon and represents a potential for amputation and gangrene.

In rheumatoid arthritis the nails become dry and brittle. Longitudinal striations become more pronounced and subungual hyperkeratosis may ensue; where onycholysis is present marked separation of the nail and nail plate tends to regress toward the root of the nail and presents a significant breeding ground for onychomycosis as well as the development of subungual hyperkeratosis. As the opaqueness of the nail increases, discol-

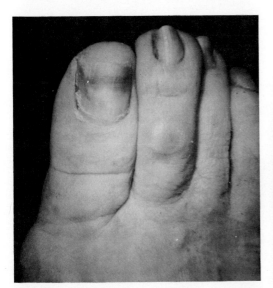

Fig. 3.13 Subungual hemorrhage associated with diabetes mellitus, demonstrating vascular hemorrhage. Pterygium of the hallux toenail is also noted with mild hallux valgus.

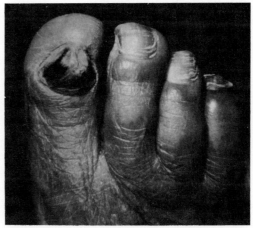

Fig. 3.14 Marked incurvated hallux toenail, subungual hemorrhage, marked trophic changes and edema of lesser digits.

oration becomes significant which may even demonstrate green, brown, and black as color changes. Adequate debridement and appropriate management of the arthritic processes tend to be required. Onychomycosis also may be more common in these types of patients than in patients without advanced arthritic changes.

With the increase of syphilis as a disease consideration, it is important to recognize that changes take place in the nail plate as a result of syphilis itself. In the early stages hypertrophic overgrowth of the nail is common. This is also present in the later stage of syphilis. As the nails become thickened they break and crumble and subungual ulcerations may be present as a result of the pressure.

Paronychia is common and is related to the development of osteomyelitis where the distal phalanx is concerned.

It should be noted that nail changes that occur in the elderly patient may be related to disease or the aging process itself. However, they do not represent a normal condition and therefore require appropriate and periodic management. It is clear that once a condition has taken place that changes in some way the root of the nail in the elderly patient, the chances of a return to normal are generally impossible. Thus, the concept of total management on a periodic basis is required and feasible to not only control the existing pathology but to prevent a more serious disease or deformity from occurring.

chapter 4

Managing Hyperkeratotic Lesions in the Elderly Patient

Arthur E. Helfand, D.P.M.

The major functions of the human foot can be classed as static and dynamic. It is an efficient organ of propulsion and locomotion. It is a relatively rigid structure, and through the years must carry a physical workload excelled only by organs such as the heart. No other portion of the human body is forced into a limiting enclosure and forced, time and time again, to contend with the hard flat surfaces which modern day civilization has inflicted upon us.

The human foot is a complex organ composed of some 76 bones, ossicles, ligaments, muscles, tendons, arteries, veins, nerves and skin. The normal foot bears weight on the triangle with the long axis being the inner and outer longitudinal arches and the base or short side being the five metatarsal heads. Weight is then transmitted from the calcaneus to the first and fifth metatarsal heads, making the angles of our triangle. However, if one looks at the foot in its anatomic shape, we find that the foot is a modified rectangle with the long sides being the inner and outer borders of the foot and the short sides being the heel and toe area. In identifying this anatomical shape, it is easy to identify the foot-to-shoe last incompatibility that provides some of the generation for the development of hyperkeratotic lesions in the elderly patient— lesions associated with deformity as a residual of younger years. Coupled with the normal physiological changes of aging, disease, and deformity, the balance of the etiologic factors become evident.

Our civilized society introduces many changes in the normal physiological functioning of the human foot. The primary concerns are the hard, flat surfaces which do not absorb shock. Paved sidewalks, streets and hard floors provide flat surfaces which do not permit weight distribution over the entire foot. This does not permit total foot function, and limits the intrinsic muscles of the foot. The prime example of this is the atrophy of the interossei and the resultant diminished function of toe action.

The primary effect is repeated tissue trauma, which creates stress on one particular area. Flat, hard surfaces further cause the foot to be maintained and function in a single attitude.

Tissue trauma results in osteitis, periostitis, synovitis, capsulitis, fascitis, myositis, arthritis and fibrositis.

Many times these pathologies and pathomechanical entities are created by an attempt to restore the so-called anatomical norm. However, correction of the anatomical attitude will not restore function. This is particularly true when an individual passes through the process of aging and his ability to adapt to change is limited.

Treatment should be aimed at eliminating the cause and redistributing weight to the nonpainful areas of the foot. We should remember that individual patients vary and so does their capacity to adjust to change. The primary aim in dealing with pathomechanical problems is to relieve pain, restore maximum normal function to the individual and to maintain that degree of normal function once it is restored.

Pathomechanical or biomechanical problems arise from the interaction between the normal morphological variations, the capacity to adapt to stress, and the stresses acting upon the foot. The terms "pathomechanics" and "biomechanics" are sometimes misconstrued, particularly in relation to the geriatric patient. The term "pathomechanics" denotes structural changes which relate to function. The term "biomechanics" primarily relates to the forces which cause change in the foot itself. The term "imbalance" is also used in the management of the geriatric foot problem dealing with hyperkeratotic lesions. The term "imbalance" relates to the inability of the individual to adjust or adapt to the alterations of stress.

There is, in effect, a related mechanical basis to the development of hyperkeratotic lesions in the elderly patient. For example, stress in various forms occurs as a result of activity. The first might be termed force, which relates to an action on the foot that tends to produce an alteration in its physical condition, either in shape or position. The second relates to a compressive stress in which one force moves towards another. The third is a tensile stress in which there is a pulling away of one part against another. The fourth is a shearing stress, a sliding of one part on the other. The fifth is friction, which is the force needed to overcome resistance and is usually associated with shearing stresses. The sixth is the factor of elasticity, which deals with weight dispersion and weight diffusion. And seventh, there is the activity of fluid pressure; the soft tissues of the body, unlike the bones, are not rigid, and attempt to conform or adapt in a relatively easy manner.

Morphologic variations may be intrinsic, i.e., within the foot itself, or extrinsic, such as changes in the physiological relationship of the legs, knees, thighs, hips and back on the human foot. These changes can be either bone or soft tissue. The common intrinsic bony changes are usually associated with the forefoot (toes and metatarsals) or the rear foot (calcaneus and talus). We can site as examples the hypermobile first segment, pes cavus, the navicular shape or a prominent

sustentaculum tali. Any or all of the above produce changes which mandate individual adaptation.

The ability to adapt to stress is dependent upon two major systems: the neuromuscular system and the vascular system. The neuromuscular apparatus controls reflexes and, in particular, conditioned reflexes of the individual. It also controls the anterior, posterior and lateral stability of the muscle actions of the foot, i.e., the prime movers, the antagonists, the synergistic and the fixation muscles.

The vascular system controls the biomedical changes, i.e., the pituitary or the adrenal cortex, which modifies and regulates the inflammatory response in tissue. An example of a hormone secreted by the adrenal cortex is hydrocortisone.

The stresses which affect the foot can be classed as those of society, those of mechanical origin and those of systemic disease.

Mechanical stresses are two in nature. The first might be termed macrotrauma, which results from sudden injuries that do not permit an opportunity for the individual to adjust to stress. An example would be a fall with a resultant fracture. The second mechanical stress might be termed microtrauma, which accounts for the hundreds of thousands of tiny injuries which result from occupational activities, overweight, poor stance and gait, and foot-to-shoe last incompatibilities.

The systemic stresses can be classed as the pedal manifestations of systemic diseases such as arteriosclerosis, the various forms of arthritis and diabetes mellitus.

It is obvious that the foot can not be divorced or segmented from the body nor can the foot itself be segmented. It is thus evident that the foot must be considered the total "end" organ of locomotion and that the resultant mechanical, rotational or positional changes comprise parts of a syndrome or a chain of events of a chronic progressive process. Once a link in the chain breaks, every effort must be made to prevent further damage and to minimize the associated complications of chronic disease.

When a change in the mechanical structure of the foot takes place, if we do not determine the etiology and prevent further alterations, the resultant series of related structural changes in the variety of objective and subjective symptoms may produce limitation of activity and further disability. The therapeutic and preventive measures depend on the particular stage in the progressive chain which is presented at the time of evaluation. The associated manifestations of chronic disease determine to a great degree the therapy, rehabilitation and preventive techniques.

Chronic disease takes many years to develop, and does not terminate rapidly unless the patient dies. To walk and move about and tend to oneself is accepted as a basic need in the care of long-term cases and chronic disease. It is evident that proper diagnosis and therapy for biomechanical foot problems play an important role in the approach to total patient management in the geriatric patient. With the increasing number of chronically ill and elderly patients, foot health has become a major community effort. Whether the etiology for an inability to ambulate is a fractured hip or a painful hyperkeratotic lesion, the end result is the same. The patient will be in pain, there will be disability and immobility. There will be an inability to maintain self-respect and dignity. There will be an inability to care for oneself. There will be psychosomatic disturbances which can result when a patient is forced into inactivity and becomes a public charge. The misconception that the management of hyperkeratotic lesions in the elderly patient represents "routine foot care" was obviously developed by individuals who have been devoid of pain, who have been devoid of discomfort, and whose families have never had a foot problem of any nature.

There are some broad basic principles which should be considered in managing hyperkeratotic lesions in the elderly patient. One of the considerations is the hyperkeratotic lesion itself. Treatment should include such principles as debridement, the use of appropriate emollients to hydrate and lubricate the skin, and the use of various modalities to remove pressure from the hyperkeratotic area. It should be noted that hyperkeratosis technically is the normal reaction of skin to pressure or force. It is only when it becomes excessive that it becomes pathologic and, in the elderly, can be significantly damaging to the total patient.

Where soft tissue atrophy is a factor, procedures must be employed to use various types of material to attempt to modify the gait and stance mechanisms to provide some soft tissue replacement through external means. Where deformity is present, principles should include the use of various orthotics to compensate for rigid deformities and to assist in rehabilitating the nonfixed deformity. Surgical consideration for the elderly patient is viable. Age itself should not be a deterrent to eliminating future pain for years. However, elective surgery as a first choice, should not be considered until other steps have been exhausted and have not produced a functionally pain-free patient. Surgical consideration should be based on the functional needs of the patient.

A tyloma or callus is a diffuse hyperkeratotic lesion commonly found on the plantar surface or ball of the foot, at the site of friction or irritation. It may also be related to abnormal weight bearing pressures. It may be directly related to a bony enlargement or anatomical abnormality, creating excessive pressure over a singular soft tissue area. Callus is a normal body reaction to pressure and friction and represents a hyperplasia of the epidermis. It is the body's own way of providing protection for areas that are under stress. The patient may complain of pain and burning, and the degree of tenderness to palpation may be directly related to the resultant inflammatory changes that occur in the soft tissues adjacent to the hyperkeratotic lesion.

Tylomas may also be present as space replacements for atrophied tissue. A common example of this would be the patient with an old rheumatoid arthritis and marked soft tissue atrophy in the ball of the foot. This characteristic rheumatoid foot presents painful lesions as a result of subluxation of the phalanges on the metatarsal heads with a prominence of the prolapsed metatarsal heads palpable beneath the hyperkeratotic tissue.

Tylomas may occur at any site on the foot where pressure and friction are continued. Examples include the marginal area of the heel, or over any other bony prominence, where irritation occurs as a result of gait or shoe last-to-foot incompatibility. Where deformity exists such as hallux abducto valgus, the head of the first metatarsal phalangeal joint and the medial plantar aspect of that area of the foot may also demonstrate a significant degree of hyperkeratosis in the form of a tyloma. Where abnormal gait patterns exist, similar lesions may be present under the first and fifth metatarsal heads. The tyloma is generally diffuse and does not contain a deeper pinpoint area of keratosis.

The initial treatment generally consists of debridement of the hyperkeratotic tissue, the use of some padding to provide tissue protection and the use of an emollient such as 20% urea cream for hydration and lubrication. Various forms of adhesive padding material are available and they include moleskin, adhesive foam, adhesive felt, and adhesive polyurethane. In addition, nonadhesive material is also available in the form of polyurethane in both open cell and closed cell varieties. In most cases, hyperkeratotic lesions in the elderly patient are generally less dense than in the younger individual but may be more symptomatic. This is probably due to general atrophy which occurs in both the soft tissues and skin. The management of marginal keratosis on the heels can be supplemented with the use of plastic or styrofoam heel cups to provide adequate control and the reduction of pressure to the calcaneal area.

Radiographic examination of the foot to determine the etiologic factors associated with tylomas generally reveals some clear biomechanical problems resulting in abnormal stress on a particular part of the foot. In addition, joint deformities and arthritic changes which are fixed in the elderly patients, tend to limit motion and therefore cause some change in gait patterns from the earlier years. The keratotic lesion in the form of tyloma will persist as long as the etiologic factor is present in the elderly patient. There is no question that foot-to-shoe last incompatibilities are a factor in the development of hyperkeratotic lesions. However, even when footwear is changed because of the biomechanical problems associated with the foot, the lesions tend to persist and require periodic management.

For the most part, orthotics generally provide a more long-range approach to the management and control of plantar tylomas and hyperkeratotic areas. A variety of materials and modifications are available in plantar orthotics. Examples include such products as Molo, Aliplast and Plastazote, used to provide changes in pressure distribution to various parts of the foot. Basic orthotic configurations generally consider the no-flange metatarsal shell, a standard flange, a Shaffer or high-flange shell, low posterior flange shells, high posterior flange shells, the Whitman type shell with a heel cup, and a molded inlay shell. In addition to these patterns, various modifications can be employed to deal with specific hyperkeratotic lesions. Examples include reinforcing the longtitudinal areas, specifically shaped metatarsal pads, full cushions, full rubber heel seat cushions, hallux leather shields, bunionette flanges, metatarsal extensions, metatarsal cutouts, combination cutouts and padding, and wedging or posting. Additional configurations include the Levy mold, the use of Spenco, leather laminates, and rigid orthotics such as Rohadur or combinations of Rohadur and other materials, to provide biomechanic control and modify the particular functions of the foot.

The choice of orthotic shape or material basically depends upon the evaluation of the patient's condition; the patient's ability to adapt to whatever modifications are prescribed; and the recognition that, regardless of the configuration, the concepts of rigidity or flexibility still apply. Most materials fall into one of these two categories and many variations exist in the basic material construction.

It should be noted that where soft tissue inflammation is significant, physical modalities such as ultrasound and whirlpool can be very useful in reducing pain and improving ambulation. Where local inflammation is associated with bursitic involvement of the metatarsal head area, local steroid injection, when not contraindicated, does provide marked relief of pain and swelling. Where extensive deformity exists, appropriate surgical consideration is a variable alternative, and procedures such as osteotomies of the metatarsal surgical necks and metatarsal bases would not be inappropriate to deal with the problem on a long-range basis. As with any elective surgical procedure in the geriatric patient, pain and the inability to ambulate, along with the absence of other contraindications, would be proper considerations to employ after conservative management has been exhausted.

Various forms of balance padding techniques have been proposed over the years, utilizing many forms of material such as felt and foam rubber. These principles generally employ the use of material in areas adjacent to the hyperkeratotic areas to provide a form of weight dispersion. Where padding materials are placed directly over the lesions to attempt to increase the amount of soft tissue replacement required to diffuse weight, these principles are generally termed weight diffusion techniques.

The second major area of hyperkeratotic lesion includes several varieties of heloma (corn) and is related to tyloma formations in view of the fact that it does consist of a more concentrated area of hyperkeratosis.

The most common variety is called heloma durum. It is composed of a hyperkeratotic area that is concentrated and cornified with a deep central portion that is highly keratinized at the site of greatest pressure, irritation or friction. These lesions generally occur on the toes or plantar surfaces of the foot where there is concentrated and continuous pressure. The color of the lesions may vary from a grayish yellow to a deeper color, including some areas of subhelomal hemorrhage. The lesion is generally dry and may appear to lack hydration and lubrication. Heloma dura

are caused by a wide variety of intrinsic and extrinsic factors. The predominant intrinsic factors include the various deformities that occur on the digits and bony prominences of the foot, the lack of fluid soft tissue protection, and abnormal gait positions as a result of pathomechanical changes in the foot which cause inappropriate weight distribution. The extrinsic factors generally deal with a foot-to-shoe last incompatibility and result from shoe irritation or irregularities in footwear that create localized continued pressure. These lesions can also occur on other areas of the foot where there is continued and concentrated pressure.

The most common sites in the elderly are those on the distal ends of the three middle toes, related to digital contractures usually associated with arthritic changes. In these cases, where the contractures are flexible, appropriate orthotics can be constructed out of silicone or other material to serve as a digital brace to raise the distal end of the digit and produce some straightening of the toe. One also notes that in these areas, as a result of digital contraction, the nail of the involved toe also appears to be somewhat hypertrophic and the hyperkeratotic area may extend around the nail, thereby increasing the level of pain for the patient. Debridement and emollients are of use, but some digital orthoses—including the silicone mold or the use of tube foam or other similar materials—are necessary to relieve pressure on a more continued basis. A prime concern in the elderly patient is to utilize orthotics that do not

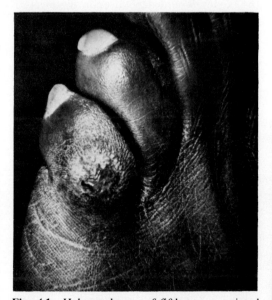

Fig. 4.1 Heloma durum of fifth toe, associated with contracture, rotational deformity, hyperostosis and enlargement of the head of the proximal phalanx of the fifth toe. Marked trophic changes noted.

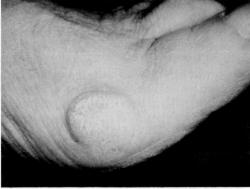

Fig. 4.2 Keratosis associated with hallux valgus and bursitis of the first metatarsophalangeal joint. Associated with deformity and shoe-to-foot last incompatibility.

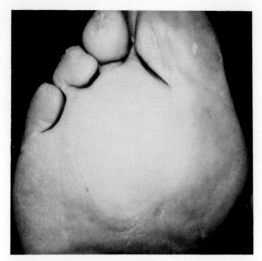

Fig. 4.3 Plantar tyloma (callus) associated with hallux valgus, displaced second toe and prolapsed metatarsal heads with continued microtrauma.

adhere to the skin for long periods of time and that are removable by the patient. It is also essential to recognize that patients who are unable to bend properly may be unable to utilize any digital orthotics, and periodic debridement of the hyperkeratosis may, in fact, be the only approach to managing the patient and preventing additional complications. Other common sites for these lesions include the dorsal aspect of all four lesser digits with the most common site being the fifth toe. This is due primarily to a rotational deformity of the digit accompanied by some change in the soft tissue configuration of the toe. In addition, there is a common bony abnormality, involving either the base or the head of the phalanges, which precipitates pressure by virtue of the rotational deformity and a foot-to-shoe last incompatibility. For example, where the foot is basically an out-flair foot and it is placed into an in-flair shoe, the incompatibility produces continual pressure on the fifth digit. With contracted toes, lesions may appear on the dorsum of the three lesser toes. With continued pressure over joints, a subhelomal bursitis may develop and may result in significant pain, swelling and the possibility of sinus formation with ulceration. In general, a similar approach in management is proper and should consist of adequate debridement, emollient therapy and orthoses to remove pressure from the area. Many forms of orthotics can be constructed, including those involving liquid Latex, silicone, foam, sponge rubber and various other materials. Local steroid therapy would be appropriate in the presence of sub-helomal bursitis. A change in footwear may be required to compensate for a last incompatibility or to provide extra depth for contracted digits. When pain and deformity are present and are unmanageable through normal means, an elective surgical procedure should be considered following radiographic examination to remove the excess bony prominence in these areas. Where ulceration is present, appropriate management of the ulcer needs to be implemented and surgical consideration should also be given, as ulceration is an early sign of severe and continued localized pressure. Heloma durum may also appear at the medial aspect of the first metatarsophalangeal joint or the fifth metatarsophalangeal joint associated with hallax abducto valgus (bunion) or digiti quinti varus (bunionette). Conservative management should consist of the methods previously outlined and would also include consideration of a bunion last shoe and/or a molded shoe if the deformity is significant. Elective surgical revision of the osseous site may be appropriate and, again, would depend upon the level of pain, the decrease in ambulation, the loss of movement and the social needs of the patient, along with a complete medical appraisal of the vascular state of the patient.

Heloma durum may also be found on the plantar surface of the foot as part of a tyloma. Where this is present, adequate debridement and appropriate management employing both techniques of weight diffusion and weight dispersion should be considered. Where the problem is pathomechanically or biomechanically induced, appropriate orthotic or surgical consideration should be considered for the elderly patient based upon a complete evaluation of the total patient. It should be noted that age and age alone should not be the total contraindication for surgical management of foot problems. If this criterion were employed in all of the other health fields, we would totally dismiss the elderly as patients and would no longer consider their needs.

Heloma miliare usually consists of small punctate hyperkeratotic lesions that may be

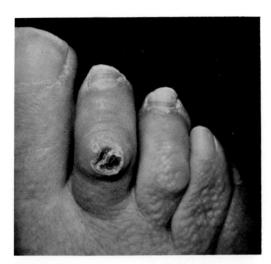

Fig. 4.4 Heloma durum with subkeratotic hemorrhage and preulcerative state. Hammer toe (digital contracture) of second toe with early bursal formation noted on the third toe.

associated with tylomas and helomas or may be isolated. They are generally extremely dry and are usually found on the plantar surface of the foot, most often in the heel area.

They are generally related to some incompatibility or pinpoint pressure from footwear or hose. They may appear to be circumscribed and may be mistaken for verruca, which are rare in the elderly patient. Treatment generally consists of adequate debridement, emollient therapy and removal of the etiologic factor involved.

Heloma molle represents a hyperkeratotic area similar to other forms of heloma that has generally absorbed a significant amount of moisture and is usually found in interdigital areas of the foot. Inflammation may occur as a result of continued irritation. Where the area is acute, pain is significant on pressure. Interdigital heloma found with the absence of excessive moisture becomes hard and dry and resembles other forms of hyperkeratotic tissue. However, the pain factor is persistent upon pressure. The etiologic factors involving the formation of heloma molle generally include the abnormal shaping of either the base or the head of the adjacent proximal phalanges, a compression factor, a lack of interdigital soft tissue and continuous irritation of subcutaneous bone against subcutaneous bone. In the elderly patient, digital contractures, rotational deformities and ar-

thritic changes generally provide most of the etiologic considerations in the evolution of heloma molle.

Where the pressure becomes excessive and atrophy is significant a continued compression factor can result in the presence of a sinus and ultimate ulceration. With significant vascular impairment and/or diabetes mellitus as a complicating factor, secondary infection, lymphangitis, lymphadenitis and osteomyelitis may be considered when significant inflammatory changes are present.

The treatment of heloma molle in the geriatric patient encompasses several phases. The initial phase is the reduction of the hyperkeratotic tissues. The secondary phase is the use of some material to act as a buffer or space replacement for the atrophied soft tissue between the digits. Examples include lamb's wool, foam rubber, polyurethane, tube foam, felt and silicone molds. Other forms of Latex or urethane orthodigital devices may also be employed. Orthodigital molds such as the silicone mold or Latex impregnated mold also tend to provide some traction, resulting in a positional change of the deformity. Many times in the geriatric patient this simple activity can, in fact, reduce the degree of pressure and provide a continuant relief of the symptom. Where a subhelomal bursitis is present as a result of a protective mechanism, local anesthesia and the local injection of steroids in small amounts can produce a significant relief of pain. Various surgical procedures can also be completed when pain and deformity are unable to be managed by conservative means. These include the revision of the offending portions of the adjacent digits, tenotamies, and/or other appropriate procedures to remove bony projections that cause the irritating effect.

Heloma neurofibrosum is a hyperkeratotic lesion that may be somewhat circumscribed and many times is mistaken for a verruca. The lesion consists of a heloma or hyperkeratotic area with some neurologic tissue invasion. The lesion is generally painful and may produce a burning or stabbing pain. The base of the lesion may appear yellowish or gray and can easily be demonstrated on debridement. These lesions are relatively rare in the elderly but may be seen at sites of continuous friction or significant direct pressure. It is not uncommon to find a small inclusion cyst under the base of the lesion which, if present, requires surgical excision. These lesions can be managed similarly to other helomas but greater emphasis must be placed on orthotic control and the use of appropriate medications to reduce somewhat the neurologic sensation. Mild applications of silver nitrate solution will tend to cauterize the area, and have proven to be a relatively safe method in management where the vascular supply is adequate to the part and when used in combination with pressure removing material such as weight diffusion and weight dispersion techniques.

Heloma vascularis is a heloma that contains a small blood vessel or some extravasation of blood into the hyperkeratotic tissue. The lesion is similar to other helomas, except for the presence of vascular elements or hemorrhage. When hemorrhage is found in hyperkeratotic tissue, it is generally an indication that there is significant direct pressure causing some rupture of the superficial capillary areas beneath the keratotic tissue. These lesions are generally associated with metabolic and endocrine changes such as diabetes and circulatory involvement of the lower extremities. The presence of vascular elements in the hyperkeratotic tissue may also be related to a previous foot infection. These lesions generally are more painful than hyperkeratotic tissue or heloma without hemorrhage and the most common sites include the dorsum of the fifth toe, and the plantar aspects of both the first and fifth metatarsal heads. Hemorrhage may be frequent during debridement of these lesions.

Treatment includes the debridement of the hyperkeratotic tissue and the use of appropriate weight diffusion and weight dispersion techniques. Where hemorrhage is encountered due to subhelomal ulceration or significant hemorrhage within the hyperkeratotic tissue itself, the use of 25–50% silver nitrate is of value. Lumicaine or Negatan may also be employed as a styptic agent to reduce the hemorrhagic area.

Porokeratosis is an obstruction by pressure of the terminal portion of a plantar sweat pore with the formation of a hyperkeratotic plug in the area. These lesions are relatively rare in the geriatric patient but may produce a significant degree of pain. Their management should include some degree of debride-

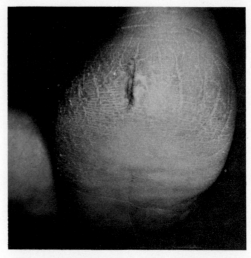

Fig. 4.5   Heel fissure with xerosis of heel.

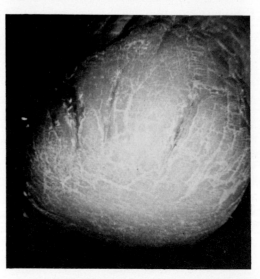

Fig. 4.6   Heel fissure and xerosis associated with arteriosclerotic changes involving the feet.

ment and a significant use of weight diffusion and weight dispersion techniques to remove pressure from the area. The use of plantar-digital urethane pads or some other soft tissue replacement material generally provides an effective means for controlling the symptoms on a regional basis.

Verrucae are neoplastic types of lesions caused by filtrable viruses. Their presence on the foot in the elderly patient is a relatively rare finding. When present, management would be based upon the location of the lesion and the degree of atrophy present in

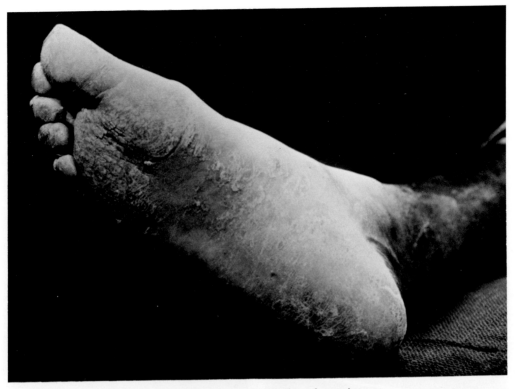

Fig. 4.7   Marked keratosis and xerosis.

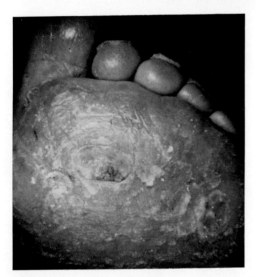

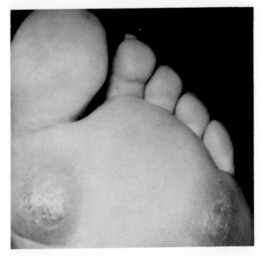

Fig. 4.8   Marked keratosis and xerosis associated with prolapsed metatarsal heads in a patient with residuals from rheumatoid arthritis.

Fig. 4.9   Keratosis involving the first and fifth metatarsal heads, plantarly, associated with biomechanical imbalance.

the patient. Electrosurgical techniques are useful when the lesions are not on the plantar surface of the foot. When the lesions are on the plantar surface of the foot, the controlled

use of Duofilm appears to be an appropriate mechanism for treatment when applied on a daily basis. The solution consists of 16.7% salicylic acid and 16.7% lactic acid in a flexible collodion base. The material should be removed prior to the next application using an appropriate solvent. Care must be exercised, however, in those patients who are diabetic and present with peripheral vascular insufficiency. The treatment of any such lesion in a geriatric patient should be carefully monitored on a periodic basis and patient compliance with instructions is essential. Where mosaic verrucae are present, a most

effective choice in management consists of b.i.d. applications of a solution containing 10% formalin, 1% rose water, and isopropyl alcohol q.s. 100%. This solution is augmented in the evening with the nonoccluded application of Keralyt Gel.

Treatment may require a long period of time but management is relatively safe and few complications are encountered. If the use

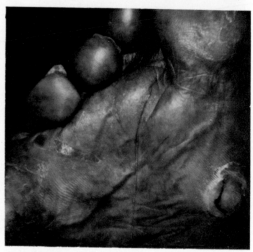

Fig. 4.12 Same as Figure 4.10.

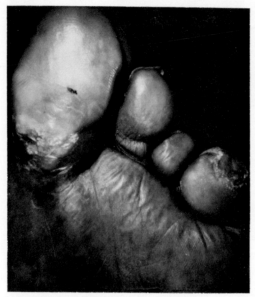

Fig. 4.10 Second-degree chemical burn as a result of self-application of a commercial "corn cure" over-the-counter product.

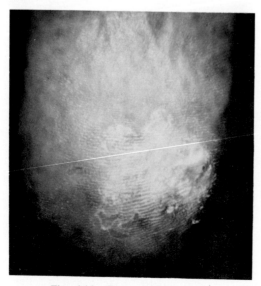

Fig. 4.11 Same as Figure 4.10.

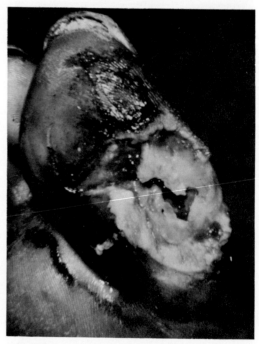

Fig. 4.13 Trauma and ulceration as a result of self-induced removal of keratotic lesion by the patient.

of the formalin solution produces too much drying or fissuring, it may be discontinued for a period of time. If the use of the Keralyt Gel produces any degree of masceration, it too may be discontinued for a period of time. Again, treatment in the geriatric patient should be closely monitored and never considered a routine activity.

Because most geriatric patients present with a significant degree of atrophy involving the skin and muscles of the foot, many of the hyperkeratotic lesions described are also atrophic in nature. Their management should be considered as essential to the geriatric patient's health as the management of any other condition which would create a disability and limit his ambulatory activity. The social ramifications of pain and limited activity in the geriatric patient are significant and far outweigh the cost in what might be considered periodic management of these chronic conditions. Their management is not routine but has been considered routine. One might liken the management of hyperkeratotic le-

sions in the geriatric patient to the management of other diseases such as hypertension, and adult onset diabetes mellitus which require periodic monitoring by the practitioner in order to maintain optimum health and prevent complications. Most foot infections in the geriatric patient, particularly in those who are diabetic and present with vascular insufficiency, can be traced to neglected or inappropriate management of hyperkeratotic lesions. In the diabetic patient, most of the catastrophic loss is the result of self-treatment of these types of lesions.

It is important to note that the management of this class of clinical entity only becomes a noncovered service when present on the foot, as of the writing of this chapter. Unless patients develop significant disease, they are unable to obtain care in a reimbursable manner that many times is the difference between remaining at home in the community and being confined to an institutional environment for their remaining days, giving up the dignity of old age.

chapter 5

Common Skin Problems Associated with the Aging Foot

Arthur E. Helfand, D.P.M.

Perhaps the most common sign of the aging skin of the foot is an associated dryness or atrophic appearance that follows a normal aging process. In addition to dryness, scaling and atrophy of the subcutaneous tissues may present a foot that has a degenerating appearance. Causes for these considerations are varied and multiple. They may be related to systemic disease, functional problems in the elderly, or occur as a result of the normal aging process. However, there is generally a diminished sebaceous activity, there is a diminished hydration of the horny layers, there are alterations in the metabolic and nutritional components associated with the skin, and there is a dysfunction in keratin formation. There is an associated loss of hair which is related both to vascular insufficiency and the aging process involving the skin. The skin of the foot loses its elasticity. Other degenerative changes and pigmentations are common. The associated involvement of the peripheral, arterial and venous systems may also produce many color changes and an increased deposit of hemosiderin in the soft tissues. This factor adds to the disturbed keratin formation.

One of the most common symptoms in the aged foot is pruritus. Its etiologic factors may include disturbed keratin formation, dryness, scaliness, decreased sebaceous activity, environmental changes, hypersensitivity and a defatting of the skin as a result of continuous hot baths. It may also be associated with chronic tinea, neurogenic and emotional dermatoses. It may be more severe in the winter and fall and may be associated with a lowering of the humidity. It may be significant in the presence of xerosis.

There is generally a scratch-itch reflex and many elderly patients generally seek over-the-counter anti-itch remedies. Many of these products, when locally applied, frequently irritate and sensitize the skin, resulting in the early manifestations of a contact dermatitis and increase the pruritus. Pruritus is also a symptom of many other common skin problems that can occur on the foot, including neurodermatitis, contact dermatitis, eczema, drug eruptions and chronic tinea. Because the foot is covered most of the time with stockings and footwear, managing itching in the elderly foot requires both a therapeutic and psychological approach. The elderly patient who is not active, for example, may tend to exaggerate or increase the symptomatology, particularly when it involves pruritus.

Where a specific etiologic factor is involved in the manifestations of pruritus, therapy should be directed to that factor. However, generalized itching of the aging foot involves some basic principles to control the scratch-itch reflex and to deal with the manifestations that are present. The use of mild antihistamines such as tripelennamine hydrochloride, 25 mg. b.i.d., or diphenhydramine hydrochloride, 50 mg. 1 capsule at bedtime, generally provides a significant initial control of itching. Where pruritus is associated with dryness, the use of techniques to both hydrate and lubricate the skin of the foot is of value. This would include the use of bland soaps, the addition of a therapeutic oil bath, bland emollients and/or 20% urea cream, and the application of emollients immediately following hydration. Other antihistamines that are effective in the management of itching include chlorpheniramine maleate, 4 mg. t.i.d., trimeprazine tartrate, 2.5 mg. t.i.d., and for more severe itching, topical corticosteroid preparations are of use.

Neurodermatitis is a localized pruritic dermatosis that may be present on the dorsum of the foot, around the ankles or immediately proximal to the ankles in the geriatric patient. It generally consists of one or more patches of chronic thickened, dry, scaly skin, which cause itching and pigmentary changes. It may be related to a primary problem, but as the itching becomes more intense, the size of the lesion tends to enlarge. In general, this condition tends to be chronic. The patient's primary complaints are those of intense itching, which generally appears to be worse in the evening. Where the etiologic factor can be established, such as contact dermatitis, psoriasis or stasis, for example, treatment should be aimed in that direction. Treatment should generally consist of a frank explanation to the patient and antihistamines to help relieve the itching. Mild bland compresses and topical corticosteroid preparations also are of significant value. Where a significant emotional or psychologic factor proves to be the etiology, mild tranquilizers should be considered, along with a controlled zinc gelatin boot application.

Contact dermatitis is a problem dermatosis in the elderly patient. For example, when the primary factor turns out to be the patient's footwear, the patient may in fact reveal that this is the only pair of shoes he has and he may not be able to afford a new pair to remove the primary irritant. Contact dermatitis in the foot is generally easy to distinguish, as it provides a clear line of demarcation in most cases. The primary etiologic factor in the elderly patient, where the problem is localized and confined to the foot or parts of the foot, tends to be from footwear, such as shoes and stockings, or some topical medication that has been applied by the patient. During the primary phase of contact dermatitis, mild redness, edema, vesicles and/or bullae may be present with some drainage. As this condition progresses, crusting may occur and secondary bacterial infection may be present. Pruritus may accompany this condition and lead to excoriations of the skin itself. Treatment should be directed to identifying the etiologic factor involved in the manifestation of the condition. Where shoes or stockings result in a positive patch test or can be clearly isolated, they should be discarded and changed to material that does not provide the same chemical base. Where topical medications can be clearly isolated, they should be eliminated.

In general, mild saline or aluminum acetate compresses following the elimination of the primary irritant will generally provide a basic relief of the symptoms. The use of a topical corticosteroid preparation will generally produce a rapid return to normally functioning skin. It should be noted that nickel seems to be a primary irritant and, coupled with excessive moisture, may result in dermatologic problems which are basically managed by removing the primary irritating factor.

It should be noted that the general configuration of senile skin may not necessarily be related to the aging process itself. One should remember that aging is an individual matter influenced by many factors, including heredity; thus, aging occurs at different rates even in the same person. The exposure to sun and other harsh weather conditions may accelerate the aging process, but generally speaking, these factors are minimized in the foot, inasmuch as there is a general tendency to provide a foot covering throughout the patient's lifetime. It should also be noted that the lessening of the arterial supply to the skin itself impairs nutrition and changes the metabolic rate which fosters some of the distinctive marks of the aging skin.

In general, the skin may appear dry and yellowish with a wrinkled, inelastic and parchment-like appearance. It has been described many times that the aging foot and lower legs may appear to be cross-hatched in appearance as the effects of glandular activity and hair follicles are decreased. The longitudinal ridging or onychorrhexis that occurs in the toenails as a striated pattern in effect represents an aging process or an onychopathy, which is accentuated by the presence of certain systemic diseases such as diabetes mellitus and peripheral vascular insufficiency.

One of the significant signs that should be noted in any minor trauma is multiple and transient ecchymotic areas which tend to resolve themselves but clearly demonstrate that the skin is undergoing an aging of the peripheral vascular system.

The changes of aging may produce some tumor-like blemishes on the skin which tend to advance with age. These include actinic keratosis, seborrheic keratosis and various types of skin tags. Vascular excrescenes and yellowish papules of hyperplastic sebaceous glands may also appear on the aging foot. Although malignancy of the foot is rare, basal cell carcinoma, squamous cell carcinoma and melanoma should be suspected when lesions are present that do not heal with proper management. Biopsy should be completed and appropriate surgical excision, radiation and/or chemotherapy utilized where indicated by appropriate specialists. With retirement, and the time available to bask in the sun, elderly patients should be advised to limit their exposure to the sunlight inasmuch as the feet may be exposed to excessive amounts of sun for the first time.

Clinicians should also be aware that little or minor strokes may occur, producing bizarre symptoms, including itching of localized parts of the skin. Where these symptoms are suspected, treatment should be aimed at the management of the cerebral vascular problem, the daily ingestion of aspirin and the management of local symptoms by the use of antihistamines and topical antipuritic agents. Care must be exercised in the prolonged use of topical corticosteroids to limit their effects on the atrophied skin of the foot.

Pigmented or purpuric dermatoses may occur on the lower extremities and may exhibit changes in the foot itself. In general, attempts should be made to provide an appropriate and definitive diagnosis. Treatment may be limited to the use of medications for symptoms. The use of bland, antipruritic emollients and topical corticosteroids has been effective in some cases, but much depends upon the ability of the patient to comply and to accept idiopathic problems.

Stasis dermatitis as a result of a complicating factor of varicose veins is common in the elderly patient. Nutritional changes in the skin as a result of chronic venous insufficiency produce a series of disturbances which usually present with a dermatitis of the ankles and feet. If the inflammatory reaction is pronounced, continued secondary injury and infection may be present. The skin presents an ulcer that tends not to heal easily. Most stasis occurs in the elderly patient in a chronic nature and generally may be found in patients who are obese and have suffered from venous disease for a long period of time. The nonsurgical management would include an appropriate evaluation of the venous system, conservative management by the use of well-fitting elastic stockings or other appropriate constricting bandages, and the use of topical treatment, including bland compresses, topical corticosteroids and antibiotics. Where topical treatment fails, surgical skin grafting should be considered, along with other surgical means to manage the varicose ulcers which may be present on the lower portion of the leg and on the foot. The morphologic picture of stasis hemosiderosis is many times clinically identical to that seen in pigmented purpuric eruptions and can be managed in a similar manner.

Ischemia associated with arteriosclerosis obliterans of the lower extremity gives rise to skin color changes on elevation, a decrease in skin temperature, atrophy and glossiness of the foot, a loss of hair over the toes, feet and legs, onychial abnormalities, dry hyperkeratotic lesions on the plantar surface of the foot, ulcers of the toes and heels, and may result in gangrene. There is frequently a coexistence between endarteritis obliterans, diabetes and arteriosclerosis obliterans in the geriatric patient. There need to be significant attempts to provide a preventive mechanism to deal with the problems of patient compliance with hygiene and concern for foot care. Patients should be advised to provide adequate care for any foot condition and to seek immediate attention for any bacterial or fungal infection that may be present.

Patients, particularly women, between the ages of 50 and 70, who have had hypertension, under variable control, for long periods of time may develop a spontaneous painful red plaque on the lateral portion of the ankle or posterior lateral portions of the leg which may involve the foot. The plaque may become purpuric. The lesion may also appear as a simple bluish discoloration of the skin. In general, a hemorrhagic bleb forms as the initial lesion, which then breaks and forms an ulcer. The ulcer tends to be pale and there is little granulation tissue present. A thick scar generally forms and the lesion continues to develop over a period of several months. These ulcers tend to be chronic. Treatment should be aimed at management of the hypertension and appropriate local measures both to control the infection and provide support to the ulcerative area.

Other ulcerative lesions that may occur in the aging foot as a result of venous disease include those associated with thrombophlebitis and sickle cell anemia. In both cases, appropriate management of the identified disease should, in fact, be adequate to provide local support for the condition itself. The elderly rheumatoid patient may present with vasculitis and skin changes which are systemic in origin. The ulcers associated with this type of condition are basically ischemic and should be managed as ischemic ulcers in conjunction with appropriate management of the arthritic process.

Erythema nodosum, erythema induratum, and other nodose lesions may appear on the foot and lower legs of the elderly patients. They may be manifestations of drug sensitivity, especially to iodides, salicylates, the sulfas, barbiturates and antibiotics. Because of the quantity and variety of medications being taken by elderly patients at any given time and because of the prevalance of streptococcal infections, thought to be the most common cause of erythema nodosum, nodose lesions in the elderly patient deserve appropriate consideration. With a history of eruption, sarcoidosis, deep fungal infections, ulcerative colitis, syphilis and other systemic diseases should be considered. Management should attempt to deal with the primary etiologic factor.

Hyperkeratotic lesions on the sole of the foot may be the result of dermatologic problems other than those of mechanical origin. Such problems include those induced by drugs, nonspecific keratosis occurring with lichen planus, psoriasis and Darier's disease. It should be noted that the presence of psoriatic lesions on the soles of the foot may appear to be widespread and many times are confused with tinea pedis. Secondary syphilis may also occur as tiny keratotic papules on the soles and may be present in elderly pa-

tients. Latent tertiary ulcerations of the foot may also be present with syphilis. Keratosis punctata may also be demonstrable in rare cases in elderly patients. These should be differentiated from heloma milliare and can be traced to familial origin, thus an adequate and thorough patient history is required.

Warts or verrucae are viral tumors and are rarely seen in the geriatric patient. They are many times misdiagnosed as intractable heloma, heloma durum or heloma miliare. They are also confused with porokeratosis which is referred to many times as a plugged-up cyst. Where plantar verrucae are clustered they are termed mosaic warts. Their diagnosis generally provides a characteristic pinpoint bleeding area when the lesions are debrided. These lesions tend to be somewhat recalcitrant to management in the geriatric patient and generally respond more slowly than in the pediatric patient or younger adult. Single or solitary verrucae can be treated in many ways. Simple dissection and curettage may be employed, provided that all of the necrotic debris is removed and the patient's vascular supply is adequate for a surgical approach. The use of electrodessication or fulgeration can also be applied, but should generally be avoided on the plantar surface of the foot.

Many acids have been tried in the management of verrucae. Many are effective. Our experience has shown that, for the geriatric patient, where the vascular supply is adequate, daily applications of Duofilm with periodic debridement tends to provide a conservative but safe approach to their management. Where mosaic verrucae are present in the geriatric patient, multiple daily applications of 10% formalin solution, followed by evening applications of Keralyt Gel for longer periods of time, tends to produce a reasonably adequate result.

Another viral disease which may affect the foot is molluscum contagiosum. This is generally rare and once the diagnosis is made, the lesions are easily removed by gentle curettage and minor styptics to control bleeding points.

Herpes zoster or shingles have been reported to occur on the foot. Pain is the predominant factor, especially in the elderly patient. Lesions following a nerve pattern assist in making the diagnosis. The condition is rarely seen on the feet but may be found if the disease is present on the lower extremity. Management consists of symptomatic control of pain and responding to the needs of the patient.

Staphylococcal and streptococcal infections are more common in the elderly patient and those associated with diabetes and vascular insufficiency. Bacterial infections of the foot are severe and should be considered potential threats involving limb loss when well organized. In the geriatric patient with diabetes, pain and swelling may not be identified by the patient due to neuropathy. An appropriate culture and sensitivity test should be employed where needed and antibiotic therapy should be instituted as soon as possible. Hospitalization should be considered if the patient is unable to manage the infection through adequate care. Pseudomonas also can be present on the foot. The Wood's light examination may reveal a greenish-like fluorescence where significant maceration is persistent in the toe webs. Appropriate culture and antibiotics should be employed and generally includes the topical use of polymyxin B, Gentamicin, and other broad spectrum antibiotics. Acetic acid soaks of 0.25% may also be helpful in managing this particular condition.

The effects of leprosy or Hansen's disease, although rare in many parts of the United States, may be present in the foot with ulcerations of the sole and disruption of the digits. Where these conditions are present, the disease should be considered. With the presence of neurotrophic ulcers or mal perforans, leprosy should be considered. In general, however, the ulcers of leprosy are usually multiple as opposed to the solitary lesions which are generally associated with diabetes mellitus, tapes dorsalis, syringomyelia and pernicious anemia.

Tinea pedis may be present in the geriatric patient and is significant in that it may occur with a secondary bacterial infection which presents a difficult problem for the elderly patient, particularly one with concomitant systemic disease. Patients with onychomycosis are commonly involved with the clinical manifestation of tinea pedis and their involvement is also supportive of the clinical evidence of a fungal infection. The most common organisms generally include the *Trichophyton rubrum*, *Trichophyton mentagrophytes*,

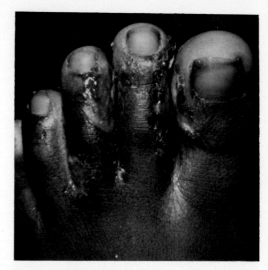

Fig. 5.1   Tinea pedis, interdigital with secondary bacterial infection.

Epidermophyton floccosum and *Candida albicans*. The condition is exaggerated by excessive moisture (hyperhidrosis), and a lack of ventilation and poor pedal hygiene. It should be noted that because of the living conditions of many geriatric patients, i.e. borderline poverty, hygiene is many times a problem for the elderly patient.

There are several clinical varieties. They include the dry, scaly or hyperkeratotic variety; a chronic interdigital manifestation; an acute or subacute vesicular pattern; and those presenting with dermatophytid reactions. With the presence of whitish plaque between the digits, *Candida* and digital psoriasis must be considered. Management of the interdigital manifestations generally include the use of topical fungicides such as clotrimazole or haloprogin and the use of tolnaftate powder to provide a degree of prophylaxis. Where hyperhidrosis may be a precipitating factor appropriate ventilation should be employed to assist in managing this condition. Where pruritus is clinically severe, systemic antihistamines may be required to relieve the itching. The dry plantar hyperkeratotic variety is characterized by an off-white coloring of the scaling aspects of the sole of the foot. In general, the *T. rubrum* generally produces a moccasin-like eruption. These conditions may respond to systemic griseofulvin. However, consideration must be given to the vascular supply of the patient and the potential for untoward reactions to the systemic drug. It has been our experience that most of these lesions can be managed topically with solutions, creams or ointments that not only assist in controlling the mycosis but also provide some degree of lubrication to the skin.

The vesicular type is generally caused by *T. rubrum*. The vesicles are often yellowish and dry to a brownish color. There may be evidence of bacterial infection which should be treated with appropriate antibiotics. Topical soaks, such as aluminum acetate solution or tepid normal saline, are useful in the management of these conditions in addition to appropriate antifungal therapy. Dermatophytids may present as vesicular lesions on the hands in an allergic reaction. Management is appropriate when the tinea pedis is controlled and antihistamines are used for the allergic response. *Monilia* may be more common in the diabetic patient and managed with appropriate nystatin therapy.

Tinea may be confused with erythrasma which is caused by a gram positive bacillus. It is common in the intertriginous areas such as the toe webs and generally provides some degree of maceration and scaling. A coral red fluorescence is noted when the area is illuminated with the Wood's light. The disease responds well to the oral administration of erythromycin and the topical application of fungicides.

Atopic dermatitis may also be present on the foot and there should be a significant historical investigation to determine the relationship to a familial tendency towards this condition. When present on the feet, the skin generally appears scaly and dry and there is a patching effect. Fissuring frequently complicates the picture along with secondary bacterial infection. Atopic dermatitis affecting the feet may also suggest some other conditions such as tinea pedis, psoriasis, contact dermatitis and localized neurodermatitis. The treatment is similar to the conditions on other parts of the body, indicating that the corticosteroid creams are generally the agents of choice. In addition, Iodochlorhydroxyquin may be useful to reduce the pruritus. Oral antihistamines are of value and may need to be dose modified based upon the age and weight of the patient.

Psoriasis is a common disease affecting many patients. When it occurs on the foot of a geriatric patient, it has usually been diagnosed before the age of 65 and has usually been under treatment for a period of time. However, there is a greater tendency for more hyperkeratosis and fissuring on the foot than on other areas of the body. The toenails may also be affected and they resemble mycotic infections. However, the classic pitting of the surface of the nail plate generally permits the diagnosis of psoriasis of the nails to be made. The arthritic changes usually associated with psoriasis generally affect the distal portions of the phalangeal joints and do produce characteristic radiographic changes.

Treatment of psoriasis of the feet differs little from the treatment of the disease on other parts of the body. The applications of corticosteroid creams and ointments generally tend to provide the best management of the problem in the geriatric patient. Generally, psoriasis of the nails is best managed by periodic debridement.

Hyperhidrosis in the elderly individual is usually associated with changes in footwear or tinea pedis. Where increased sweating results in a disagreeable odor bromhidrosis is the term utilized to designate this condition and is generally related to the bacterial involvement and decomposition. For the most part, 10% formalin and the use of topical foot powder again tend to be the most helpful in the geriatric patient. Where hyperhidrosis presents with vesicles, it is known as dyshidrosis. The vesicles may be become bullae and erythema may be present. The treatment should include the use of mild soaks and topical corticosteroids. Decreased sweating on the soles is generally never a clinical problem except when excessive dryness is associated with xerosis, tinea, psoriasis or excessive fissuring. The use of emollients preceded by hydration generally proves to be the most satisfactory treatment for this condition in the elderly patient.

As indicated earlier in this chapter, the various neoplasms, both benign and particularly malignant, may be present in the geriatric patient. Their diagnosis should include appropriate biopsy and management consistent with current treatment of the particular lesion.

There are some general principles which should be included in the management of skin problems involving the aging foot. Pa-

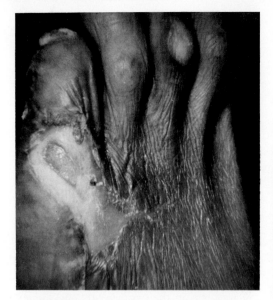

Fig. 5.2   Traumatic ulcer, pretreatment.

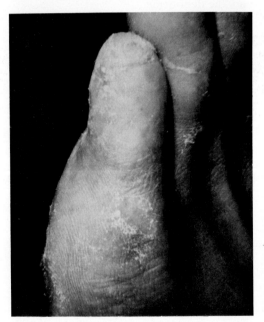

Fig. 5.3   Traumatic ulcer, as shown in Figure 5.2, post-treatment.

tients should be advised to cease using all medications, both topical and systemic, when drug-eruptive types of lesions are present. Appropriate coordination between all of the practitioners managing the patient is imperative if drug eruptions are suspected. Secondary infections, both bacterial and mycotic,

should be appropriately managed with the systemic use of antibiotics. For the most part, erythromycin, tetracycline, cephalosporines, or any other broad spectrum antibiotics generally are the choice. Mycotic infections can be confirmed by the use of culture and mi-

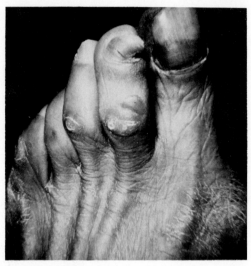

Fig. 5.4   Traumatic bulla associated with shoe trauma. Note digital contractures, bowed tendons, keratotic lesions and nail deformities. Hallux valgus and digital deformities associated with residuals of rheumatoid arthritis.

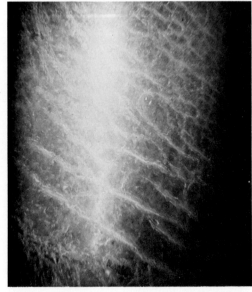

Fig. 5.5   Xerosis associated with diabetes mellitus.

croscopic examination. However, clinical judgment and a significant historical background may prove to be a good starting point in the management of these conditions. Patch testing and biopsy should be utilized where appropriate. A diagnosis should be made prior to the use of medications to relieve symptoms such as pain and itching. When soaks or compresses are suggested, care should be taken that the foot does not become macerated. Thus may lead to secondary bacterial infection, as most geriatric patients are poor compliers. The same guidelines should be used in prescribing occlusive dressings.

Patients with foot skin conditions, should be urged to wear cotton socks as much as possible and to keep a record of the various types of footwear and stockings worn daily.

Patients should be warned against wearing tight shoes or athletic shoes for long periods of time.

Skin problems in the elderly patient involving the foot represent a varied diagnostic and therapeutic approach. The physical location of a patient in either an independent activity or a long-term care facility many times provides the key for treatment and management. It is extremely important to remember that the geriatric patient may have no other occupation other than to deal with his skin condition which is both physical and touchable. Many times dealing with a patient as a whole both mentally and physically provides the best key to the management of common skin problems on the geriatric foot.

chapter 6

Orthopedic Surgical Considerations of the Aged

Frank A. Mattei, M.D.

Each generation has succeeded in increasing its longevity. Individuals who were considered "old" forty years ago are now actively enjoying their added years until their "old age" dawns upon them. We now see an increasing number of geriatric patients replacing our "cradle-to-the-grave" younger patients. These individuals have survived the test of time. Usually they have suffered from one or several degenerative diseases. They should be evaluated physiologically, not chronologically, as to their candidacy for surgery. Persons reach middle age in better physical condition than they used to because of our added knowledge from other fields of medicine. Tissues as well as organs are more adaptable to stress than they were in previous generations. Patients are now more suitable candidates for surgery because of their improved physical as well as mental condition; their attitudes are more mature, and thus they are more understanding and more cooperative in their approach to surgery. With informed consent, they now share the burden of responsibility as to the surgical adventure they are undertaking. The very nature of what surgery can serve them must be clearly understood. The surgical procedure is carefully evaluated—whether it is to be performed for the relief of pain, to gain locomotion, or to save his life—and is chosen in light of what is best for the patient.

After we have arrived at a careful understanding of the problem, and what our final goal is as to our results, we must explain the necessary complications that may develop, for we cannot forecast a prognosis with certainty, but can only go by our past experience.

In foot surgery, in the aged, careful consideration of the patient's entire physical condition is of the utmost importance. The ultimate prognosis in the aged group must rest entirely on the proper medical attention. Today, with the geriatric specialty as we have developed it, we can call on these specialists to properly evaluate the general factors of nutrition, the cardiopulmonary status, and the general urinary status, as well as the mental and emotional states of our patient, thus reducing the medical risk of surgery.

From Dr. Helfand's excellent article "Keep Them Walking," we have the theme of this book. As we know, the old story for want of a nail, the shoe was lost," etc., certainly applies when we are considering foot surgery. We must look upon the patient not only from the foot but the entire extremity in relation to the foot and then to the entire body mechanism so as to gain proper insight into our problem, and to the solution of our problem in performing foot surgery. Thus, our theme of "keeping them walking" is utmost in importance from the general standpoint of the entire body as well as the foot.

We must understand the proper mechanism of locomotion in order to gain a maximum result when we concentrate on one local entity such as the foot and ankle joint.

Whereas deformities that occur associated with dynamics are usually due to complications resulting from a disease process, such as rheumatoid arthritis, gout, or collagen diseases, they usually resemble so-called static deformities and disabilities that result from osteoarthritis, or are related to trauma, resulting in a deformed foot.

In general, the problem found in the arthritic foot is different from the problem found in that of the static disability. That is, the arthritic foot shows a general condition such as a general inflammation, severe damage, and progression of the deformity with resultant changes that resemble a static deformity. We have severe articular damage, with joint deformity of the forefoot and hindfoot, resulting in ankylosis and severe deformities that are not usually found in static conditions. The changes found in progressive rheumatoid arthritic conditions are the most serious and the most complex in our approach to treatment. During the advancement of the disease in the geriatric patient, the pathological changes have now completed their course and are "slowed down" in their rapid progression to a total disability. Pallor, pain and muscle spasm occur. This is Mother Nature's way of telling the patient to rest the joint and to try to protect the joint, i.e., muscle spasm, to insure against any further trauma. However, as we know, all muscle spasms contract and flex the joints, leading to the severe deformity that we see in a rheumatoid arthritic. In the early stages there is an inflammation of the joints, with marked thickening of the synovial tissue and a growth of panus over the cartilage of the joint. With this pain and swelling of the joint, motion is limited, thereby causing muscle atrophy and progressive weakness. Here, the vicious cycle begins and we have less motion, more pain and deformity, and fibrosis of the joint. Here we see the relaxation of the articulating capsules and ligaments of the joints, with resultant marked hallux valgus, a splaying of the entire forefoot at the metatarsal phalangeal joints, with beginning subluxation leading to luxation of the metatarsal phalangeal joints of the foot and eventual heel valgus and equinus of the ankle joint. It may be noted that these conditions progress to a static form with partial destruction, subluxation and ankylosis of the ankle, tarsal and metatarsal phalangeal joints. It should also be noted that there is a definite appearance of the skin, which becomes "tissue paper" thin, smooth, glassy, and tender to palpate.

It should be also noted that rheumatoid nodules and inflamed bursal sacs develop at the flexion points of the foot and heel and around the Achilles tendon. It is these conditions and the position of these nodules that may cause pain and put pressure on the foot when the patient wears shoes. This progression leads to congestion with a change in the vascular channel of the foot and the ankle, with resultant ulcerations, limited vascularity, loss of proper muscle function, and wasting of the areas involved. X-rays reveal marked changes in the bone structure and a loss of mineralization. It is amazing that these patients are able to bear weight and at times are symptom free. Ambulation is somewhat limited. However, with this decrease in pain, usually the patient becomes more resistant to pain. On weight bearing, the unpadded loss of tissue around the bony components of the foot leads to the development of painful callouses and bursal sacs. Ulcerations may develop at the flexion points and complete breakdown of the skin may result in osteomyelitis.

However, in the majority of patients who have developed rheumatoid arthritis, the diagnosis is usually made from an examination affecting other joints of the body, and early treatment is attempted to bring the arthritic involvement under control, to prevent any other disabilities of the feet before terminal deformities occur. This is done usually with discontinuation of weight bearing and exercises. If the patient is able to bear weight, proper fitting shoes with crepe soles, fewer pressure points, and padding, aid the patient in ambulation unless the symptoms are severe enough to limit ambulation.

When the pain becomes too severe the patient should not be allowed to walk until the pain has subsided. A foot support may consist of a cast, of soft type material, or eventual hard casting, applied from the toes and to the knee joint, with the foot being held at a right angle to the leg with the arch of the foot molded into the cast. These casts are usually bivalved so that the patient can usually remove the cast for exercising.

These are supervised exercises, and the use of physical modalities to relieve pain and swelling of the feet are also utilized. They are continued until the pain subsides. It must be noted that the supervised exercises should be done within a painless arc, and if pain becomes too severe, they should be discontinued. However, if there is little or no discomfort, these exercises are started with proper setting of the flexors and extensors of the toes, so we can have a balanced foot which will aid in ambulation. We have not advised any foot massages or any other form of physical modalities which cause irritation to the foot. However, in the aged, if the disability does not respond, weight bearing should be stopped and the foot should be manipulated and recast. When this disorder is resolved the cast is bivalved and the patient resumes his active supervised exercises. The aged patient may not respond to conservative measures because of the long-standing deformities that have been established; therefore, he must resort to surgical intervention to correct the deformities and offer a stable weight bearing support. It is almost impossible to restore a normal foot when these changes occur. The most common deformity that is not corrected with conservative measures is usually marked depression of the metatarsal heads. Here the fat pads are lessened and the skin is directly encroaching on the metatarsal heads.

Also, marked deformities of the forefoot occur at the proximal interphalangeal joints, forming so-called "hammer toe deformities." As we stated previously, surgery can be quite radical here to gain a stable weight gaining support. As stated, the removal of a metatarsal head through a dorsal incision relieves the marked pressure that occurs on the metatarsal heads. Hammer toe deformities are usually corrected by removal of the cartilage on both sides of the proximal phalangeal joints. Firm wire is then drilled through to hold the phalanges in a normal position. The wire is then allowed to remain until there is fusion. However, if there is a severe subluxation of the metatarsal phalangeal joint, removal of approximately ½ of the proximal phalanx is a preferred procedure and is much simpler and the results obtained are usually better, with better patient tolerance. For the hallux valgus deformity, a simple procedure is done where a capsular revision is performed and the exostosis is removed. All impingements of the articulating head, both superiorly and inferiorly are also removed.

Then the first toe is brought into adduction with a stretching of the capsule and brought down to its new base of the metatarsal osteotomy site. Upon completion, immobilization is approximately 3–6 weeks, with the use of a surgical shoe so that the patient can be ambulatory under supervision. It is interesting to note that in certain cases, where there is a marked displacement of the angle of the first metatarsal, with displacement of the first phalanx laterally, correction with a simple exostosectomy and capsular revision would not correct the deformity. If one adds an osteotomy of the first metatarsal to correct the deformity to bring it into proper alignment, a modified Keller or Aiken procedure should be considered. After convalescence is completed, the patient is placed on an exercise program and proper shoes are worn. This is done to train the patient in proper foot balance and strengthen the muscles to insure satisfactory results and the return of function.

Soft tissue lesions may develop and become rheumatoid nodules. These include tenosynovitis, ganglions and other cystic enlargements of the tendon sheaths. They usually respond to conservative treatments. If they are large and painful, surgery should be performed to remove these masses. If the invasion of the tendon by a rheumatoid nodule leads to a rupture of the tendon, it must be repaired. But one must recognize that this is a diseased tendon and may recur. Here again the area involved may be best repaired by bony fusion of the affected portion of the foot.

Another inflammatory entity which will cause foot discomfort with resultant surgery is that of gout. This usually begins with middle age, with an acute articular change affecting the metatarsal phalangeal joints. Other sites may be affected. The patient is usually affected in the morning hours with pain becoming unbearable on weight bearing and quite disabling. The skin of the joint is edematous, red, hot, and tender, somewhat resembling an infectious joint. This condition may subside, particularly when treated medically. However, in the geriatric patient, after repeated episodes of a gouty arthritis, changes that may occur in the toes and joints of the foot are usually at the first metatarsal phalangeal joint, and result in a breakdown of the cartilaginous area, with marked deformity.

X-rays usually demonstrate punched out lesions of the bony components with obliteration of the joint. When the area involved is so disabling, surgery is indicated. Removal of the mass and the tissue surrounding the area is to be considered. Attempts should be made to remove only the urate crystals and the deformity, sparing as much of the tendon, blood vessels, nerves, soft tissue and nonaffected areas as possible. However, the treatment of gout is usually a medical problem and at the present time, with early recognition and treatment, we see less and less gouty arthritis in the aged.

Another common disorder found in the geriatric patient is that of osteoarthritis of the foot. Many of the patients that we see who have osteoarthritis of the foot are asymptomatic. This condition differs from rheumatoid arthritis in its inflammatory nature and is less progressive, less inflammatory and less disabling. There is only a small percentage of patients who develop symptoms that we see and treat in the office. This condition is due to a decreased function of the foot with articular changes in all joints, degeneration of the cartilage, thickening of the ligamental structures, and a loss of elasticity. The foot is seen with bony overgrowth throughout the margins of the joints. Once again Mother Nature is attempting to protect the joint from additional destruction by trying to eliminate the motion by this bony overgrowth. However, less pain develops because of this pathological change. The most common sites of osteoarthritis are usually at the first metatarsal phalangeal joint. Spurs develop and interfere with dorsiflexion of the first metatarsal phalangeal joint, leading toward a condition called hallux limitus or hallux rigidus. Other spurs usually occur at the Achilles tendon and at the insertion of the plantar fascia, just beyond the medial tubercle of the os calcis. These bone spurs are along the ligamentous and muscle planes.

In an asymptomatic foot as well as a symptomatic foot, prevention of any additional deformity of the joint is done by proper support to limit joint motion, and to delay the eventual fusion of the joint. During this time the arches of the foot are protected and the patient is given a program of foot care with exercises to strengthen the supporting structures. In the past, injections of the first meta-tarsal phalangeal joint have been used for the relief of pain and to reduce articular swelling. These injections were given directly into the joint and not in the tendon sheath. It is only when the foot becomes totally disabled and the patient cannot move his foot in a spring-like manner that one must resort to surgery to relieve this deformity. Most problems are usually relieved by proper support, proper exercises, and weight reduction, to prevent any further trauma to the foot. When surgery is indicated, it is usually chiefly to remove the bone spurs and exostosis that may develop.

At the present time, procedures that produce a short toe have been replaced with implants at the area of the proximal phalanx to communicate with the head of the first metatarsal. While we are still at a preliminary stage, our results have generally been good.

Heel spurs that may develop are helped by a heel cup to remove shoe irritation and reduce pressure. If the condition does not improve, then we may resort to a simple removal of the spur with partial resection of the interfacial plane, but this condition is only surgically considered when the pain is too severe and conservative care provides little relief. Spurs that occur on the phalanges should also be removed to eliminate any friction points on the opposite toes.

As we pass from the inflammatory conditions of the so-called dynamic disabilities of the foot, it must be said that these conditions that occur from deformity are usually associated with friction and pressure related to external incompatibilities. They are most commonly caused by an ill-fitting or incompatible shoe that exerts continuous pressure on existing deformities. These conditions, such as hallux valgus, hammer toes, etc., are mechanical in nature and degenerative, and limit ambulation.

Hallux valgus deformity, or bunion, is a deformity of the first metatarsal phalangeal joint with the phalanx pointed in the lateral direction, and the probable formation of an exostosis on the first metatarsal head with a bursal sac developing over the exostosis. Symptoms usually begin with pain over the dorsal medial aspect of the first metatarsal head or over the "bunion pocket" itself. The great toe becomes enlarged and is tender to palpate. Also, the second toe may override the first toe, causing callous formation over the great toe on the medial side and under the plantar surface of the metatarsal head. Many times the patient thinks that cosmetically she wants to have this condition corrected. If asked if she has any pain, she says "no, but it looks terrible."

In evaluating hallux valgus deformity, a careful history, as well as an examination of the total patient, is essential. Does the patient have any loss of motion of the joints of the feet? Is there any disturbance of circulation? Does the patient have any pinpoint tenderness? Does the patient have any neurological deficits in respect to the great toe? Is the range of motion in all planes normal? What is the degree of deformity in relation to other foot segments? Is there any deformity and are there pressure points over the toes? Is there any subluxation of the metatarsal phalangeal joints?

Muscle tone and function should be demonstrated. Weight bearing and nonweight bearing x-rays should be studied. Following this evaluation, the patient should then identify what she is looking for: "to relieve pain," or to improve appearance of the foot, or both. Will the patient try conservative measures? Will the patient resort to surgery? If the patient decides on conservative measures, a proper shoe should be utilized to help relieve pressure. Orthotics may also be employed. The patient is placed on a program of exercises for muscle strengthening and stretching. If the patient states that she is willing to resort to surgical measures, and certain criteria are met, such as pain, inability to ambulate without difficulty, or that the condition has been progressive, surgery can be considered, and the proper operative procedure selected, following proper medical evaluation and postoperative planning.

A review of the literature demonstrates that approximately 150 procedures have been prescribed for correction of this deformity. We are not advocating any one particular surgical procedure but only that the clinician remember the principles involved and follow these principles to gain good results. Following surgery, a vigorous postoperative care program should be followed to prevent infection and strengthen muscles, and proper shoes should be used to prevent any further deformities. To the patient it seems like a long drawn-out affair, but she must follow the postoperative course to the limit.

Another entity that produces disability is a hallux rigidus or hallux limitus. The term rigidus was first described as a dorsal bunion. This condition is a degenerative osteoarthritis of the first metatarsal phalangeal joint which is usually due to trauma or other mechanical means. On examination and manipulation, there is restriction of motion, both flexion and extension, of the metatarsal phalangeal joint. There is usually a marked amount of pain after passive motion. X-ray evaluation demonstrates narrowing of the joint with possible spur formation and a flexion of the joint. Treatment is directed towards the prevention of any further destruction of the first metatarsal phalangeal joint. This may be done by conservative measures such as a rigid orthotic applied to the shoe to restrict motion at the metatarsal phalangeal joint. Intra-articular steroids may be given to relieve pain. Orthotics and support are also appropriate.

If the pain is severe and the patient cannot ambulate with comfort when he walks because of the pain, surgery may be considered, and only considered after conservative measures have failed. Again, in this condition, there are many operative procedures considered. However, the most popular is a Keller operation which relieves the joint surface by removing part of the proximal phalanx to allow a greater range of motion. The second most popular procedure is complete arthrodesis. The third is to remove all of the excessive growth of bone around the metatarsal head and phalanges, and attempt to maneuver the joint in flexion and extension. However, this condition requires a continued amount of rest to the joint to relieve any swelling for the period of approximately 6–8 weeks. And finally, the insertion of a joint prosthesis into the phalanx should also be considered. Here again, postoperative care is quite important.

Another deformity is the hammer toe, which is a contracture of the interphalangeal joint. It may be treated conservatively by different paddings and braces to prevent any pressure over the area involved. Surgical revision is usually successful. One procedure that should be considered is a partial phalangectomy of the proximal phalanx. The postoperative course is usually uneventful and the patient usually gets very good relief from this simple operation.

A tailor's bunion or bunionette involves

the fifth toe and metatarsal. It may become quite painful due to a callous formation over the fifth metatarsal head. A partial ostectomy of the fifth metatarsal head may be considered for this condition.

GANGRENE AND INFECTION IN THE FOOT

Two of the most common causes of arterial insufficiency of the foot are occlusive arterial disease, due to diabetes, and arteriosclerosis. In our experience, these two conditions may lead to ischemic gangrene and infection in the foot.

Care must be provided in the treatment of the diabetic foot. The majority of the patients we have seen with diabetes have clinical evidence of arterial insufficiency of the foot at the time corrective surgery is to be performed. It must be understood that diabetes must be kept under control before any attempt at foot surgery can be considered regardless of how small the procedure is. Instructions should be given to the patient on proper foot care in order to prevent patients from self-treating any superficial lesion. We stress that when you are dealing with a diabetic foot, it should be treated as a potentially infected foot as soon as the skin is broken. Care must be taken to prevent such infections from developing which may eventually lead to gangrene if unproperly cared for. When the complications of infection develop in the diabetic foot, following surgery, great care must be taken to eliminate any possibility of gangrene developing. However, once gangrene develops, care must be given to the foot from a surgical standpoint for proper drainage of the infection to allow a proper line of demarcation. However, the decision to amputate a part of a toe, the whole toe, the foot, or the leg depends on the progression of the gangrene and the vascularity of the leg. We must remember, in dealing with the aged, that they do not tolerate the prosthesis of the limb as well as the young, and it is disabling for them to manage without their joints and foot sen-

sation to the ground. This should be taken into consideration when one attempts to eliminate gangrene by amputation. In dealing with the patient with arteriosclerosis who has had an injury to the circulation of the foot, one must evaluate the entire lower limb as to whether there is a sound indication of a major vessel blockage which usually affects the toes and the foot, and progressively moves up to the ankle joint and the lower leg.

Once necrosis has been established and diagnosed properly, there is little alternative but to amputate the limb and use a prosthesis for ambulation.

Arteriosclerosis that may affect the blood flow, resulting in an ischemic limb, may be due to thrombosis with vascular changes to localized areas of the foot. The problem is one of a line of demarcation. Noting that there is usually no infection, or if the infection is controlled, an amputation may be performed at any proximal level consistent with good function, provided the skin at that level is warm and demonstrates good blood supply. The patient must be observed following surgery to eliminate causes of infection. This is the major enemy of the limb following amputation. All steps must be taken to control infection before the amputation is done. In the foot that is gangrenous and has evidence of infection, you can rest assured that the gangrenous area will become progressive and any attempt to operate at the level of the gangrenous site only results in the need of further surgery because of the progressing gangrene associated with ischemia. Therefore, with evidence of infection all areas must be open sufficiently to allow proper drainage regardless of the area involved. All necrotic tissue must be removed. If done inadequately, this only results in further needless surgery. The entire period may take many weeks. When the lesion is stabilized, additional decisions can be made. If dealing with ischemic gangrene of the foot, one must always control the infection for a successful end result.

The most important factor is proper diagnosis, proper criteria for care, and a total team approach to patient management.

chapter 7

Common Orthopedic Problems in the Geriatric Foot—Part I

Neil J. Kanner, D.P.M.

More than any other segment of our population, members of the geriatric community are dependent upon their feet. Geriatrics who can walk comfortably are able to lead an independent lifestyle. They are able to care for themselves, shop for themselves and socialize with friends and relatives. Geriatrics who are unable to walk because of a foot problem become dependent upon friends and relatives. The basic necessities of life—caring for themselves, shopping for themselves and socializing—become a tiresome burden. These people then lose their independence and in many cases become dependent upon society. Institutionalization is then required to care for them. Studies have shown us that the geriatric who is capable of independent ambulation has a much higher quality of lifestyle. These patients are much less susceptible to physical and mental problems which will develop in the geriatric who is kept immobile. The geriatric patient is keenly aware of how debilitating foot pathology can be, and for this reason readily seeks podiatric care.

One of the most exciting and challenging aspects of podiatric practice is the dealing with orthopedic foot problems of the geriatric patient. These problems can be quite complicated and many times difficult to treat. There are many and varied factors which come together and serve a direct part in causing orthopedic problems in the geriatric patient. The aging process, which causes degeneration in the health and quality of the skin, fat, muscle, and osseous structures of the foot, is one of the most contributing factors. Vascular and nutritional changes occur, having a deleterious effect upon the geriatric foot. Common orthopedic deformities can usually lead to abnormal pressure points. One of the most common complaints that the geriatric patient will present in the podiatrist's office is a "painful corn or callus." These structural abnormalities of the foot will result in an abnormal weight bearing pattern, which will usually result in the formation of hyperkeratotic lesions. As mentioned before, due to aging and vascular changes that take place, the geriatric skin cannot tolerate these abnormal pressures to it. The result is that the skin often breaks down and forms an ulceration. Infections can and do develop quite rapidly in the geriatric patient. In many cases it may take many weeks of pain and suffering until the infection is healed. Because of the dependent attitude of the foot, treatment of a pedal ulcer can be quite involved and, in many cases, may require hospitalization of the geriatric patient.

Concomitant problems such as rheumatoid arthritis, degenerative joint disease, wear and tear effects upon the joints of the foot that occur after 50, 60 or 70 years of age, coupled with the normal changes that occur with the aging process, all add up to making treatment of orthopedic problems in the geriatric quite challenging.

In geriatric foot orthopedics we are not as concerned with the etiology of the structural foot deformities as we are with alleviating their symptoms. With younger populations, we are much more concerned with the biomechanics of the foot. By understanding and investigating the biomechanics of a foot we can detect any early abnormalities of the musculoskeletal system, especially osseous deformities of the foot. However, with the geriatric foot, we are dealing with a foot that has been functioning for the last 5–7 decades and the abnormal biomechanical forces have done their work in causing the fixed structural deformities. In addition to biomechanics, we also have to deal with the forces that the many years of wearing certain styles of shoes have done to the foot, as well as the types of environmental surfaces and uses to which the foot has been subjected to. We also have to deal with the systemic medical factors that can also affect the foot, as was said before, such as the arthritis, gout, aging, peripheral vascular disease, and neurological disease entities.

HEEL PAIN

A geriatric patient will often present with a chief complaint of pain in the heel. The clinician will first have to determine what part of the heel is painful and second, what is the cause. The pain may be secondary to an acute fascitis or a calcaneal bursitis. It may be secondary to a Haglund's deformity, or ankylosing spondylitis. It may simply be caused by significant loss of the fat pad beneath the heel, subjecting the plantar surface of the calcaneus to an abnormal amount of pressure. This loss of fat is commonly found in many long-standing cases of rheumatoid arthritis. The pain in the heel may simply be caused by shoe pressure of long standing.

One of the most common heel problems is that of the painful heel spur. Many theories have been presented as to the etiology of the heel spur. My feeling is that the pain associated with a heel spur is not always caused by the osseous spur. The spur is actually a shelf of bone that usually forms along the entire width of the plantar surface of the medial calcaneal tubercle.

We know that in many cases of painful heels there is no bony spur visible on x-ray. We also know that many times, upon examining a lateral radiograph of a foot, we find heel spurs and there is no associated pain.

This type of heel spur is found on x-rays as an incidental finding. The pain experienced with the heel spur is due to an inflammatory process that occurs at the attachment of the plantar fascia and soft tissue structures to the plantar tubercle of the calcaneus. I explain the etiology of this disorder to my patients by comparing the foot to an archer's bow. This analogy makes it very easy to explain how both the inflammatory process and the formation of the actual shaft of bone (heel spur) occur. The osseous structures of the foot resemble the bow, and the soft tissue structures attached to the heel resemble the bow string. As we know, the attachment of the soft tissue structures to the heel is limited predominantly to the area of the plantar calcaneal tubercles. The soft tissue structures run distally and attach to many different areas of the forepart of the foot. With an associated hypermobility syndrome of the foot such as excessive pronation, there is a lot of pulling at both ends of the "bow string." The pulling at the distal aspect is hardly noticed since there are many and varied points of attachment. The pulling at the proximal area is concentrated at the tubercle of the calcaneus and this is where all the force occurs. Soft tissue structures pulling on the periosteum of the bone set up an inflammatory process. The pulling also ruptures small parts of the periosteum away from the bone with the eventual formation of the bone spur. As we can see, the primary etiology of this problem is mechanical in nature, i.e., excessive pulling of the soft tissue structures upon the intracalcaneal tubercle of the heel.

The patient will usually present to the office with a history of the heel being very painful upon weight bearing. The pain is usually greatest upon initially stepping upon the foot, such as on arising first thing in the morning, or after sitting and resting for awhile. With walking, the pain seems to lessen somewhat. Yet, with continued sitting or walking there seems to be an exacerbation of symptoms. Usually the symptoms are relieved with rest. In severe cases pain will be quite severe and constant. This constant pain may be quite disabling to the geriatric patient, making him unwilling and unable to do much walking.

On evaluation of the patient, we find, in most cases, an excessive amount of pronation or hypermobility occurring at the subtalar joint. The treatment therefore should be based on and geared towards etiology. Initially we want to immobilize or stabilize the subtalar joint against excessive motion. This may be done initially by the use of an adhesive Low-Dye strapping, or other such modality. We usually like to incorporate a scaphoid pad or Carleton saddle pad. The strapping is applied holding the joint slightly inverted. This will prevent the excessive amount of motion or pronation at the subtalar joint. In acute cases the use of injectable corticosteroids with local anesthesia is indicated for the patient's immediate relief. The heel should be palpated thoroughly and the greatest point of pain is the trigger area and that is where the injection should be performed. After injection of the corticosteroid, physical therapy should be applied to that area. The physical therapy modalities can include ultrasound, and/or a form of hydrotherapy. The immobilization can then be applied. The patient is usually given a prescription for a nonsteroidal anti-inflammatory medication. Patients are also instructed to apply heating pads to the foot for 20 minutes twice a day. It is advisable to warn a geriatric patient to put a towel between the foot and the heating pad and to check the temperature occasionally, to make sure that it is not too warm. The patient should be reevaluated in approximately 5–7 days. If there is still any tenderness left upon palpation of the heel, the strapping should be reapplied after physical therapy is given. It should be explained to the patient that long-term stabilization is going to be needed of the subtalar joint to prevent recurrence. This is most efficiently accomplished by the use of a semi-rigid or rigid orthotic device placed in the shoe. If the patient has the joint motion to accommodate a functional orthotic, this of course will give the greatest amount of stability to the subtalar joint. However, it has been my experience that most of the geriatric patients are unable to tolerate such a rigid device. We then go to the use of a semi-rigid orthotic. There are many different types of devices that can be used to stabilize the subtalar joint. The basic philosophy is the same: stabilize the foot and prevent the abnormal pulling at the calcaneal tubercle. Whether we use a heel cup, semi-rigid orthotic, Carleton saddle pads or rigid orthotic is immaterial. What is important is that stability is accomplished. We also give the patient a prescription for an oxford shoe with a rigid shank and counter to again increase the maximum degree of stability. Important in treating any painful symptom on the geriatric foot is the taking of weight bearing biomechanically positioned radiographs of both feet.

Plantar Fascitis

Sometimes a patient will present with pain in the heel radiating distally into the arch of the foot. Pain radiating into the arch can occur with or without concomitant heel pain. Upon palpation it will be noticed that the pain appears to occur along the course of the plantar fascia. As stated, plantar fascitis can occur with or without concomitant painful heel. The problem with plantar fascitis is likewise a mechanical problem and is treated in a similar fashion, i.e., stabilization of the subtalar and midtarsal joint. Initially treatment is instituted via the application of a Low-Dye strapping, incorporating a scaphoid pad. In acute cases if a trigger point can be located the injections of corticosteroids and local anesthesia can afford significant relief of pain. Likewise the use of oral nonsteroidal anti-inflammatories and physical therapy modalities will usually provide the patient with an almost immediate and dramatic relief. Following resolution of the acute symptomatology the patient should be followed up with an orthosis to stabilize the foot and to prevent excessive pronation. Needless to say, weight bearing and biomechanically positioned radiographs should be taken, since the pain in the heel can also be caused by Paget's disease, arthritis or stress fractures. Among the degenerative changes that occur with the aging process, there is in some cases a loss of the adipose tissue that is found beneath the calcaneus. This is a common occurrence in the long-standing rheumatoid arthritic patient. When this occurs the "shock absorbing" effect of the fat pad is lost. Without this fat pad the calcaneus can become sore. In many cases the patient will develop a thick callus beneath the calcaneus. Treatment for this condition is to attempt to supplement the loss of the shock absorbing quality of the fat pad. This can be accomplished in many different ways. The use of plastic heel cups can be quite helpful in this condition. Urethane or styrofoam molded heel cups also can be constructed to protect the plantar surface at the calcaneus. In very mild cases the placement of a 1 to 2-inch urethane foam heel pad may be sufficient to prevent any symptoms whatsoever.

Haglund's Deformity

Pain in the heel can also occur at the posterior aspect of the calcaneus. The pain may be caused by pressure on an enlargement of the posterior superior aspect of the calcaneus at the area of the attachment of the tendo achillis. This osseous enlargement is commonly called "pump bump," or Haglund's deformity. Over the years as a result of this osseous deformity, a bursal sac may form due to the constant pressure and friction from the counter of the shoe. Continued irritation of this osseous deformity and the bursal sac can establish an inflammatory process on the bursal sac leading to an acute bursitis. In chronic cases there may even be a thickening callus forming over the entire area. The pain associated with this deformity can occur either from irritation to the bone or, as I said before, from an adventitious bursal sac that can form in the area. Bursae may form between the calcaneus and tendo achillis or between the tendo achillis and the skin.

Treatment

If we are dealing with an acute bursitis the treatment of choice would be aspiration of the bursal sac and injections of a corticosteroid and local anesthesia to reduce the inflammation.

Physical therapy modalities to the area such as ultrasound, hydrotherapy, and/or hot packs can also be implemented. Follow-up with nonsteroidal inflammatory agents is again indicated in acute inflammatory stages. As the initiating factor in this problem is irritation of the counter, it is imperative that the patient remove all irritation from the shoe counter to this part of the heel bone. We instruct the patients to either take an old shoe and cut the counter or wear a counterless shoe, such as a slip-on, slipper or sandal. Once the acute stage has passed attempts should be made to prevent further irritation

from the shoe to this area of the foot. This can be accomplished in several different ways. One, simply using a heel lift to elevate that part of the heel above the counter in many cases is quite helpful. In addition, we can modify the shoe to prevent the counter from irritating the foot. Removable orthotic devices can be constructed to fit directly over the calcaneus to protect the enlargement of the posterior aspect of the calcaneus from irritation of the shoe. Needless to say, radiographs should be taken of the area to determine the extent of the osseous pathology involved. Shoes should be chosen that have either a very low-cut counter or, at best, a very soft, nonrigid counter. Obviously, a very rigid and stiff counter shoe is one to be avoided. In severe cases, or when the patient does not seem to be responding to conservative modalities, surgical intervention may have to be considered.

Equinus Deformity

Over the years of wearing shoes with high heels, female patients tend to develop a shortening of the tendo achillis and/or the gastrocnemius-soleus muscle group. This shortening or equinus deformity can cause significant symptoms and problems for the patient. The patient is unable to wear shoes with flat heels, as they cause too much strain at the posterior attachment to the calcaneus. The patient can feel the symptoms of strain and pain at this attachment of the tendon to the calcaneus or to the tendon itself or in the muscle belly or in all three places. In cases where there is sufficient motion in the subtalar joint, the patient may pronate excessively in an attempt to compensate for this equinus deformity. This excessive pronation can cause fatigue and strain symptoms in the foot.

In acute cases, the use of a heel lift to relieve the stress is indicated. Likewise, the use of physical therapy modalities, such as warm compresses, ultrasound, and/or hydrotherapy will afford the patient great relief. In addition, the short-term use of the nonsteroidal anti-inflammatories or muscle relaxants, as indicated, is also effective in relieving the symptoms. When the acute symptoms have been resolved, the patient can begin exercises in an attempt to stretch the gastrocnemius-soleus muscle group. In most cases, with the geriatric patient, however, the use of a heel lift incorporated into the shoe to relieve the stress is probably the best for long-term relief of symptoms. When pedal symptoms are also present, a heel lift can also be incorporated into a semi-rigid orthotic to relieve the stress and stabilize the subtalar and midtarsal joints.

MIDFOOT PATHOLOGY

Most of the pathology and symptomatology that we see in the midpart of the geriatric foot is caused by stresses and strains placed upon the foot. With the aging process, the ligamentous and musculoskeletal structures of the foot lose their strength. Hypermobilities will occur predominantly in the subtalar and midtarsal joints, causing abnormal and excessive muscle pull and ligament strains. These hypermobilities will in time cause actual deviations in the osseous structures. It is not uncommon, therefore, to see, in many geriatric feet, an enlargement around the head of the talus as it bulges along the medial side of the foot. Commonly, callus formations are found above these lesions secondary to shoe rub. Another area commonly subjected to this motion is the first metatarsal cuneiform joint. There is often found an exostosis or enlargement of bone dorsally at this area. This becomes painful to the geriatric patient, secondary also to shoe rub. With prolonged irritation an adventitious bursal sac may form over the area giving rise—in addition to bone pain—to an acute bursitis. There are also symptoms over the medial side of the navicular where, in some cases, an os tibial externum may be found.

In addition to the above-mentioned factors, abnormal motions will, in time, cause degenerative joint disease to develop in the affected joints. Another area that can become symptomatic is the base of the fifth metatarsal. Whether due to hypermobility in the foot or an enlargement of the base itself, the area can be subjected to a great deal of pressure and therefore causes the geriatric patient discomfort on ambulation.

Treatment will be based upon determining the etiology of the pain. Is it shoe rub, acute bursitis, or inflammatory changes of the joints themselves, secondary to degenerative joint disease? Weight bearing biomechanically po-

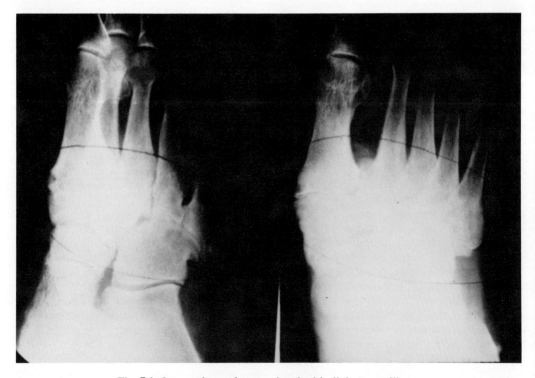

Fig. 7.1 Osteoarthropathy associated with diabetes mellitus.

sitioned radiographs should be taken in an attempt to arrive at an exact diagnosis. If overlying plantar hyperkeratosis is present, it should be shaved down, as the thickened dead skin itself can, in time, become a pressure point. Pressure dispersing pads can be applied to enlargements of the osseous structures in an attempt to afford immediate relief. In cases of acute inflammatory processes either in bursal sacs or in joints themselves, injections of corticosteroids and local anesthesia will afford prompt relief. This can be followed by applications of physical therapy, such as ultrasound, hydrotherapy or hydroculator packs. The use of the nonsteroidal anti-inflammatory agents is also indicated for these problems. Long-term therapy is going to require stabilization of both the subtalar and midtarsal joints. This will therefore require orthotic devices, either rigid or semirigid fitted foot gear. When dealing with fixed, rigid deformities the use of pressure dispersing orthoses would then be indicated. Modification of the shoe will also be necessary. It is quite difficult to relieve the symptomatology of an acute inflammatory process in the dorsum of the foot in the area of the first metatarsal or cuneiform joint when a tight-fitting shoe is constantly irritating the area. In cases of severe deformities and degenerative joint disease, especially in the subtalar and midtarsal areas, where the foot is in such abnormal alignment that the normal-last shoe cannot be properly fitted upon the foot, the use of a custom molded or space shoe should be considered.

FOREFOOT PATHOLOGIES

In my experience the greatest number of painful symptoms on the geriatric foot seem to occur within the forefoot segment (metatarsal heads, distally). The major functioning joint in the forefoot, needless to say, is the first metatarsal phalangeal joint. This joint appears to be subjected to many deformities. An enlargement found at the medial aspect of the first metatarsal medial or dorsomedial aspect of the first metatarsal head is called a bunion. Commonly found with the bunion deformity is a migration of the larger toe towards the lesser digits called a hallux val-

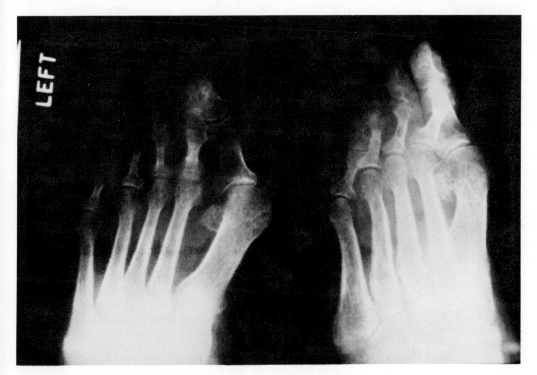

Fig. 7.2 Hallux valgus: demineralization and subluxation of second toe associated with the residuals of rheumatoid arthritis.

gus. Although with a hallux valgus deformity there is always a concomitant bunion deformity, the converse is not always true. In other words, one can find a bunion deformity without a concomitant hallux valgus deformity.

The enlargement of the first metatarsal head can occur in several ways. First, it can be due to degenerative changes with osseous proliferation. There can be an enlargement of the metatarsal head itself. As mentioned before, the enlargement can occur dorsally and/or dorsally medially, and/or medially. There can also be a metatarsus primus varus deformity where the entire metatarsal shifts medially away from the other metatarsals. This will likewise cause a medial bulge on the side of the first metatarsal phalangeal joint. The majority of symptoms that occur with this bunion deformity are caused by the fact that the vamp part of the shoe irritates the enlargement. Concomitant to bone pain an adventitious bursal sac generally forms in this area. Whether the bunion deformity and the concomitant hallux valgus deformity, if present, are caused by pathomechanical abnormalities, tight shoes or whatever etiological factor you may believe proves to be a moot or academic point. What is important at this time is not what has caused the deformity, but how we can alleviate the geriatric patient's painful symptoms.

When dealing with the geriatric foot we are dealing in most cases with the end results, i.e., the deformity. Our main concern at this point should be to afford the patient the maximum degree of comfort and not be quite as concerned about what has caused the deformity. It is important at this time to determine exactly where the pain is occurring that the patient is experiencing. Is the pain occurring at the head of the first metatarsal? Is it occurring in the joint? Is it occurring at the adventitious bursal sacs that may have formed overlying the enlargement of the metatarsal head?

The important aspect in treating this problem is to remove the initial exciting agent, in other words, the shoe last incompatibility. Except in cases where we are dealing with an acute inflammatory process in the joint itself, the major cause of pain in this area is shoe rub. One only has to look at the shoe that the patient is wearing to see how much the shoe can deform the foot. With a large outpock-

eting on the medial aspect of the vamp of the shoe we can realize how much irritation the metatarsal head must be receiving. There is no possible way to relieve the pain and inflammatory process that may develop in this area as long as the shoe constantly rubs the metatarsal head. It must be kept in mind that with a tight-fitting shoe in this area, pressure dispersing pads may not be of help. The more padding applied the more room is going to be taken up in the shoe, causing it to appear tighter with more constriction and pressure upon the metatarsal head. In acute inflammatory conditions we strongly suggest that a patient take an old pair of shoes or slippers and cut out the vamping area to relieve all pressure of the first metatarsal head. With an acute inflammation of the bursal sac and/or joint, injections of corticosteroids into the joints or bursal sac will produce prompt and long-lasting relief. With large amounts of fluid accumulating in the bursal sac, withdrawal is indicated before injection of the corticosteroid. The use of physical modalities such as ultrasound, hydrotherapy and hydroculator packs is also indicated. Follow-up with nonsteroidal inflammatory drugs affords the patient continual relief to this area. The use of adhesive felt bunion pads, removable dispersion pressure pads, such as tube foam, Latex shields or silicone shields, likewise affords the patient a maximum degree of comfort. Attention must be paid to modification of the footgear. Bunion last type shoes should be prescribed. In cases of severe deformity, the use of custom made, molded or space shoes should be indicated. In cases nonresponsive to conservative palliative methods, then surgical intervention should be considered. With an associated hallux rigidus, a steel plate between the insole and outsole will reduce dorsification and reduce pain.

Metatarsalgia

Metatarsalgia is a nonspecific term referring to pain in the metatarsal heads. This pain can be secondary to atrophy of the fat pad where the plantar aspect of the metatarsal heads are now bearing all the weight without the afforded protection and shock absorbing properties of the plantar fat pad. Metatarsalgia may be found concomitant with a hallux valgus deformity where the lesser digits are

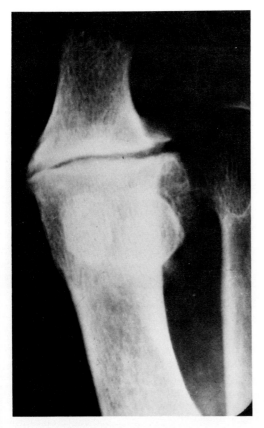

Fig. 7.3 Hallux limitus.

contracted dorsally in an extended manner, causing a plantar-grade force on the metatarsal head. This causes an abnormal amount of pressure to be born by the specific metatarsal head. This abnormal pressure can set up an acute bursitis, capsulitis or arthritis in the joint surrounding the metatarsal head. With abnormal pressure will also come thickening of the keratin layer of skin, forming a painful corn or callus.

Treatment should consist of attempting to determine what is causing the abnormal weight bearing pattern by the metatarsal head and correcting it. Weight bearing biomechanical radiographs should be taken. In cases of fixed deformities attempts should be made to redistribute the pressure off the offending metatarsal head. Many of these metatarsal conditions are found in conjunction with subtalar and midtarsal joint hypermobility. In these cases the use of a semi-rigid orthotic to stabilize the subtalar or midtarsal joint is indicated. Sometimes the need for forefoot

extensions to protect the metatarsal heads is indicated. Materials such as Molo or Spenco can be used quite successfully to give the metatarsal head an additional cushioning. Another means of therapy is the use of cutout accommodative forefoot devices which, again, can be incorporated into the orthotic to relieve the abnormal weight bearing pattern of the offending metatarsal head and redistribute it to the other metatarsal. In acute conditions the use of corticosteroids and local anesthetics injected into the joint or bursal sac will afford the patient immediate relief. The use of adhesive cutout pads will likewise redistribute the weight pattern until the acute inflammatory stage is over.

LESSER DIGITAL DEFORMITIES

The lesser digital deformities include hammer toes, overlying and underlapping digits, and rotation of the digits.

Hammer toe formation with or without overlapping and underlapping can occur frequently in conjunction with a hallux deformity. The lesser digital deformity can also occur as an entity in itself. The etiology may be one of congenital origin. The geriatric patient may come into the office with a deformity of a lesser digit which he will relate as having had all his life. He may even relate a family history of the deformity. Some hammer toe

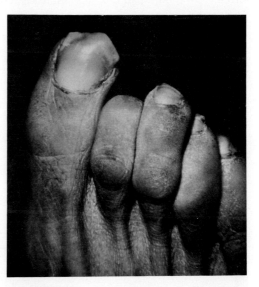

Fig. 7.4 Mallet toe with hammer toes. Bowstring tendons and nail deformities.

formation may be an acquired deformity either via biomechanical abnormalities or abnormal external forces. Again, dealing with the geriatric foot, determinant of the etiological forces causing the deformity of the digit is not as important as finding a way to relieve the symptom.

Most of the symptoms of the digital deformity are caused by shoe pressure. With a hammer toe or cocked up toe there is usually hyperextension of the proximal phalanx upon the metatarsal head. In more severe cases there may be even a subluxation or complete dislocation of the digit upon the dorsum of the metatarsal head. There is usually a concomitant flexion deformity at the proximal interphalangeal joint. When inside a shoe this area would be irritated by the vamp of the shoe and cause a painful tyloma at the proximal interphalangeal joint. In some cases a bursal sac can form in this area and an acute bursitis can add to the pain.

Flexion deformities can occur at the proximal interphalangeal joint alone causing weight bearing upon the distal aspect of the toe instead of upon the fat pad which is found beneath the plantar of the distal phalanx. This "mallet toe" deformity causes a painful hyperkeratotic lesion at the tips of the toes and/or subungually.

With varus rotations of the digits the weight bearing portion of the digits is transferred from the fat pad on the plantar aspect

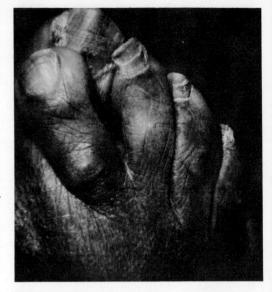

Fig. 7.6 Hallux valgus with overlapping second toe.

of the toe to a portion of the toe where there is no fat pad or to a portion of the toe which is not afforded the fat pad protection. Again, a painful hyperkeratotic lesion will develop as a result of the abnormal pressure on that part of the digit. One of the more common areas of the foot to be affected is the lateral side of the fifth digit and the lateral nail groove. Enlargement and deformities of the joint of the lesser digits can cause abnormal rubbing and pressure forces between two adjacent digits. This will usually result in the formation of a "soft corn." In most cases this abnormal pressure on the digits will cause an inflammatory process to develop in the area, resulting in pain and swelling.

Treatment should be directed towards redistributing the pressure away from these abnormal areas to the normal weight bearing areas of the digit. Weight bearing biomechanically positioned radiographs should be taken to evaluate the extent of the osseous or structural deformities and any joint involvement. There are many different types of digital orthotics that can be constructed by the podiatrist to redistribute the weight. Something as simple as an adhesive felt or foam pad on the digit or a removable tube foam can in many cases provide the patient with a great deal of comfort. Traction devices likewise can be employed in certain instances to help redistribute the weight bearing aspects of the

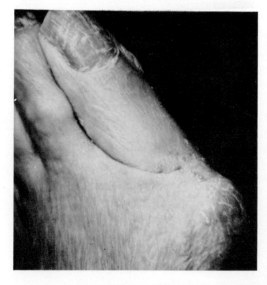

Fig. 7.5 Hallux valgus.

digit. The use of injectable corticosteroids in acute inflammatory processes, as stated before, can be quite effective in affording the geriatric patient quick and long-lasting relief. The use of physical therapy and nonsteroidal anti-inflammatories can be used as needed and indicated to further relieve the symptoms.

In the case of subluxed or dislocated hammer toes, therapy can become more involved. As a primary cause of symptoms is shoe rub upon the digit, the shoe must be modified to accommodate the deformed digit. No matter how sophisticated the digital orthotic may be, if the patient can't wear it in the shoe, it is ineffective. In some cases the vamp area of the shoe can be modified. Stretching the shoe to allow for the deformity may be helpful. The exact area to be stretched is easily found, as the patient's hammer toe has most assuredly deformed the shoe. In severe cases the patient can take the shoe to the shoe repair shop and have the vamp area of the shoe out and an "outpocketing" of leather sewn in place to give a toe box of greater height to the shoe. If the deformed digit cannot be satisfactorily housed in a conventional shoe, then the use of a custom made molded or space shoe should be considered.

Once again, if all attempts at conservative therapy fails, then surgical intervention should be considered.

As we stated earlier, the normal aging process that occurs with the geriatric foot in itself can cause problems. With the progression of osteoporosis in the geriatric foot, the osseous structures become more susceptible to stress and pathological fractures. It is, therefore, imperative when a geriatric patient presents to the office with the diagnosis of pain and/or swelling in the foot that biomechanical weight bearing radiographs be taken. There is no way possible to diagnose or rule out a fracture without the use of a pedal radiograph.

Treatment of orthopedic problems in the geriatric foot presents a challenge, but successful treatment of the above mentioned problems can be extremely gratifying and rewarding to the practitioner. The patients are very appreciative of all the efforts brought forth in their behalf, and are quite patient, and will work with you in an attempt to relieve their symptomatology. In our youth oriented society geriatric patients—and geriatrics as individuals—are usually cast aside and forgotten. It is up to us to make sure that this does not occur in the care of their feet.

chapter 8

Common Orthopedic Problems in the Geriatric Foot—Part II

Arthur E. Helfand, D.P.M.

There are many inflammatory lesions involving the bones and joints that produce pain in the geriatric patient. Periarthritis is a complicating factor of joint change in the elderly patient, demonstrating localized joint pain, which may be present on motion and on palpation. Radiographically, there may be clear evidence of some degenerative joint change and hyperostosis involving the articular surfaces. For the most part, these complaints represent limiting factors in ambulation. Treatment generally is directed towards local steroid injections accompanied by supportive measures such as ultrasound and immobilization. For the most part, these conditions tend to resolve with local management and may recur with stress placed upon the particular joint involved.

Geriatric patients who have had aseptic necrosis in younger years may demonstrate with a monoarticular degenerative change of the joint involved. The most common site is that of the second metatarsal head resulting from an old Freiberg infarction. Treatment should be directed towards removing pressure from the area and the use of orthotics to control weight distribution to the second metatarsal phalangeal joint. Local steroid injections and physical modalities also tend to relieve the symptoms of pain. Where the joint change is significant enough to preclude ambulation in a comfortable manner, surgical consideration should be given to this type of residual disease.

Continued microtrauma to the medial sesamoids beneath the first metatarsal head may produce an inflammatory change commonly called sesamoiditis. The condition results from an inflammatory reaction involving the tendon as well as the osseous structures themselves. There is soft tissue inflammation and swelling associated with this. The most common treatment in the elderly patient represents a removal of pressure from the area by the use of a felt pad or other similar modality in the form of what is termed a "dancer's pad." This consists of a cutout involving the first metatarsal head to remove weight from the area totally. This method of weight dispersion, accompanied by physical modalities, tends to provide relatively significant relief.

Where the condition persists, an appropriate orthotic should be constructed to remove pressure from the area. Changes in footwear may be appropriate based upon the needs of the particular involvement of the elderly patient.

Elderly patients many times complain of pain along the dorsum of the foot involving the first metatarsal cuneiform articulation. The primary problem results from a degenerative osteophytic formation involving a hypertrophy of the joint involving the tarsal metatarsal area. The problem is exaggerated by footwear, is often more significant in the female patient, and is the direct result of metal eyelet irritation. An associated tendonitis or tenosynovitis of the extensor hallucis tendon may be associated with this condition. The simplest treatment in the elderly patient is to remove the eyelet and remove pressure from the hypertrophied area of bone. Rarely does this require surgical intervention, but when it is to be instituted, it can be done with a minimal amount of trauma to the patient.

Alterations in the normal metatarsal length pattern can easily be demonstrated in the geriatric patient. For the most part, these generally are residuals of structural deformity accompanied by occupational pressures in younger years which have produced keratotic lesions, anterior metatarsal bursitis and hyperkeratotic lesions.

In general, Morton's syndrome represents a shortening of the first metatarsal ray and as well as some degree of hypermobility. The lateral segments may also demonstrate similar changes. Treatment generally consists of a mechanical approach to provide either weight diffusion, weight dispersion or balance therapy to redistribute weight to provide a more normal metatarsal parabola.

Calcaneal spurs may be present in many geriatric patients. Their primary symptoms of pain represent an associated plantar fascitis, subcalcaneal bursitis or periostitis. Treatment is mechanical and medical for the most part, dealing with the use of anti-inflammatory agents, physical modalities and mechanical activities to relieve pain and pressure from the area.

Tenosynovitis and tendonitis are closely related to the formation of ganglionic cysts in the geriatric patient. For the most part, the elderly patient with a ganglion has had the lesion for many years and it rarely becomes symptomatic in advancing age. The cystic formation involving the long tendons, usually on the dorsum of the foot, only produces pain when aggravated by footwear. Treatment consists of a change in footwear, surgical excision of the ganglionic mass, the use of ultrasound and the use of injectable steroids to reduce the inflammation and effectively remove the gelatinous fluid from the cyst.

With advancing years, there is a significant loss of the plantar fat pads. For the most part many patients complain that they feel as though they are walking on the bones of their foot. The most appropriate management is to use some material by weight diffusion to provide some soft tissue replacement to the anterior metatarsal area, to compensate for the loss of the metatarsal fat pad. The choice of material and the exact mechanism should be determined by the clinician based upon the particular needs of the patient. They may consist of orthotics or polyurethane foam to relieve pressure from the area and provide some cushioning effect for the patient.

Synovitis and bursitis in the geriatric patient generally occur in the anterior metatarsal area and are the direct result of continued microtrauma. They respond exceedingly well to mechanical therapy, the use of injectable steroids, systemic anti-inflammatory drugs, physical modalities and efforts to redistribute weight away from the affected area of trauma.

Peripheral nerve entrapment in the elderly patient, commonly known as Morton's neuroma, is the primary end result of continued microtrauma and compressive stresses on the nerve sheets as they relate to the anatomical structures of the metatarsals. They may occur interdigitally between any of the metatarsal heads. Their treatment in the geriatric patient may include the use of injectable local anesthetics and steroids and some mechanical therapy to provide a metatarsal blocking effect. However, a true neuroma or entrapment neuropathy responds best to surgical excision.

Trauma in the elderly patient can be difficult to manage. For the most part, fractures involving the foot itself tend to be closed unless they are a result of a direct trauma and many times are the result of pathologic or march types of fractures. Dislocations in the elderly patient tend to be rare per se but are many times demonstrable on x-ray and as a result of previous bone and joint disease. For the most part, digital fractures, when in good position, can be easily managed with the use of moldable silicone compound molds to maintain a fixed position of the digit. Fractures involving the metatarsals and rear foot should be appropriately managed with a short leg cast if there is significant difficulty on ambulation and if there is significant pain. However, many times the geriatric patient is limited in his ambulatory ability and the use of a rigid, surgical shoe with an appropriate source of local immobilization, such as an elastic bandage may provide the best functional management for closed fractures in good position. For the most part this permits the geriatric patient to ambulate to some degree, thereby reducing the period of post-fracture osteoporosis and fracture stiffness. In addition, it provides the maximum degree of exercise tolerable to the patient.

An additional feature in the surgical shoe is that it permits the foot to be bathed on a daily basis, thereby maintaining appropriate hygiene and thus reducing the possibility of a circulatory embarrassment to the extremity.

Patients with the residual forms of arthritic disease present with a significant variety of foot deformities in the geriatric years. These are generally best managed by the use of physical modalities, local anti-inflammmatory agents, systemic anti-inflammatory agents, appropriate footwear and orthotics to maintain a degree of support for the involved joints.

The deformities of rheumatoid arthritis usually demonstrable in the elderly patient include the residuals of hallux rigidus, arthritis of the first metatarsal phalangeal joint, hallux valgus, cystic erosions, sesamoid erosions, metatarsal phalangeal dislocations, and hyperostosis, digitus flexus, fused interphalangeal joints, phalangeal reabsorption, cuneonavicular arthritis, extensor tenosynovitis, rheumatoid nodules, bowstring extensor hallicus longus tendons with hallux valgus, lateral displacement of the extensor tendons, ganglions, and a rigid or pronated foot. Arthritic changes involving any of the mid- or rear foot joints may also be demonstrable.

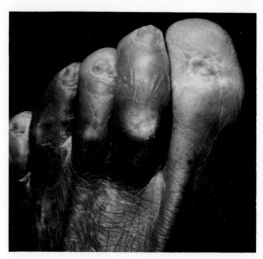

Fig. 8.2   Hammer toes, postsurgical onychial excision and early digital ulcer related to contracture and pressure.

Early morning stiffness characterized by pain, fibrosis, ankylosis, contracture, deformity, impairment and a loss of the ambulatory status of the individual many times is the result of severe rheumatoid arthritis.

Osteoarthritis or degenerative joint disease in the elderly patient may be associated with or secondary to trauma, inflammation, metabolic changes, chronic microtrauma, strain, obesity, osteoporosis and postmenopause. Many changes occur in the weight bearing joints of the foot. They include plantar fasciitis, spur formations, periostitis, osteoporosis, stress fractures, tendonitis and tenosynovitis, and tend to magnify existing deformities such as pes planus, pes cavus and digital deformities.

Gout or the residuals of gout may be present in the elderly patient. During the acute phase the joint may appear inflamed, red and swollen and exhibit significant pain. During the chronic phase the joints may be painful and stiff and atrophy may be evident.

There is generally a loss of bone substance, and gouty arthritis may be demonstrable on x-ray with urate crystal deposits both in the cartilage and synovial membrane. Gout should be managed metabolically and should be managed in the foot by supportive measures to include orthoses as well as physical modalities to assist in alleviating pain and maintaining maximum joint function.

Adequate footwear gives proper support

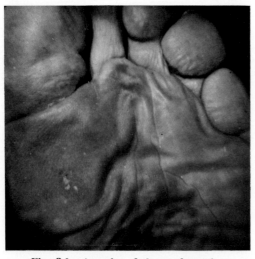

Fig. 8.1   Atrophy of plantar fat pad.

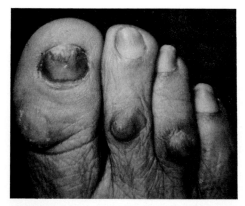

Fig. 8.3 Hammer toes with adventitious bursa formation.

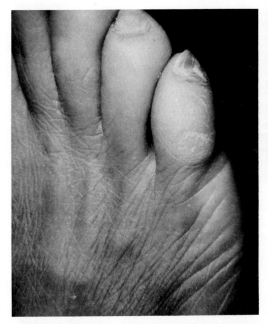

Fig. 8.4 Rotational deformity of fifth toe with heloma formation, bursitis and osseous enlargement.

activities or the person who is confined to limited activity in an institution or in some other limiting environment. The patient who is living at home and is maintaining his usual normal community activities should procure shoes that provide adequate protection and support to meet the occasion for which they are being used. In the case of an older patient,

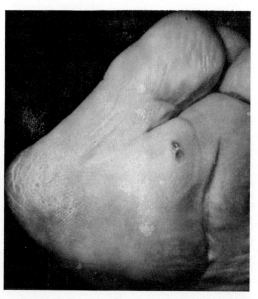

Fig. 8.5 Marked hallux valgus with early ulceration and keratosis.

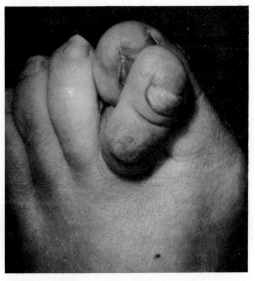

Fig. 8.6 Hallux valgus with overlapping second toe and dislocation.

and protection and is valued and important for the geriatric patient. It may need to be augmented by the use of molds, inlays and shields, which diffuse, disperse and redistribute the various pressures and weight from painful conditions.

In recommending a shoe for the aging patient, one of two different problems should be dealt with: the person who lives at home and goes about with his usual community the problem may be quite different from that of the young, because of the differences of physical demand.

It is of prime concern that shoes and stockings be acquired to fit the requirements of the patients. Shoes should be tried on in the shoe store and feel comfortable. Shoes should also conform to the shape of the individual's foot where feasible. Where deformities such as callus or bunions exist, special shoes or modifications should be utilized which compensate for these deformed or older foot contours. An extra depth inlay shoe is also another appropriate means to provide additional room for deformities that occur in the foot. The older person should be warned about wearing someone else's shoes, and with the current economy placing serious strain on limited incomes, there is a tendency for elderly patients to wear used shoes which can result in significant foot problems due to foot-to-shoe last incompatibility.

Most women wear high heels in their earlier years. Depending upon the height of the heel, the last and the length of time worn, a short or tight heel cord can be created. High heels also change the weight bearing surface of the foot and reduce the total area in contact with the plane of support. This reduction in contact causes greater stress on the contact areas. It is observed that many older people still need some heel height and this should be limited to a medium heel, which offers greater stability to the foot. At times modifications are made in the heel such as lateral extensions to offer greater contact with the heel.

Additional shoe modifications useful in managing the elderly patient's foot problems include medial and lateral sole wedges to compensate for equinus and varus static or fixed deformities. A medial sole wedge will restrict subtalar motion to minimize the effects of localized joint change. Lateral and anterior-lateral sole wedges can be utilized to compensate for the residuals of youthful gait changes. Metatarsal bars can be utilized, depending on the type and placement, to transfer weight over the metatarsal heads and prevent supination.

The Thomas heel and reverse Thomas heel can provide additional support to either the medial or lateral longitudinal arch areas. Long medial counters add to inner support but care must be taken when used with old prominent navicular areas. Heel flares, as identified, provide additional support to medial or lateral ankle instability.

A shank filler or wedgie is utilized to provide full contact and add support to the entire plantar aspect of the foot.

A steel plate placed between the insole and outsole on the medial aspect of the shoe may be utilized in the management of hallux limitus. The limitation of dorsiflexion or extension of the hallux will eliminate the irritating factors caused by the mechanics of the condition and help reduce future pain.

Rocker bars can be utilized to prevent flexion and extension of the shoe. Cork buildups may be required to compensate for a short limb. In addition, bracing may be utilized as a means to assist gait whenever paresis follows a stroke.

Internal shoe modifications include longitudinal medial arch pads for support; metatarsal pads for support and weight transference; cutout pads for sensitive areas and ulcerations; medial heel wedges for support; calcaneal bars for weight transference; heel pads and lifts for calcaneal spurs and bursitis; and tongue pads to prevent the foot from riding forward in the shoe.

Special soles may also be employed for additional weight diffusion and/or dispersion, as indicated.

The orthopedic shoe per se is not a corrective device but is intended to compensate for some preexisting condition, deformity or weakness. The shoes should be used and/or prescribed following adequate evaluation, including radiographic studies when appropriate. It is here that extended cooperation between all members of the patient's health team must prove beneficial to the patient and the overall health of the individual should be considered. Many times, because of the very weight of the so-called orthopedic shoe, patients are limited in their ambulatory ability. It should also be noted that many elderly patients, by virtue of their inability to bend or use their hands properly, may not even be able to tie shoes.

Mention should also be made of the "molded shoe," a made-to-order shoe which may resemble a standard shoe with special sizes or modifications built in. A molded shoe generally conforms to the shape of the foot, and the sole or inner surface conforms to the total weight bearing of the foot. Its basic advantages are to reduce shock, provide a shape to fit the foot, and provide a greater distribution of stress to help compensate for painful conditions. Judicious evaluation and prescription should be employed and commercialism should be avoided to protect the safety of the patient. For the most part, care must be exercised in the geriatric patient even in the casting sequence to avoid excessive heat of setting plaster and to compensate for elongation on weight bearing.

Patients confined to institutions usually do little in the way of physical activity. Their periods of ambulations are limited, but even so, care should be maintained in the selection of appropriate footwear to meet the occasion. In these instances, the basic purpose of the shoe is to afford protection and the upper should be of a soft, flexible material to eliminate undo pressure. Inasmuch as many elderly people are unable to bend and tie laces, a slip-on and a long shoe horn will enable many patients to do for themselves. It is suggested that in order to add more stability to the foot during ambulation, full foot coverage with counter and full upper be provided, as opposed to an open sandal. Care should be exercised in shoe fitting in geriatric institutions, as people's feet do change with advancing years and an effort should be made to have all shoes properly fit rather than guessed at in the area of sizing.

There are many types of orthotics that can be employed for the elderly patient. For the most part, two basic principles are involved: the use of (1) a rigid orthosis, or (2) a flexible orthosis. The final determination as to shape and modifications would depend upon deformity of the patient, the weight of the patient, the functional means of the patient, and the ability of the patient to adapt to the corrective or supportive device that has been prescribed. Our experience has demonstrated that there is no firm rule which could reflect either rigidity or flexibility for the geriatric patient. The choice would depend upon the individual practitioner's evaluation of the patient and his particular condition. Some of the types of materials include Plastazote, Spenco, Alimed, Molo, Korex, sponge rubber, felt and other soft tissue supplements. Rigidity today generally involves the use of plastics, metal, or the use of leather with Celastic reinforcement. Rubber butter, which may be a combination of ground cork or ground leather and liquid Latex, is also used as a filler material to provide both dynamic and static redistribution of weight to conform to the configurations of the shell or foot itself.

Some of the types of modifications that occur in most geriatric orthotics include the following: Celastic longitudinal reenforcements, specially shaped metatarsal pads, protective top covers, full rubber cushions, full rubber heel seats, hallux leather bunion flanges, tailor's leather bunion flanges, padded cup, heel seats, lateral longitudinal flanges, medial or lateral heel levelers, metatarsal head extensions, cutouts for point relief, combination specialties, metatarsal and cutout pads, saddle pads, full tarsal balancing, Dutchmen wedges, tarsal elevations, full insole extensions, heel elevations and the use of material to provide total weight diffusion to feet that have lost their normal soft tissue and elastic function.

In conclusion, it would seem essential to emphasize that many neuromuscular diseases that occur in younger years present with residual deformities in the geriatric foot. Patients who have been institutionalized for long periods of time, due to mental retardation or other neurologic diseases, do present with specific foot problems that cause both pain and deformity and create a limiting factor in the individual's ability to adapt and function within an institutional environment. Studies that have been completed on a longitudinal basis have clearly demonstrated that the foot deformities of youth become degenerative deformities in the elderly. Institutionalized patients still deserve the right to adequate care and the right to remain pain-free and ambulatory during their declining years. To the individual who has been institutionalized for a long period of time due to mental illness, foot pain may be the only factor that prevents his involvement in out-of-bed activities, to whatever degree that may be. All institutionalized patients should receive appropriate evaluation and treatment that is as high in quality as those provided to patients in the general population. Perhaps there needs to be a greater degree of compassion in dealing with this type of patient. However, it has been clearly demonstrated that because of the current lack of funds in delivering care to this population segment, foot health is often a low priority. Efforts should be made to institute an appropriate foot health service for all patients in this category.

chapter 9

Podiatric Surgical Consideration of the Aging Patient

Vincent N. Tisa, D.P.M.

This chapter addresses itself to those surgical problems peculiar to the elderly patient with foot complaints. At present there are 25 million individuals 65 years of age and older, and their numbers are expected to increase by about 50% in the next three decades. Although longevity is increasing, the greatest advances are being made in the quality of life of the elderly. Federal legislation, health science curriculum changes and increased social concern reflect a growing public awareness of the quality of life and the health needs of our senior citizens.

The elderly person is well aware that, with time, comes an accumulation of long-term disease such as arteriosclerosis and disabilities such as joint trauma. The primary concern, however, is for retention of functional mobility. For the elderly, loss of mobility means loss of independence and, ultimately, a decline in physical and mental well-being. Thus, the most important physical sign in geriatric orthopedics is to see the patient walk.

In the past, these considerations were not thought to be of much importance since average life span rarely exceeded 65 years of age. More recently, however, clinicians have become cognizant of the fact that when a person reaches the age of 65 he may have 10–15 more years of life remaining. Accordingly, when 60- to 70-year-old patients present themselves with painful deformities, they should not be denied possible relief by operation on the assumption that they are approaching their life expectancy. Obviously, the older patient represents a special problem when elective surgery is considered, but in view of the fact that less than 50 years ago any elective surgery in the aged was felt to be unwarranted, it seems remarkable that today we can predict very satisfactory results in most cases. Remarkable advances in all areas of surgery have made available a broad range of corrective and reconstructive procedures that would have been considered impossible even a few years ago.

When contemplating any procedure, the clinician must reflect upon the balance between the benefits and risks of the procedure, the likelihood of poor toleration of intraoperative complications, and the significant incidence of postoperative complications. Despite the increased risk, advanced age no longer is an absolute contraindication to elective operation, but simply becomes one factor to be balanced against the benefits to be gained. Justification for surgical consideration should be based upon the symptoms present, the functional needs of the patient, and the general medical condition presented. If the patient is physically able, and conservative measures have failed, surgical revision may be considered when the deformity is marked, when pain is persistent and when such consideration can prevent future complications and further extension of the impairment.

One of the factors that must be weighed in the final decision is the patient's life expectancy in comparison to the natural course of the disease. An example of how this may produce a balance against surgery is the case of a 70-year-old patient with significant heart or lung disease who develops a bunion deformity. Since the primary disease process carries a life expectancy of 2 or 3 years and the bunion may take up to 5 years to prove disabling, the treatment of choice should be conservative. The quality of the patient's remaining life would not be greatly improved by incuring the pain and risks of operation. However, in a case involving a patient with severe arthritis of the feet so crippling that life is intolerable, reconstructive surgery should be considered provided no other major disease is present, even though the operative risks are higher than in the first hypothetical case. The quality of life to be gained makes the risk worth taking.

Another factor to be weighed is how much comfort is to be gained by the patient in comparison to the risk of complications that in the elderly tend to escalate quickly to life- or limb-threatening proportions. The patient developing an infection following a bunionectomy may require a second operation, the lengthened hospitalization increasing the risk of thrombophlebitis, pulmonary embolism, and pneumonia. Several complications may be tolerated by younger patients, but not by the elderly, who often lack physical reserves. Therefore, every effort must be made to avoid the initial complication. The essence of effective surgery for the geriatric patient may be summarized briefly as "Do as little as necessary to solve the patient's problem." However, the preoperative and postoperative role of the clinician is not so readily stated.

In spite of the limitations we acknowledge in the aged patient, we must recognize that careful preoperative assessment and treatment, well conducted anesthesia with expeditious surgery, and meticulous postoperative care with early ambulation will result in a successful outcome in most of our elderly patients. They have the resources to respond to good surgical care and we cannot offer them anything less. The approach to patients who are often in their seventies raises some philosophical consideration. We have been conditioned to think about surgery in terms of young or middle-aged adults. So many patients to whom surgery was not offered because of age have spent the next 15 or 20 years in a wheelchair. Serious consideration should be given to any patient who is in general good health and who is strongly motivated, regardless of age.

"Will to live" or "motivation" plays an important role in controlling postoperative complications. The elderly patient reacts differently to disruption as his age progresses, and he has established certain ideas over the years. A hospital, for example, presents a different environment and the practitioner must give him time to adjust, and in so doing, gains his confidence and cooperation. The properly motivated patient will work with the doctor toward a common goal. In treating the patient as a responsible adult, the clinician should clearly define the diagnosis, prognosis and treatment options in detail. The patient is much less receptive in the postoperative period due to the effects of anesthesia, analgesics and pain. This is often complicated in the geriatric patient by confusion, so it is imperative to advise him preoperatively of what you expect of him postoperatively. Any questions the patient may have, including length of hospital stay, expected period of rehabilitation, and restrictions in postoperative activities, must be answered concisely in terms of the patient's understanding. Remember always to speak slowly and clearly and to face the patient in a well-lit room. The aging process takes it toll and hearing is no exception.

Special attention must be given to the diagnosis and management of concurrent metabolic diseases and to nutrition in general. The geriatric patient undergoing an operative procedure presents special nutritional and metabolic problems. This group of patients may have nutritional deficiencies as a result of poor dietary habits, chronic illnesses, malignant disease or socioeconomic factors. These deficiencies, often subtle, become clinically significant in any preoperative plan, since abnormalities of hydration and nutrition must be corrected before surgery.

Maintenance of a positive nitrogen balance and a hemoglobin of 12 gm. or more is essential. This can be accomplished by the administration of a high protein diet, vitamin and protein supplements, adequate fluid intake and iron preparations. A patient who is dehydrated may show an elevated hemoglobin and hematocrit and false results in serum protein and electrolytes. The goal of nutritional support is to provide sufficient calories and nitrogen to meet required metabolic demands. If hypovitaminosis is present it should be corrected preopertively. Deficiency of vitamin C may delay the healing process while low levels of various members of the vitamin B complex may inhibit carbohydrate metabolism and the utilization of protein. In the elderly patient whose nutritional state is acceptable, maintenance therapy may be sufficient. In other cases, support is geared toward restoring an acceptable nutritional state wherein the appropriate supply of protein, calories, vitamins, trace elements and minerals is immediate. Optimal preoperative preparation is a worthwhile investment, and improvement in nutrition, hydration and respiratory status pays large dividends in the postoperative period.

PREOPERATIVE EVALUATION (WITH REGARD TO JOINT SURGERY)

It must be recognized that the evaluation of the arthritic patient at any one point in time is related both to the past and to the future. The clinician must establish what course the disease process has taken so far, and what it may be expected to do in the future.

Many questions must then be considered. First, what characteristics is the condition manifesting in this patient? Is there joint destruction? What can be anticipated without surgery? Postoperatively, can an extended period of bed rest and delayed ambulation be expected? Lastly, is the patient really up to the challenge of surgery?

The clinician must then evaluate whether or not every available form of treatment is being utilized. The approach to any joint destructive disease may be divided into three therapeutic approaches. First is the basic approach of rest, physiotherapy and palliation. The second approach involves the use of analgesics or steroids, which do not ultimately solve long-range problems, but may make a projected operation unnecessary or less im-

mediate. The third approach is elective surgery. The art of geriatric foot orthopedics lies in the wise application of these three approaches; not employing them sequentially, but simultaneously, with emphasis shifting back and forth as the occasions demand. There is always available treatment for a patient with a joint related foot disorder; it is merely a question of how much to do now and how much you should postpone until later.

Assuming that all approaches are in effect, the clinician must then establish what part the proposed surgical procedure plays in the total plan. Surgical intervention in the geriatric patient should be aimed toward relief of symptoms. It is important that the overall goals be discussed preoperatively between the clinician and the patient. Reconstructive surgery designed to restore and correct deformity in the foot of the geriatric patient often fails to meet the patient's needs and expectations. For example, a patient presenting with a primary disease process that minimizes or eliminates ambulation has little or no need for bilateral bunionectomies in the realization of his long-range goals. However, surgery designed to restore or retain present functional capacity in the future is a more realistic goal. Unless properly prepared however, the patient may feel after surgery that nothing has been accomplished. Again, emphasis rests on clear definition of goals, both immediate and long-range, preoperatively.

Finally, we come to the question of whether the patient is physically prepared for surgery. Of course, the usual general medical considerations must be taken into account. Before surgery, the following lab studies are usually necessary; electrocardiography, chest x-ray, urinalysis, 2-hour postprandial blood sugar, blood urea nitrogen, creatinine, hemoglobin and hematocrit, leukocyte count, blood volume, serum protein determinations and liver function tests. Always keep in mind, of course, that these values may be altered simply by the aging process. Since a primary disease process in the elderly is often complicated by a urinary tract infection, diabetes or an altered cardiovascular status, the clinician utilizes appropriate medical consultants. However, when all data has been collected, judgment should not be too strict. These patients cannot be compared to young, healthy individuals. One must consider their status with surgery as against that without surgery.

These are just some of the considerations which arise during the preoperative evaluation of the geriatric patient. The questions that have been raised are often easier to ask than to answer, but in attempting to answer them the clinician accumulates valuable knowledge of the patient, the presenting disorder and himself.

Thorough preoperative assessment of the geriatric patient's status and his ability to withstand stresses associated with anesthesia, surgery and the postoperative period are of paramount importance. The status of the aged patient is often complicated by several degenerative diseases affecting vital systems and thereby necessitating the ingestion of multiple medications. The high morbidity and mortality rates associated with surgery in the aged, as well as the ultimate prognosis, are primarily related to these preexisting diseases and their complications. The primary presenting disease process must always be considered in relation to these superimposed illnesses in order to get a true picture of the patient's condition.

Selection of patients for operation requires careful evaluation both of the patient's vascular status and of his general condition. Significant collateral disease complicates the evaluation of geriatric candidates for foot surgery; surgical risk is known to rise strikingly with the severity of the collateral disease. Keeping this in mind, there are certain instances, in which, in the interest of the patient, it is best that elective surgery be avoided or at least delayed. One of these situations is any patient who has or is recovering from an upper respiratory tract infection. Aging affects all systems and the lungs are no exception. With loss of elasticity, muscle atrophy and joint sclerosis, mobility of the thorax decreases. Almost every elderly patient has some degree of pulmonary dysfunction. In the aged, a cough of long-standing may be associated with chronic lung disease, smoking or congestive heart failure. However, when there is evidence of an active infection process, surgery should be delayed 7–10 days to avoid possible intraoperative complications.

The status of the heart as a pump and the adequacy and competency of the blood vessels to carry oxygen to vital organs and tissues must also be determined. With aging, there is a decrease in smooth muscle elasticity in blood vessels, and a rigidity forms in the vascular bed, making it incapable of reacting to stress. Atherosclerosis often follows, going unrecognized until it causes occlusion. These pathological processes may lead to another, relatively frequent risk factor, that of myocardial enlargement. The possible complications associated with operating on a patient recovering from a recent myocardial infarction are almost endless; in fact, major surgery performed within 3 months of an infarct brings a mortality rate of 40%. However, the longer the interval between surgery and the time of the infarct, the better the prognosis. Since the risk tends to stabilize by 6 months, surgery should be delayed for at least that amount of time whenever possible. Prior to 6 months, regional anesthesia is not a positive alternative, since there is often a high level of patient anxiety and emotional strain with this method of anesthesia.

Baseline electrocardiograms should be obtained in elderly patients, followed by consultation and evaluation by an internist or cardiologist to review any questionable cardiac reserve. Patients with established cardiovascular disease must take multiple medications, which often include digitalis. This drug is known to have a narrow therapeutic margin; however, digitalis toxicity is even more common in the elderly patient because of the aging renal system. If serum digitalis levels are in the toxic range, elective surgery should be postponed.

Another group of medications frequently used in the treatment of the cardiac patient are diuretics. These generally serve two purposes: to manage congestive heart failure and to control hypertension. The most significant effects relative to preoperative evaluation are the changes in blood volume and electrolyte balance. It must be remembered that orthostatic hypotension is pathognomonic of hypovolemia, but is not specific for that diagnosis. Unfortunately, electrolyte imbalance, a possible result of the drug therapy, tends to remain asymptomatic until it becomes relatively severe. A low potassium level at the time of anesthesia increases susceptibility to digitalis intoxication and to the development of ventricular arrhythmias, hence, preoperative replacement is the rule.

The existence of liver disease rarely limits the choice of anesthesia technique in the elderly, since hepatic reserves are great. One exception to keep in mind is regional anesthesia utilizing large amounts of local anesthetic agents. This may be hazardous due to dependence on hepatic function for metabolic disposal. Understanding that liver disease tends to be a chronic process, it is not usually necessary to delay elective surgery. However, if there is associated hypovolemia or dehydration, these should be corrected to insure a more stable course.

The elderly diabetic patient presents with multisystem disorder. Special attention to the competency of the cardiovascular system is essential. Hyperglycemia must be controlled and ketoacidosis corrected before elective surgical prodedures can be undertaken. It is important to be well acquainted with the individual patient's treatment plan, and to alter this routine as little as possible. One generally followed rule on the day of operation is to administer a smaller dose of insulin and then cover that by an intravenous glucose solution. It is unusual for the elderly patient with unrecognized or untreated thyroid dysfunction to come to surgery. The hypothyroid patient generally needs less preoperative sedation. The patient with uncontrolled hyperthyroidism may develop a "thyroid storm" due to surgical stress and should not be considered for elective surgery until a euthyroid state has been established. When evaluating a patient receiving corticosteroids, the drug of choice in this case, the dosage schedule and duration of therapy must be ascertained. In most cases, the usual dosage may be continued and, if necessary, the route of administration changed.

The precise impact of age on operative mortality and morbidity is difficult to assess. The geriatric patient usuually presents with a complex medical and drug history, and the importance of careful assessment and correction of any physiological imbalance cannot be overemphasized. Foot surgery is primarily an elective procedure and adequate preoperative preparation is the rule. It has been found that mortality rates of elective procedures are actually less than 25% of those reported for emergency procedures with inadequate assessment and preparation. A preoperative medical evaluation requires a thorough and thoughtful history, a careful physical evaluation, and a review of the patient's medical record. At times, a short walk down the corridor will reveal signs and symptoms that the patient was unable to communicate.

It is often easier to rush past an elderly patient for whom a history may be slow or difficult. These patients often feel threatened or anxious in the presence of a surgeon, but a little extra time and reassurance may prevent unforeseen postoperative problems. The choice of an anesthetic technique is too often a compromise based on the procedure to be performed. To avoid this situation, preoperative consultation between the clinician, the internist and the anesthesiologist is essential.

When evaluating the geriatric patient in whom inhalation anestheisa would be poorly tolerated, regional anesthesia should be strongly considered. A distinct advantage of this method is the lack of direct effect on pulmonary and cardiac function, thus greatly decreasing anesthetic mortality and morbidity. Regional techniques, especially spinal and ankle nerve blocks, are effective and reasonably well tolerated by the patient.

Many surgical procedures may be performed under spinal anesthesia. A small dose of local anesthetic agent deposited within the subarachnoid space has little direct effect on cardiac function. There is also minimal effect on respiration unless the level of anesthesia is unusually high, which would not be the case in foot surgery. The major disadvantage of spinal anesthesia is its indirect effect on the circulatory system. Sympathetic blockade, with its resultant vasodilation, may cause precipitous decreases in arterial pressure and decreased cardiac output. Therefore, it is contraindicated in patients with hypotension, hypertension, coronary artery disease and cardiac decompensation. Relative contraindication would be in those patients who are hypovolemic, who have central nervous system diseases, systemic infections or spinal anomalies, either acquired or congenital. When evaluating any patient for spinal anesthesia, epidural anesthesia should also be considered. One major advantage of this method is that the patient is relieved of the possibility of developing a spinal headache, nausea and vomiting postoperatively. However, there are certain possible complications that must be kept in mind. These include total subarachnoid block, for example.

Some degree of hypotension is to be expected in epidural anesthesia due to peripheral vasodilation and decreased cardiac output resulting from a block of cardioaccelerator fibers. However, a reaction more often seen in geriatric patients is hypertension, especially when a vasoconstrictor agent is part of the anesthetic agent.

A systemic reaction to the local anesthetic agent is encountered more frequently after an epidural than after a spinal due to the larger amount of medication used and the stronger possibility of an intravascular injection into the peridural plexus of veins. Unsuccessful anesthesia occurs in 2–6% of cases, but failure in geriatric patients is four times greater due to fibrosis or calcification of interspinous ligaments. However, in comparison to spinal anesthesia, an epidural has a longer duration and a more well defined area of anesthesia. Also, since spinal fluid is not removed from the canal, the need for bed rest is eliminated, and depending on the surgical procedure, ambulation may be almost immediate.

Usually foot surgery can be performed with regional ankle block anesthesia. Peripheral nerve blocks seem to be well tolerated by elderly patients and cause little morbidity. The dose of local anesthetic agent must, by necessity, be larger than that used for spinal anesthesia, and as a result there is greater systemic reaction. The local anesthetic agents may cause vasodilation and cardiac depression.

Allergic phenomena are extremely rare and when systemic reactions do occur they are generally due to overdosage or improper administration. Direct trauma to the nerve from the injection itself is also very rare. Nerve block anesthesia may be combined with intravenous sedation to eliminate the psychological and physiological effects of regional anesthesia. Ankle block may be preferred in most cases, except in instances where surgery will involve one metatarsal or the forefoot, in which case a field block will usually suffice.

In choosing local anesthetic agents, when anticipated postoperative pain is minimal, a short-acting agent such as lidocaine may be used. When pain is expected following an extensive procedure, a longer-acting agent such as bupivacaine that can provide anesthesia up to 7 hours is desirable. A long period of anesthesia could provide the patient with freedom from pain and thereby allay much postoperative anxiety. The vasodila-

tion from temporary local sympathectomy achieved with nerve blocks has the corollary benefit of a concomitant increase in circulation in the anesthetized area. This in turn may improve wound healing in the postoperative period. These considerations, plus excellent patient acceptance of this method of anesthesia, enhance the use of spinal, ankle, metatarsal and digital nerve blocks in the elderly patient. An in-depth description of regional ankle block and metatarsal block anesthesia is presented to further familiarize the clinician with these procedures by detailing their techniques.

Premedication includes a drug such as diazepam to decrease possible lidocaine activity and anxiety reactions, as well as the potential for vomiting or convulsions. The patient is placed in the supine position with a sandbag under the calf and the foot slightly extended.

The ankle is cleansed and the regional anesthesia is administered using 1% lidocaine without epinephrine. With a 25-gauge, 1-inch needle, lidocaine, 5 ml., is injected in a fan-like manner about the posterior tibial nerve, which is approximately one fingerbreadth posterior to the medial malleolus. The needle is directed inwardly at a 45° angle towards the malleolus. Next, lidocaine, 4 ml., is injected into the deep peroneal nerve at a point just proximal to the level of the tibiotalar joint and just medial to the extensor hallucis longus tendon. The needle is directed at right angles pointed slightly toward the fibula and anesthetic solution is deposited to the region of the periosteum. It is then redirected and injected in a fan-like manner between the extensor digitorum longus tendon and the tibia. The sural nerve is blocked by introducing lidocaine, 4 ml. lateral to the Achilles tendon at a level approximately 1 cm. above the lateral malleolus and directed toward the fibula.

After injection of lidocaine into these nerves, the cutaneous nerves are anesthetized by a subcuticular injection of 0.5% lidocaine without epinephrine circumscribing the ankle joint, just proximal to the malleoli.

This anesthetizes the many sensory nerves and the area where the tourniquet will be applied. It is not essential to locate the nerve precisely by eliciting paresthesias with the needle when the individual nerve blocks are performed. Following a 10-minute surgical scrub of the foot and the ankle proximal to the level of the local block, the foot is draped in the usual fashion and the distribution and effectiveness of the block are tested with a needle.

Prior to the skin incision, an Esmarch bandage is applied under moderate tension, starting at the toes and proceeding proximally to the site of the block in the ankle region. Here four turns of the bandage are applied and it is then looped under itself. The distal bandage is then removed by unwinding it back to the ankle and tucked under a fifth turn loosely applied about the ankle. The tourniquet may be applied proximal to the ankle block without the patient experiencing discomfort. The judicious use of tourniquets is advised in most older patients, especially those with a history of phlebitis, because of the danger of traumatizing arteriosclerotic vessels. Arterial damage may precipitate gangrene due to dislodged emboli and venous damage may cause thrombophlebitis. The use of a tourniquet is contraindicated when there is any question about the vascularity to the foot or in the presence of arterial calcification or severe varicosities.

The metatarsal block technique is as follows: 1% lidocaine without epinephrine is injected subcutaneously on the dorsum of the foot on each side of the metatarsal shaft. Extending the injection plantarly through the skin wheals, branches of the superficial peroneal nerve dorsally and the nerve branches of the posterior tibial nerve plantarly are anesthetized. The needle is angled slightly so about 3–4 ml. of anesthetic solution at each intermetatarsal space is sufficient to completely circumscribe the metatarsal bone with the anesthetic solution.

Indications for regional ankle block anesthesia include multiple or complex forefoot procedures and mid- or rearfoot procedures. Simple bunionectomies, metatarsal resections, bunionette resections, digital amputation, plantar neurectomy and hammertoe procedures are a few of the indications for metatarsal block technique.

Ankle block and metatarsal block injections cause only minimal discomfort to patients. We prefer this method of anesthesia to the Bier block because it avoids intravenous administration of lidocaine, early tourniquet pain, and the delayed pain frequently arising from prolonged tourniquet use. Because both ankle and metatarsal blocks wear off slowly, the patient recovers from the surgical procedure and adjusts to pain gradually outside the operating room. This aspect of postoperative management allows short procedure surgery or discharge with minimum stay for those elderly patients who are in good health and are undergoing uncomplicated surgical procedures. Rapid ambulation and discharge are extremely important in the geriatric patient to prevent the problems associated with immobilization, such as thrombosis, pneumonia, urinary tract infection, negative protein balance and pressure sores.

The aim of surgical intervention of the geriatric patient is to do the least amount of surgical trauma to effect the maximum result. In the older patient, the type of procedure is therefore of extreme importance. Functional corrections are of less value than surgical procedures aimed at relieving the source of pain and trauma. Surgery should be definitive and may mean the use of destructive as opposed to reconstructive procedures. The former type of surgery is feasible in the presence of degenerative joint disease of the involved joint, while the latter procedure would be contraindicated. Joint destructive procedures are indicated when there is evidence of articular degeneration, as disease cartilage cannot support normal function. Performing a joint preservation procedure when there are indications for a joint destructive procedure cannot yield a successful result, and may in fact present a greater propensity for complications due to the greater trauma and stress in the operative approach.

A further consideration is the time it takes to perform the surgery and the length of recovery. The elderly patient is more prone to surgical complications and there is an even greater potential for these in a lengthy procedure. An increased surgical time may also result in greater patient susceptibility to infection, cardiovascular distress and pulmonary complications.

The prudent clinician will "stage" his surgical procedures when multiple deformities exist, rather than attempt a lengthy "total forefoot reconstruction" at a single session. While an operation in the elderly should be expeditious, meticulous surgical technique must never be sacrificed for speed. In general, most foot surgical procedures are completed within 1 hour. This concept is of particular importance in our geriatric patients, who generally tolerate poorly any procedure lasting an extended period of time.

The length of recovery time is also of importance to the older patient. As was mentioned earlier, loss of function in the elderly means loss of independence. The older patient is worried, not by the loss of full range of movement, but by the loss of function commensurate with their general activity in their declining years. Thus, it is important that the surgical procedure be not so complex as to keep the patient at bed rest or nonambulatory for a prolonged period of time. It is far better for the patient to achieve independence and a speedy recovery than to have an extensive postoperative course, complicated by the risk of thrombophlebitis or pulmonary emboli.

An arthroplastic repair of a bunion deformity should allow the patient to be up the next day. Extensive bed rest after such an operation can undo in general all the good that the operation has achieved locally. The best surgical procedure on an elderly patient is one that affords immediate ambulation and a quick return to normal routine.

Against this background, let me now turn to some specific surgical approaches. Our purpose is not to be encyclopedic, but rather to cover enough of the range to give a sense of geriatric strategy.

NAIL SURGERY

The geriatric patient's most common minor foot lesion is the ingrown nail. The infection which so frequently accompanies this condition must be eliminated. However, this is not always possible if the ingrown toenail is of long-standing duration and is deeply imbedded in the soft tissues on either or both sides of the nail. Treatment must be directed toward eradication of this constant source of irritation in order to alleviate the infection. When an elderly patient suffers from obliterative peripheral vascular disease and diabetes mellitus, the usual procedure of excising a portion of the nail on one or both sides, together with a section of matrix and soft tissue, constitutes a hazardous operation. These patients have a lowered resistance to infection, so it is unwise to open up new tissue spaces. In addition, the arteries which are partially obliterated in the toes are end arteries, and it is not possible to increase the blood flow from other vessels to assist in the healing of the wounds which have been established. The edema which usually develops after making such a defect in the soft tissue of the toe further embarrasses the depleted blood supply available for the toe to remain viable.

Thus, gangrene can develop. For these reasons, it is far better to carefully remove the nail in its entirety, being careful to avoid trauma to the matrix, nail bed or soft tissues during this process. With drainage established, the infection subsides and the toe heals. As the new nail grows out, it can be accommodated to its proper place and away from the soft tissues on either side. In the healthy geriatric patient surgical correction of the chronic, incurvated nail condition should include sharp surgical excision of the matrix for permanent success. A surgical technique which permits excision of matrix tissue without skin incision seems to be the best procedure. Chemical matrix destruction may also be employed. As a result of minimal surgical trauma, healing is by first intention and it is usually rapid.

DIGITAL SURGERY

A hammer toe deformity consists of fixed flexion at the proximal interphalangeal joint of the toe, a compensatory hyperextension of the terminal joint, and eventual hyperextension of the metatarsophalangeal joint. The concept of the pathomechanics of hammer toe deformity is based on anatomic and functional considerations. This deformity occurs in a digit that has undergone changes in its intrinsic musculature over an extended period of time. Failure of the intrinsic muscles to stabilize the metatarsophalangeal joints of the lesser toes results in the hammer toe deformity, in which the proximal phalanx becomes displaced dorsally on the metatarsal, and the intermediate phalanx is plantar flexed in relation to the proximal phalanx.

Once the intrinsic muscle stability is impaired, function of the long flexor muscle and its tendon is altered, producing a buckling at both the metatarsophalangeal and proximal interphalangeal articulations. The long and short extensor muscles accommodate by contracting, and thus maintain this contracted position. In the elderly, shortening of the dorsal capsule of the metatarsophalangeal joint, and ankylosis of the proximal interphalangeal joint have also taken place. A related effect is seen in which the dorsal subluxation of the proximal phalanx pulls the plantar fat pad from beneath the metatarsal head area, relocating it in the sulcus area of the foot. With loss of the fat pad, metatarsalgia and hyperkeratosis will eventually develop under the metatarsal heads. This is usually found in the geriatric patient as the hammer toe deformity has now fully developed.

The primary indications for surgery are painful digital deformities that cannot be managed by conservative treatment. Additional indications are those deformities severe enough to prevent the wearing of sensible footwear. Therefore, surgical intervention should be directed toward elimination of pain and repair of the deformity. Surgical treatment should be simple and direct. Complicated reconstructive procedures such as those involving pin fixation or tendon transfers should be avoided. Prolonged postoperative immobilization, whatever the reason, is usually unwise in the geriatric foot.

Repair of the hammer toe deformity is accomplished by a variety of surgical techniques. One of the most widely used techniques is that of resection of the head of the proximal phalanx and cutting and suturing of the extensor tendon and joint capsule with the toe in the corrected position. At times, a capsulotomy of the metatarsophalangeal joint and tenoplasty of the extensor tendons are also necessary to avoid excessive cock-up deformity of the remainder of the proximal phalanx. It is rarely necessary to perform an arthrodesis or transfix the phalanges with a Kirschner wire.

The presence of a "flail toe" is not seen following this procedure. With removal of the head of the proximal phalanx, the tissue of the joint area heals by fibrosis, and stubbing of the toe operated upon does not take place. There is no rigidity of the interphalangeal joint as seen in an arthrodesis procedure. The absence of complications and the short postoperative morbidity make it the operative method of choice.

A mallet toe consists of a fixed flexion deformity of the distal interphalangeal joint. Its etiology of muscle imbalance involves the contraction of the flexor tendons to the toe. Surgical correction is accomplished by resection of the head of the middle phalanx or excision of the terminal phalanx, as cosmetic appearance is not a factor. Other minor digital deformities, such as interdigital helomas, are best treated by partial resection of the involved osseous structures.

The results of surgical treatment of digital deformities in the geriatric patient are usually gratifying to both the patient and surgeon. Careful surgical management will provide most patients with freedom from pain and the ability to wear shoes.

BUNION SURGERY

Osteoarthritis is one of the degenerative afflictions in the middle-aged and elderly. It is a progressive disorder insofar as individual joints are concerned.

Palliation is unlikely to affect the course of joint degeneration very much, although it will occasionally be found to give relief of surprising extent and duration. Rest for an inflamed joint, exercise for weakened muscles, and local heat to decrease painful spasm are all worthy of trial. One cannot discount the psychological benefit of these conservative measures. Systemic medication with nonspecific analgesics of the aspirin group and anti-inflammatory compounds like indomethacin should be considered for all patients. Intraarticular injections of cortisone or one of its derivatives have produced impressive symptomatic relief, but repeated injections have produced disastrous disintegration of abnormal cartilage, particularly in weight bearing joints. Pain from degenerate joints of the feet may be relieved considerably by use of orthoses. Only the overzealous clinicain will undertake surgical treatment of a patient with osteoarthritis before most or all of these palliative measures have been properly tried.

The objective of surgical treatment in osteoarthritis is the relief of crippling symptoms. Operative treatment is undertaken primarily to relieve pain, the most significant symptom, with secondary considerations being restoration of movement and correction of deformity. Joint stiffness and deformity only rarely are the presenting symptoms, since they are usually slow to develop and can be compensated for. Any surgical procedure on an arthritic joint must have pain relief as its prime objective; increase in joint movement and correction of deformity are only worthwhile if pain relief is held to be of prime importance.

Each patient must be considered individually since the intensity of the symptoms and the patient's general state indicate the magnitude of surgical treatment. The patient deserves to be considered for surgical correction despite his age, since regional anesthesia and conservative joint operations can be performed in patients 70 or 80 years of age.

Gross deformity and arthritis of the first metatarsophalangeal joint is an indication for arthroplasty—that is, resection of the diseased joint with or without replacement by an artificial joint. Keller described a resection arthroplasty with removal of the proximal portion of the proximal phalanx of the great toe and Mayo described a resection of the first metatarsal head. Both procedures produce relief and mobility; the Mayo operation often has the edge cosmetically, but has to be carried out with more precision and skill to produce a functional result comparable to the Keller procedure. There is both a functional and cosmetic improvement if the great toe can be kept out to length; also the sesamoids do not displace, the muscles maintain good mechanical advantage, and there is less shift of stress onto the lateral metatarsals. Arthroplasty seems the obvious and logical solution to the problem that arises when a natural joint is irreparably diseased, and the question of how to best form a painless, stable and freely movable joint has exercised the ingenuity of surgeons for many years.

The so-called conservative operations, Silver and McBride procedures, are suitable for the older individual who is not as concerned with the correction of the valgus deformity of the great toe as he is with relief of pain from the bunion. In the geriatric patient with a fixed arthritis of the medial cuneiform-first metatarsal joint, one does not anticipate continued adductus of the first metatarsal and, hence, a recurrence of the medial bony prominence.

Resection of the medial eminence with soft tissue release of adductor tension on the lateral side of the joint and shortening of the capsule on the medial side will allow the hallux to be brought into a more corrected position with only minimal osseous remodeling. This simpler procedure will provide satisfactory relief of bunion pain with the least surgical trauma. When osteoarthritic changes accompany a moderately severe bunion deformity with hallux valgus in an elderly patient, the resection arthroplasty is the most satisfactory procedure.

In resection arthroplasty the principle is to resect one or both of the opposing joint surfaces and thus to form a gap between the articulating bones. This gap is preferably filled with a flap of soft tissue, which acts as a cushion to prevent the raw surfaces from coming together. Such a false joint (pseudoarthrosis) is usually painless and may gain a surprisingly good range of movement. There is a drawback, however, that some shortening and instability are inevitable. This type of arthroplasty is still the procedure of choice in the geriatric patient afflicted with degenerative joint disease of the metatarsophalangeal joints.

Resection arthroplasty, which usually involves resecting the base of the proximal phalanx, rather than resecting the metatarsal head, has many advantages contributing towards its present popularity. Foremost among them is that it is a relatively simple procedure requiring little or no immobilization time and gives motion at the metatarsophalangeal joint, thereby allowing the patient to wear varying types of shoes. Pain is relieved in most cases.

The most widely accepted resection arthroplasty technique of the first metatarsophalangeal joint is the Keller procedure. This has been successful, for the most part, as far as relief of pain and obtaining motion in a previously rigid joint; however, it has not been without problems. A painful, stiff pseudoarthrosis may follow insufficient removal of bone. Excessive bone removal may result in shortness and instability of the toe with migration proximally and laterally, thus reversing an initially good cosmetic appearance, and occasionally, forming a recurrent bunion deformity.

Specifically, there are four principal reasons for the occasional unsatisfactory result of a Keller procedure.

1. *Metatarsalgia.* Although the relationship between the Keller procedure and increased

metatarsalgia postoperatively remains controversial, the operation clearly cannot be expected to relieve it. Metatarsalgia following the Keller procedure may be due to the effects of releasing the flexor hallucis brevis muscle by the excessive removal of the base of the proximal phalanx. Some patients who undergo this operation will be dissatisfied if they expect relief of metatarsalgia, but this should not prevent a Keller operation from being performed when painful bunions are present as well as metatarsalgia. Keller's procedure performed for metatarsalgia in the absence of symptoms from the hallux valgus is sure to lead to dissatisfied patients and, consequently, disrepute the procedure.

2. *Inconvenience or disability related to the great toe.* Shortness, floppiness, excessive valgus, dorsiflexion contracture, medial rotation or dorsal subluxation are associated with removal of over one-third of the proximal phalanx. This is an avoidable technical error. Also, following excision of the base of the proximal phalanx, the sesamoid-phalangeal ligaments are lax, which results in retraction of the sesamoids and decreases the flexor power of the hallux. To obviate this complication, suture the tendon of the flexor hallucis longus to the sesamoidal pad. In this manner, retraction of the sesamoids is prevented and the force of the intrinsic muscles through the long flexor is transmitted to the great toe.

3. *Cosmetic result.* In the geriatric patient, the cosmetically unsatisfactory great toe should not be a ground for dissatisfaction. However, if a Keller operation is performed for the correction of hallux valgus becuase it was cosmetically unsatisfactory to the patient, then dissatisfaction will clearly arise if this is used as an indication for operation.

4. *Shortening of the hallux results in flexion deformity of a comparatively long second toe.* This condition could be avoided if the hallux is not excessively shortened by removal of more than one-third of the proximal phalanx. If the second toe is already long, then shortening of the proximal phalanx of this digit to bring it to the level with the hallux following the Keller bunionectomy is advisable.

Therefore, a Keller procedure performed for metatarsalgia in the absence of symptoms from the hallux valgus is sure to lead to dissatisfied patients. The most common technical error in the operation is the excising of more than one-third of the proximal phalanx which produces a short, rotated, floppy toe and a relative projection of the second toe which often develops a hammer toe deformity.

In hallux rigidus, the reverse seems to be true. Unsatisfactory results are associated in those cases in which less than one-third of the proximal phalanx had been excised and were all due to metatarsalgia.

The Mayo procedure encompasses soft tissue and metatarsal surgery in effecting arthroplasty. Basically, it is a resection arthroplasty of the metatarsophalangeal joint involving the resection of the medial eminence and the distal three-eighths inch of metatarsal head. There is no disruption of the weight bearing portion of the metatarsal or the sesamoids. The site of bone resection leaves a surface for reattachment of the capsule on the medial surface in a shortened postion to aid in reestablishing the more normal tendon alignment. It has been modified in various ways in an attempt to substantiate its utilization in the correction of hallux valgus and hallux rigidus. Concern that partial resection of the first metatarsal head will cause metatarsalgia has brought the procedure into disrepute.

The criteria for the Mayo operation are as follows: (1) elderly, sedentary individuals; (2) severe hallux abductus angle with subluxation of the first metatarsophalanageal joint; (3) positive (preferably) metatarsal protrusion distance; and a proximal phalangeal base with minimal degenerative changes.

Comparison studies of the functional and anatomical results of the Mayo and Keller procedures seem to indicate that satisfactory end results can be obtained with either procedure. From this study, it is apparent that there is no discernible difference between the two operations in regards to metatarsalgia. This problem may be solved either by some form of an orthotic or selected lesser metatarsal surgery.

The Mayo-type arthroplasty should be viewed as an effective procedure of choice in the geriatric patient with severe deformity and discomfort. Foremost among its advantages is a short convalescence as compared to the Keller procedure. After the Keller procedure the toe is unstable, so that interposition and immobilization with pins for varying periods of time to prevent proximal migration is frequently employed. In a Mayo-type operation, the bones are held apart by a proximal soft tissue flap. This means a simpler type of support, quicker healing and earlier ambulation for the elderly individual suffering with severe hallux valgus deformity.

Replacement arthroplasty entails the cutting away and discarding of one or both of the opposing joint surfaces, and replacement by an artificial part or prosthesis made from suitable silicone rubber, plastic or other substance known to be inert and harmless to the tissues. If only one of the joint surfaces is replaced the term "hemiarthroplasty" is sometimes used, whereas if both joint surfaces are replaced, the operation is known as total replacement arthroplasty. The Silastic[a] Great Toe Prosthesis (Swanson design) and the Sutter[b] total joint replacement are widely used prostheses for hemi- and total replacement arthroplasty procedures of the first metatarsophalangeal joint, respectively.

Swanson developed a silicone prosthesis for the first metatarsophalangeal joint, replacing the base of the proximal phalanx, acting as a hemiarthroplasty. This solved the problem of a shortened great toe with poor function, as was often seen with the resection arthroplasty. The stability of this procedure relies heavily on the soft tissue reconstruction of the medial capsule, as there is no inherent stability in the prosthesis. This prosthesis acts only as a dynamic spacer for the resection. This relative mobility adds up to a probable recurrence of the deformity.

A relatively recent fault of the hemijoint prosthesis is bioincompatibility secondary to microscopic silicone debris in the periarticular tissues. A wearing of the prosthesis in time results in a microscopic foreign body reaction with ultimate clinical evidence of total rejection.

The disadvantages of the resection arthroplasty and hemiarthroplasty appear to be lessened utilizing a total joint prosthesis. Toe propulsion power is near normal. There is good correction of any deformity regardless of severity due to inherent stability of the prosthesis. There is no pain and no evidence of bioincompatibility.

---

[a] Dow Corning Corporation, Midland, Mich.
[b] Sutter Biomedical, San Diego, Calif.

In the geriatric patient there remains one disadvantage of either replacement arthroplasty as measured against a resection arthroplasty. Whereas there is a much greater margin for error in performing a Keller-type arthroplasty, with hemi- or total joint replacement particular attention must be given to the skin and soft tissues, for if there is any devitalization and breakdown, infection with a foreign body implant becomes a real possibility, with resultant ultimate failure.

It is frequently asserted that either the hemi- or the total joint prosthesis arthroplasty will improve cosmesis and push-off power as opposed to the Keller arthroplasty alone. Unless the insertion of the flexor digitorum brevis is preserved, this is not true. Either component requires a fair degree of proximal bone resection. If the brevis insertion is cut, then push-off is considerably weakened.

Arthrodesis or joint fusion is a time-honored method of dealing with a severely disabling arthritic joint and one that is likely always to retain an important place. Arthrodesis should not, of course, be recommended unless arthritis is severely disabling and at the same time not readily amenable to more conservative methods of treatment. The great advantages that it offers are that it eliminates all possibility of pain in the affected joint, and that the relief is permanent. This is more than can be said of any other operation for degenerative joint disease. Its disadvantages, apart from loss of mobility, are that convalescence after the operation is rather prolonged, and that it is sometimes technically difficult to achieve sound fusion.

In the geriatric patient, the surgical treatment of osteoarthritis of the ankle, subtalar and midtarsal joints is rarely indicated, as palliative care in the form of orthoses usually suffices. In the forefoot, resection arthroplasty is preferred to arthrodesis for surgical treatment of the arthritic first metatarsophalangeal joint seen with hallux valgus and hallux rigidus and of the arthritic interphalangeal joints of the toes. The prolonged pin fixation and plaster immobilization before arthrodesis is solid relegates this procedure to a younger age group.

The operation described by Keller, in which the base of the proximal phalanx and the medial eminence of the first metatarsal head are resected, results, of course, in a pseudoarthrosis. This remains the standard procedure in the surgical treatment of hallux valgus or rigidus with superimposed osteoarthritis in the elderly.

METATARSAL SURGERY

Metatarsalgia with callosities is common in the older patient. Loss of intrinsic tone leads to dorsal subluxation of the proximal phalanges of the toes, which claw. The metatarsal fat pad migrates distally, and the metatarsal heads come to lie subdermally. The epidermis undergoes a compensatory hypertrophy and cornifies in response to the excessive stress,

Most patients describe their initial symptom as pain under the metatarsal heads accentuated by walking and, in particular, with the forefoot push-off. Some patients state they consciously inhibit any flexion of the toes while walking to avoid increasing pain. Such inhibition of plantar flexion results in a combination of intrinsic muscle imbalance and mechanical pressure forcing the toes into dorsal subluxation.

Examination usually reveals tender callosities underlying single or multiple metatarsal heads. The metatarsophalangeal joints are frequently dislocated, so the base of the proximal phalanx comes to lie on the dorsal or lateral aspect of the metatarsal head. The dislocated head lies very close to the plantar skin which, on occasion, can ulcerate with the excessive pressures.

In patients with a less severe degree of metatarsalgia, it is frequently possible to make them comfortable by fitting specially constructed footwear or orthoses designed to distribute the body weight over a large surface area of the foot. If this procedure, combined with palliative care, fails to provide adequate relief, then surgical management is indicated.

Local excision of callosities or resection of the metatarsal heads has proved unrewarding or afforded only temporary relief since, if the problem is confined to one or two metatarsal heads, resection of these will transfer an increased load on those remaining. An oblique telescoping osteotomy of the neck of the metatarsal, thereby displacing the metatarsal head dorsally and proximally, has helped in dealing with the problem. Not infrequently after osteotomy of the most depressed meta-

tarsal, another may feel quite prominent, and osteotomy of this metatarsal is recommended through the same incision. If more than two osteotomies are indicated, a second incision is recommended and the additional surgery adds little to the morbidity. If the procedure is confined to any or all of the middle three metatarsals, the patient is allowed out of bed within 24 hours. Surprisingly, little discomfort occurs on weight bearing, which helps in correctly displacing the metatarsal heads.

Metatarsal osteotomy is not the solution to all cases of metatarsalgia. In the geriatric, the metatarsal head resection is still the procedure of choice in instances of a laterally or plantarly prominent fifth metatarsal head. When frank dislocation of the middle three metatarsophalangeal joints is present, then partial, rather than total, metatarsal head resection will prove more successful.

In the rheumatoid foot or where severe degenerative arthritis has caused subluxation of all the metatarsal heads, then the Clayton technique, consisting of a resection arthroplasty of the metatarsophalangeal joints, is indicated. To accomplish this, the depressed metatarsal heads are removed and, in the more severe deformities, the proximal portions of the proximal phalanges of the medial four toes are likewise resected. Resection of the proximal phalanx of the fifth toe is rarely indicated. Experience has shown that it is better to resect all of the metatarsophalangeal joints if three or more are involved, rather than to preserve one or two relatively normal joints. When all are resected, the toes can be aligned completely. If one or two metatarsal heads remain, when weight bearing is begun, the major portion of the weight falls on the surviving metatarsal heads, and almost invariably they become symptomatic and require surgery.

A Clayton resection is a radical procedure, and when indicated in the selected geriatric patient, it can be done with less trauma and dissection by the use of three dorsal longitudinal incisions or a single plantar transverse incision rather than a single transverse incision across the dorsum of the foot. Although it is not a simple operation, its postoperative management is usually uneventful, healing is fairly rapid and needs no fixation of any kind. These patients are remarkably comfortable, but the thickened soft tissue incident to the bony resection frequently requires several weeks to shrink enough to permit definitive shoe fitting. In the meantime, accommodative footgear is employed.

Painful deformities of the foot are common in geriatric patients who have severe degenerative arthritis, and should be corrected surgically in selected patients after conservative measures have failed to provide relief of pain. Patients generally rate the results of these operations as the most successful of all the surgery performed as the treatment of degenerative joint disease.

FRACTURES

In fractures which involve displacement in the geriatric patient, closed reduction should be attempted as the primary treatment of choice. This is best accomplished under general anesthesia. If the initial reduction is unstable and the fracture/dislocation can be displaced with ease, then fixation with smooth Kirschner wires or Steinmann pins is indicated. This can be accomplished either percutaneously (preferred) or by open technique, depending on the clinician's ability and experience. Whether the reduction is accomplished by open or closed means, it must be acceptable. Good surgical technique is mandatory in handling the soft tissues during open reduction, since these tissues necrose if handled roughly.

Internal fixation in the tarsus is seldom indicated. The opinion that rigid internal fixation of marginal fractures in the forefoot is more effective than traditional treatment is beginning to gain ground. However, because of poor vascularity in the geriatric, the healing of such fractures treated by this method has the potential of pseudoarthritis.

Fracture complications in the elderly frequently require operation. Here, internal fixation may be applied as the benefits of open reduction outweigh the possible complications. Such instances are those where closed reduction would not be possible or where secondary operations are indicated.

Pseudoarthroses in the forefoot are rather common. They are usually situated in weight bearing areas such as the proximal phalanx of the great toe and the fifth metatarsal. Because of poor circulation in this area, metal fixation alone is insufficient as a rule. It is recommended that bone grafting also be undertaken either by a bone peg or by a compressed bridging graft. As these tubular bones are so short, operation may be required, especially in the great toe.

In comminuted articular fractures, either a primary or secondary arthrodesis is required. Kirschner wire fixation is indicated in this age group rather than internal fixation with plates or screw fixation.

POSTOPERATIVE COMPLICATIONS

After surgery, the elderly patient requires careful intensive care to prevent postoperative complications and to detect the first sign of any complications that may develop.

Every caution must be taken to prevent venous thrombosis, which is particularly likely to occur in older persons subjected to surgical trauma because of associated decreased cardiovascular activity and changes in the vascular system. Application of compression bandages to the lower extremities is of value not only to control postoperative edema, but because they compress the superficial veins and thus shunt the blood into the deep system and increase blood flow. Active mobilization of the legs, particularly active, forceful plantar flexion of the foot against resistance, is of importance. As soon as possible, the patient should be gotten out of bed and made to walk. Undoubtedly, one of the reasons for the incidence of venous thrombosis and pulmonary embolism is that patients are kept in bed for a long time, the lack of activity predisposing to venous thrombosis. Deep breathing exercises or use of intermittent positive pressure breathing devices in the immediate postoperative period is important to aeration of the lungs and in decreasing the incidence of atelectasis.

Emptying of any secretion from the tracheobronchial tree immediately postoperatively is absolutely imperative. Unless the bronchial secretions are eliminated, atelectasis and pneumonitis are likely complications. Usually it is possible to make the patient cough, but in patients who cannot cough, the tracheal secretions must be removed by suction.

In elderly surgical patients the cardiovascular system must be carefully monitored.

History of myocardial infarction is important, particularly if it is of recent origin. Coronary occlusion can occur intraoperatively or postoperatively, and often as a result of sudden hypotension. If hypotension develops, adequate fluid replacement is necessary, but must be controlled to prevent cardiac decompensation.

For reasons unknown, preexisting cerebrovascular disease carries less risk of postoperative complication than does preexisting cardiac disease. However, diminished cerebral blood flow may produce difficulties in the geriatric patient postoperatively, particularly when there is minor body temperature elevation. Every effort must be made to avoid fever or to find and correct its cause quickly. Indeed, geriatric patients generally should be watched postoperatively for mental changes indicative of deterioration in blood flow, electrolyte balances and other factors such as adverse drug reactions.

Diabetes mellitus may alter the patient's postoperative course on several counts. There is an increased tendency to infection (wound, urinary, pulmonary or systemic) among diabetics, and their ability to overcome infection is lower than that of nondiabetics. The diabetic patient is prone to arterial disease.

Many older men have prostatic hypertrophy with resultant partial urinary retention, which can be compensated for preoperatively, but may become acute after operation. If the patient has difficulty in emptying the bladder postoperatively, catheterization is indicated to prevent infection. Women are also catheterized because of incontinence. For these and other reasons, the incidence of chronic bacteriuria is high in both sexes in the elderly. Whenever possible, urinary tract infections should be resolved prior to surgery, and every precaution should be taken to prevent new infections.

The incidence of postoperative wound infection increases with age, regardless of the classification of the wound (clean, contaminated or dirty). Fortunately, the frequency of wound infection in clean surgery is relatively low. However, the likelihood of infection increases with prolonged preoperative hospitalization, which should be kept to a minimum. Clean wounds should be closed, primarily, and drains should be avoided.

Prophylactic antibiotics do not alter the incidence of infections in the vast majority of types of clean wounds. Antibiotic use in heavily contaminated wounds is probably not true "prophylaxis" but rather treatment of infection early. Should a clinically apparent wound infection occur, antibiotic choice should be as specific as possible. A gram stain of wound drainage permits the most judicious selection of initial therapy. Subsequently, the antibiotic should be continued or changed, depending on the results of bacterial cultures and susceptibility tests. Wound infection is associated with an increased incidence of wound disruption, and an open wound is more likely to become infected. There is no substitute for aggressive and meticulous local care; thus, systemic antibiotics should be used only when necessary. As previously noted, nutritional supplementation prior to surgery may be beneficial.

Wounds and the management of their complications are no different in the aged than in any other patient. Because it is not possible to accelerate wound healing, it is imperative that the surgeon know and avoid those factors that retard wound healing.

The local management of wounds should and must be meticulous, as the incidence of complications is greater in the aged, even under the most ideal circumstances. This means proper choice and use of suture material, gentleness, avoidance of tension, preservation of a good blood supply, hemostasis, asepsis, obliteration of dead spaces, careful approximation, and the judicious use of drains, irrigation, debridement and antibiotics.

In surgical management of foot infections in the elderly, adequate drainage and excision of infected bone and necrotic tissue are crucial. Gangrenous infection confined to one toe without involvement of the tendon sheath can be treated with simple amputation and, usually, reconstruction of a functional foot. However, if the infection has involved the fibrofatty pad of the toe and spread via the tendon sheath to the deep space of the foot, more radical surgery is needed. The standard procedure is excision of the phalanx and a portion of the metatarsal bone, using a long vertical incision that is extended to the deepest point of infection on the plantar aspect to provide adequate drainage. Since supportive exudate tends to pool in the proximal portion of the central plantar space, dependent drainage is crucial. The least collection of suppurative material on the bottom of the pocketlike space can lead to destruction of the plantar skin and fascia.

Infection on the dorsum of the foot that invades via the lumbrical area to the deep space of the foot is treated with a longitudinal incision along the involved ray that extends plantarly into the foot to expose the deepest point of the infection. The wound is packed and left open to heal by secondary intention, which requires from 2 to 4 months.

Perhaps even more crucial than the surgical procedure is proper management of the consequent wound. The wound should be dressed once or twice daily with gauze moistened with normal saline to absorb exudate. Systemically given antibiotics are questionably effective in treating deep-seated foot infections in those patients whose circulation is defective.

Clearly there are many unique problems to be considered when dealing with the geriatric surgical patient. Age per se is no longer a contraindication to surgery; it is merely a matter of good judgment on the part of the surgeon.

Successful surgery in the aged must be a combined effort between the surgeon, internist, anesthesiologist, nurse, therapist and others. Whenever possible, alterations of normal physiologic function due to chronic and degenerative diseases should be corrected. Careful evaluation of the effects of coronary diseases on the postsurgical course should be considered.

Fifty years ago, an elective operation of major proportion in a patient older than 50 years of age was not justified. Modern day advances, however, have made it possible for the elderly patient to tolerate surgery and anesthesia. Today it is recognized that the well-being of the patient cannot be measured by a statistical figure, but rather by his capacity for mobility, independence, and his relative freedom from pain.

The most importance principle to follow in the management of the elderly is to perform with minimal interference. This often means settling for relief of symptoms in order to cope with a disease, rather than to cure the disease entirely. The older the patient is, the less disturbance in his lifestyle that can be tolerated. This places the surgeon in a paradoxical position: he must bring a certain amount of disruption to the patient's routine, but he must do so in an unhurried, supportive manner. Rather than discussing surgery as the definitive answer, explain it as a possibility and then give the patient a reasonable amount of time to think about it. Explain procedures as you go along and repeat as many times as necessary. Finally, work with the patient with gentleness and understanding to achieve the anticipated results. Our older patients need quiet kindness rather than excessive urgency and an atmosphere of unrushed care and personal contact.

Old age is characterized by a sense of losses; loss of reproductive activity, loss of a companion, loss of physical beauty and mental speed, and a widespread variety of physical losses, including vision, hearing, memory and the capacity for mobility. These losses briefly describe what old age means: a progressive state of dependency. Provided the clinician recognizes that without walking the patient is doomed to a loss of independence, then he will realize that to achieve walking is the most important aspect of rehabilitation in the elderly. Also, he will realize that if walking is lost for any length of time it becomes difficult to achieve thereafter. If a geriatric patient continues to walk almost without interruption during the hospital stay, all will be well, because in the elderly the return to function is the return to independence. The clinician only begins to understand the geriatric patient when he appreciates what old age really means to the elderly.

These individuals have proven stamina to have reached an advanced age and the clinician should take up the challenge to use their available resources to bring about a successful surgical experience, physically as well as mentally. If surgery can afford the geriatric patient greater mobility and independence it will truly be a worthwhile experience.

chapter 10

Gout and the Arthritides

Jay H. Davidson, M.D.

In a discussion of this type, the author is placing emphasis on the practical, clinical and diagnostic features of the disease processes, as well as the management of these processes. This chapter is designed to give the reader a general overview of the entities covered and practicalities in dealing with the pathology encountered, as well as the implications of the pathology as it refers to the rest of the bodily economy. As has been oft repeated in the past, pathology of the lower extremities is intimately related to the rest of the body. The lower extremities cannot be dealt with in a vacuum. For more detailed information the reader is referred to the numerous excellent textbooks of medicine, metabolic disease, neurologic disease and vascular disease, as well as to the many textbooks of rheumatology, including the excellent primer on rheumatic diseases available through the Arthritis Foundation. The author's innate conservatism is reflected in his use of salicylates and the various modalities of physiotherapy.

GOUT

While in the past gout has been said to be a single entity, it is now considered a syndrome resulting from a number of different biochemical alterations. Accordingly, gout is termed a metabolic disease with which the individual is born, or at least activated. There is a secondary form, which is an acquired one associated with hyperuricemia due to a number of other disorders which produce the hyperuricemia.

The hyperuricemia associated with gout may be a result of overproduction of uric acid or underexcretion of uric acid or may be a combination of both.

Clinical Course and Manifestations

The clinical course has been described as consisting of asymptomatic hyperuricemia, acute gouty arthritis and, finally, chronic gouty arthritis. The characteristic clinical features of the disease, which occurs primarily in the male (but the postmenopausal female now shows an increased incidence) has been that of acute attacks with symptom free intervals and increasing severity and duration of each attack as well as shortening of the interval between each attack. An acute attack is usually that of a peripheral joint and, as frequently depicted in the past, involves the great toe. It would appear that it usually develops at night. Even contact with the bed sheets is most disturbing. A current concept holds that the nighttime attack is a product of increased concentration of urate in the joint as a result of absorption of fluid from the joint, in the course of recumbency.

Stress in the form of physical or emotional factors may induce an attack. The disease often has been called a rich man's disease in the past, as the older members of society who acquired wealth tended to overeat and overimbibe.

Early in the course of the disease, as indicated previously, the interval between attacks may be quite long, but as the disease progresses, the interval becomes shorter and, as indicated, the severity more pronounced. Attacks may be polyarticular.

In the past, so-called chronic gouty arthritis was frequently seen with visible prominent joint changes, and tophi. The tophi are a product of the increase of the urate pool and subsequent crystalline deposition in various portions of the soft tissues and cartilages.

Kidney stone constitutes a significant complication and manifestation of the disease. Impaired renal function has been described frequently in the presence of gout, with deposition of crystals in the kidney.

Diagnosis

The clinical features of acute sudden onset involving a peripheral joint in the presence of hyperuricemia and a rapid response to colchicine usually make for a satisfactory clinical diagnosis. The presence of tophi and punched out destructive lesions, as seen typically on x-ray, all suggest the diagnosis.

Tapping the synovial fluid and finding leukocytes with needle-like sodium urate crystals, showing strong negative birefringence to polarized light microscopy, is quite diagnostic. In this regard it should be noted that pseudogout will present the same finding, except that the pyrophosphate crystals present will demonstrate positive birefringence.

Tophaceous material may be obtained from its site by a variety of techniques. Microscopic identification is carried out as indicated above, and biological identification is carried out by degradation with uricase. All of the above diagnostic techniques are described as pathognomonic. However, many physicians will rely on less specific but highly reliable elevation of the serum uric acid, an acute presentation of a peripheral joint, and most importantly, a dramatic response to colchicine.

Treatment

In the acute attack, colchicine is of specific therapeutic as well as diagnostic value: 0.6 mg. every hour for a maximum of 12 doses usually suffices and gives dramatic relief. If no relief occurs within this interval, the drug should be stopped. Many physicians give paregoric along with the colchicine to prevent the diarrhea associated with its use. Usually, however, the cessation of pain and the onset of gastrointestinal symptoms occur concomitantly. Colchicine has been given intravenously in a dose of 0.1–0.3 mg. in 20 ml. of saline slowly. Great care should be exercised, since extravasation will produce a slough. Patients who recognize the prodromal symptoms of an acute attack can abort it by taking colchicine 0.6 mg. three times a day over 2 or 3 days. They do not require the full course described above. Phenylbutazone is likewise very effective in the treatment of an acute attack, after the diagnosis has been established.

A dose of 200 mg. three times on the first day, followed by a dose of 100 mg. four times a day for several days may be employed. Indomethacin, 100 mg. four times a day for the first 24 hours, followed by 100 mg. daily has also been employed effectively. A number of additional anti-inflammatory agents have been effective.

Beyond drug therapy, the avoidance of weight bearing during the acute attack is obviously indicated. When the pain is severe enough, the patient will do it himself, but with less severe pain, the physician should so advise. When pain is gone, mobilization is indeed advisable. During the interval, some dietary limitation is probably indicated but not the severe limitation often imposed. In the presence of severely impaired renal function, this perhaps may be wise. Patients with gout who are obese should be advised as to a weight reduction program. This should be gradual, since rapid weight reduction may precipitate an attack. High fluid intake is used to maintain a large urinary output with the hope that less crystal formation will take place. Alcohol in the form of beer, ale and wine should be avoided whenever possible. It is said that alcohol obtained by distillation has much less influence on the gouty process. A maintenance dose of 0.6–1.8 mg. of colchicine is effective in controlling many patients.

Probenecid, 0.5–3 gm. daily in individual doses, starting with the smaller dose, is an effective drug blocking tubular reabsorption of urate as its mechanism. Salicylates should never be used at the same time as probenecid.

An additional approach is to block the production of uric acid. This is accomplished with allopurinol, 100 mg. three to four times a day. This drug in particular may be extremely useful in the patient with asymptomatic hyperuricemia with a family history of gout. However, periodic and careful clinical observation is essential.

Other Sources of Hyperuricemia

These conditions may result in what has been called secondary gout. It is associated with hematologic disorders such as polycythemia vera, secondary polycythemia, leukemias, myeloma and in chronic hemolytic anemias. Obviously the hyperuricemia is the result of an increase in breakdown of amino acids in cells. Cardiacs and hypertensives treated with commonly used diuretics may develop elevation in the uric acid, with achy joints and acute attack. Discontinuance of the drug will usually lead to relief.

OSTEOARTHRITIS

Osteoarthritis is also known as degenerative joint disease, atrophic arthritis, and also old age arthritis. As can be seen by some of the titles by which it is known, it is a disease found commonly in the older age group. This increased population represents a sizable number who, while surviving, must learn to accept the burden of the discomfort of the disease.

It is a chronic disease characterized by degeneration of articular cartilages and bony hypertrophy. Pain is associated with movement of the joints, and will subside with rest. In addition, it may occur as a result of joint injury. Biomechanical changes are thought to be the source of the cartilaginous destruction, but no specific etiologic factor has been determined.

In the lower extremities, the joints most frequently involved are the hip, knee and first metatarsal phalangeal joint. Symptoms are usually insidious with pain, primarily, and some degree of stiffness. The pain is relatively mild and usually will disappear with rest. Some stiffness may be associated, but not always. Stiffness may be present after the part has been rested, usually disappearing with activity. On examination one may find no abnormality of the joint. With a symptomatic patient, one does not usually feel any heat, nor is there any redness about the joint area. There is no specific laboratory abnormality associated with the disease. X-ray findings of narrowing of the joint space, subchondral bony sclerosis and osteophyte formation are the characteristic findings. It should be pointed out however, that patients with early disease have no x-ray changes. With moderate pain, there may be only minimal x-ray changes. When the pain finally becomes fairly severe, the x-ray changes will be only moderate.

The treatment of the patient with this condition, as in the treatment of any patient, is primarily the reassurance on the part of the treating physician. Informing the patient that the disease is not serious, while uncomfortable and certainly annoying, generally not causing severe pain nor significant disability, is most helpful. The management of the condition is primarily supportive and symptomatic. In obese patients with involvement of a weight bearing joint, a weight reduction program is certainly indicated. Avoidance in the use of the joint by a periodic rest period during the day is helpful. Analgesia with salicylate is useful. Physical therapy and corrective exercises are extremely useful in the management of this condition. Most patients are readily managed this way. In far advanced disease, surgical management has been employed and has been helpful in patients who have marked loss of joint function with significant restoration of mobility accomplished. However, this approach should be reserved for the most severely immobilized patient.

RHEUMATOID ARTHRITIS

This condition, which is generally considered to be found predominantly in the younger age group in females, is now known to occur in the older age group up to the ninth decade. Over the age of 60, the incidence of the disease is approximately equal in both sexes. In contradistinction to osteoarthritis, which is considered to involve individual joints, rheumatoid arthritis is considered to be a systemic disease with joint manifestations as well as other areas of involvement.

Current concepts consider the disease to be related to some alteration in the immunologic mechanism. The exact nature of this mechanism is yet to be clearly defined. Clinically, the usual case will begin with systemic symptoms with no specific joint involvement. It consists primarily of loss of appetite, weight loss, occasional fever and ease of fatigue. The patient notices aches and pains in muscles and joints. It is at this time the patient may then seek help. This is particularly so after swelling or redness and heat develop in the joint areas. In the lower extremities, the knees and feet are the most commonly involved. Rheumatoid arthritis (RA) tends to involve multiple joints and tends to involve them so that, while the involvement may appear to be migratory, the effect is one of addition. The duration of involvement may be from weeks to years. Joint deformities are a clear-cut indication of intrinsic articular disease as well as connective tissue and muscle involvement. The skin may appear to be cool and clammy, with evident pallor. Sweating of the soles and palms is frequent.

As indicated previously, the disease is systemic with involvement of multiple other areas, including the blood vessels, the pleura, lung and the eye.

The American Rheumatism Association (ARA) has proposed a set of diagnostic criteria. It is said to be a classic disease if 7 of the 11 criteria are met and last 6 weeks. It is said to be definite if 5 of the 11 criteria last 6 weeks, and finally, it is said to be probable if 3 of the 11 criteria last 6 weeks.

The criteria are as follows:

1. Morning stiffness in at least one joint.
2. Pain on motion and tenderness in at least one joint.
3. Swelling in at least one joint.
4. Swelling of at least one other joint—swelling should occur within 3 months of the swelling of the previous joint.
5. Symmetrical joint swelling—bilateral involvement of the midphalangeal, metacarpophalangeal joint, or metatarsophalangeal joints is acceptable without absolute symmetry. However, terminal phalangeal joint involvement will not satisfy this particular criterion.
6. Subcutaneous nodules over bony prominences or extensor surfaces. Almost all of these patients will have a positive RA latex fixation test.
7. X-ray changes typical of rheumatoid arthritis include bony decalcifications in or around the involved joint.
8. Positive agglutination test.
9. Poor mucin precipitation from synovial fluid. This is with shreds and cloudy solution.
10. Characteristic histological changes in the synovial membrane with at least three of the following: marked villous hypertrophy; proliferation of superficial synovial cells, often with palisad-

ing; marked infiltration of lymphocytes and plasma cells; and the tendency to form lymphoid nodules.
11. Characteristic changes in nodules, including granulomatous foci with central zones of cell necrosis, surrounded by proliferated fixed cells and peripheral fibrosis.

Criteria 2, 3, 4, 5 and 6 must be observed by a physician.

Laboratory Findings

Hypochromic anemia unresponsive to iron and other therapy is common; the white cell count is variable; the sedimentation rate elevated during the active phase of the disease is used as an index of the degree of activity. Serologic tests for rheumatoid factor are positive in a high percentage of cases which, as indicated above, is part of the "classical" or "definite" arthritis as defined by the ARA. C-reactive protein and elevation of the serum globulins often occur with the active disease. Lupus erythematosus cells are found in some cases, as are antinuclear antibodies. As noted above, tapping the synovial fluid will reveal it to be turbid with reduced viscosity and impaired clot formation. Polymorphonuclear leukocytes are found from 10 to 50,000 cells per cubic centimeter of fluid.

X-ray examination of the affected joint shows soft tissue swelling with osteoporosis, periosteal elevation, erosions of the joint margin and some narrowing of the joint space. Later on, the osteoporosis becomes diffuse. The marginal erosions are said to be most diagnostic.

A small percentage of patients may present with a fulminant form of the disease with fever, marked elevation in temperature, intense joint inflammation and a very rapid evolution of deformities.

Management

Psychologic reassurance and support should be given in large doses and frequently. At the same time, the patient has to be prepared for the realistic probabilities of his or her disease. If the patient is febrile and has acute multiple joint manifestations, bed rest is in order. As far as drugs are concerned, the salicylates again are the drugs of choice. Adequate serum salicylate levels of up to 30 mgm.% are required for control of pain and reduction of joint swelling. This frequently requires more than the usual two aspirins every 4 hours. While gastrointestinal symptoms are not uncommon, they can frequently be controlled by the use of antacids taken on an hourly basis. Other anti-inflammatory drugs may be tried but 4–6 weeks of adequate salicylate therapy will achieve the goals. Antimalarial therapy has been tried, but ocular side effects of the drug have been reported. Therefore, periodic eye examinations are in order if this is employed.

Gold salts were employed many years ago and have now again begun to find increasing use. Trials of new oral preparations supplanting the previous parenteral use are now going on.

Steroids have been employed but do not alter the basic course of the disease. Short term use may be used and obviously long term use offers little other than the problems of side effects. In this regard, alternate day therapy may be useful in avoiding some of them as well as protecting the adrenal gland. Local therapy consisting of aspiration of joint effusion and the instillation of steroids intra-articularly should not be used more than two

to three times a year. The use of steroid preparations with sound judgment has given significant symptomatic relief.

Physiotherapy

Physiotherapy plays a very large role in the management of patients with rheumatoid arthritis. It is begun when the acute painful attack shows signs of subsiding, and helps in the prevention of loss of joint motion and contracture deformities. Daily exercises can also help. Sleeping splints can be devised. Heat is useful and will often permit increased range of motion. Canes, crutches and walkers are particularly useful when the lower extremities are involved. The role of the physiotherapist in this regard is invaluable, and can never be too highly recommended.

Surgery

Surgery in the form of synovectomy has been employed. Surgery for the hip, knee and ankle are best left for patients with longstanding disease who have been able to maintain some degree of muscle tone. However, this is a mechanical solution for a disease that is systemic.

chapter 11

Vascular Diseases of the Feet

Stanley N. Cohen, M.D.

ARTERIAL DISEASES

Arteriosclerosis Obliterans

The most important vascular disorders of the feet are those involving the arteries; the most significant is arteriosclerosis obliterans. While primary involvement of the arteries of the toes and the feet do occur, notably in diabetes mellitus, ischemic foot lesions are more commonly the result of occlusive disease of the aorta, iliac, femoral, popliteal and tibial arteries.

Pathogenesis

The pathogenesis of the atherosclerotic lesion is the subject of considerable investigation and speculation. Cellular changes can be identified histologically and correspond to four stages: injury, cell proliferation, necrosis and repair. Three hypotheses have evolved as the mechanisms initiating arterial cell changes that result in the atherosclerotic lesion. In the lipogenic theory, abnormal, circulating serum lipoproteins and specific receptor sites on the cell surface of arteries may result in the accumulation of lipids and cell damage. The myogenic theory suggests that focal endothelial injury allows the entry of stimuli that result in proliferative changes. The mutagenic hypothesis theorizes that fibrous plaques are derived from a single smooth muscle cell and that proliferation begins with the mutation of a single cell following an injury. These three theories may well be interrelated, suggesting that atherogenesis is multifactorial in its etiology.

While the atherosclerotic lesion in diabetes mellitus is similar in all respects histologically to that of the nondiabetic, a further dimension is added in the diabetic foot where end arteries become occluded. Without the formation of a collateral circulation, tissue supplied by the end artery dies. In addition, the small skin vessels and capillaries of the diabetic foot are involved in the microangiopathic process so common in the diabetic and characterized by basement membrane thickening. When exposed to trauma or infection, these vessels become obliterated and gangrene appears.

Presentation

Atherosclerosis is both intriguing and beguiling in its presentation. Its individual varieties are related to sex (the male predominates) and geography (Western civilization), while risk factors include hyperlipoproteinemia, hypertension, cigarette smoking and diabetes mellitus. Arteriosclerosis obliterans presents anatomically in many variations. The disease may be localized to the aortoiliac segment with the occlusive process beginning at or near the origin of the common iliac arteries, ultimately occluding both, and spreading upward to the origin of the renal arteries. This is commonly known as the Leriche syndrome and may result in intermittent claudication and sexual impotency.

Complete or incomplete occlusion of the superficial femoral artery and patency of the popliteal artery and its major branches is a second common presentation and may be combined with aortoiliac occlusion. A third pattern is involvement of the popliteal artery

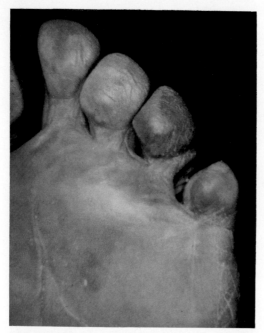

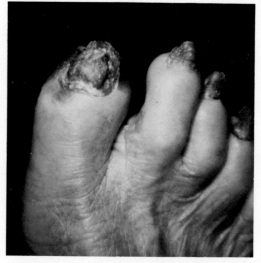

Fig. 11.2   Early thrombosis of hallux.

Fig. 11.1   Marked cyanosis and vascular impairment of lesser digits.

and its major branches, more commonly, but not exclusively seen in the diabetic.

These distinctive patterns of presentation appear to have both an age and sex relationship. Hence, patients develop predominate aortoiliac occlusion at an earlier age than distal femoropopliteal disease and have a sex ratio of 10 males to 1 female. The progression of disease is variable in femoral artery disease and may be rapid (1–3 years), moderate (5–8 years) or slow (10 years or more). In the latter group, disease may occur years later after corrective surgery in the same arterial bed or elsewhere, as in the carotid or coronary arteries. This variability in the presentation and progression of disease has led to the suggestion that specific etiological factors may be involved in the occurrence of a specific pattern.

Arterial Insufficiency

In addition to the vascular lesion itself, other factors may play significant roles in the ultimate clinical picture of arterial insufficiency. Foremost are the heart and the qualitative and quantitative makeup of the blood. If heart function is compromised and cardiac output is decreased, blood flow to the periph-

ery is diminished. Decreased oxygenation of blood may occur with disorders of pulmonary function, thereby limiting the amount of oxygenated blood flowing to the feet.

The oxygenation of blood may also be decreased if there is a limitation in oxygen-carrying capacity due to anemia or hemoglobin abnormality. An increased viscosity of blood as seen in polycythemia and other blood dyscrasias may also lead to the slowed passage of blood and resultant thrombus formation.

Diabetes Mellitus

Diabetes mellitus must be considered and appreciated as a special entity in peripheral vascular disease. Not only are arterial lesions more commonly seen in the diabetic foot and leg, but these lesions appear earlier. The absence of pedal pulses is so descriptive of the diabetic foot that this diagnosis must be sought if it has not otherwise been made.

The diabetic foot may be further compromised by the presence of neuropathy, expressed by the absence of knee and ankle reflexes, hypesthesia and the loss of position sense. The neuropathic ulcer, commonly on the plantar surface of the toes and foot, results from the loss of tactile sensation. Infection finds a rich medium in diabetic tissue, and the diabetic is limited in his response to infection by a delay in early local cellular response to infection, a reduction in migration

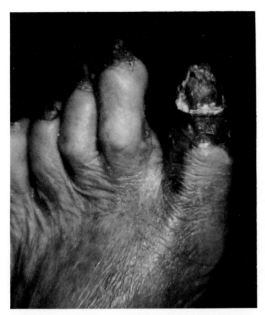

Fig. 11.3 Gangrene of hallux as a result of thrombosis.

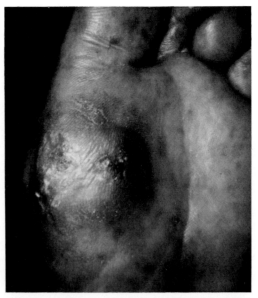

Fig. 11.4 Subcallosal hemorrhage and ulceration associated with thrombosis of small vessel.

of leukocytes, and by an impairment in phagocytosis.

Signs of Arterial Insufficiency

Rubor of the feet on dependency and pallor on elevation are specific signs of arterial insufficiency. Inspection of the legs and feet may reveal a smooth shininess to the skin, and absence of hair, brittleness, deformity, pigmentation of the nails, or frank skin ulceration. The observation of dermatophytosis is of particular significance. Muscle atrophy both in the foot and calf may be present. Calf atrophy is best appreciated by examining the patient from the rear while the patient is standing.

The skin may be cool or cold to the touch and should always be determined by the use of the more sensitive dorsum of the examiner's hand rather than the fingertips. The palpation and recording of pulses are important and offer an objectivity that can be compared in subsequent examinations. The dorsalis pedis pulse may take an aberrant anatomical course in the foot of a small percentage of normal feet (5–12%) and may not be palpable. A pedal pulse may be palpable in the case of arterial occlusion such as the popliteal artery, thereby indicating a functioning collateral or secondary circulation.

Neurological examination may reveal an absence of deep tendon reflexes of the knees and/or ankles, particularly significant as a sign of neuropathy in the diabetic. Sensation may be diminished or exaggerated in the toes and feet of the patient with the polyneuropathy of diabetes mellitus. Neuropathy may ultimately result in damage to the normal foot architecture with hyperextension of the proximal phalanges, the so-called "cock-up" toe deformity. Abnormal pressure points result and are the sites of callous formation and ulceration. While more common in the metatarsal areas, neuropathic ulcers occur also on the toes and plantar surface of the heels. Advanced and long-standing neuropathy may result in the Charcot foot deformity in which ankle joint function becomes useless.

A bruit is a vibratory disturbance which results from the production of eddy currents as a column of blood flows from a channel of normal caliber into a channel of reduced caliber. This turbulence is heard as a murmur with the diaphragm of the stethoscope placed lightly over the partially occluded artery, most commonly the abdominal aorta, femoral and popliteal arteries.

Noninvasive Vascular Examination

While careful history taking and examination will provide the clinician with the bulk of information necessary for a diagnosis of arterial insufficiency, laboratory testing is indicated to give an objective measurement.

The oscillometer is useful in recording the objective volume of pulse flow and is particularly helpful when pulses are not palpable. It is useful for the comparison of repeated studies over a period of weeks or months. Since the oscillometer is not sensitive enough to detect oscillations in the collateral circulation where pressure is lower than in the major arteries, its clinical value is reduced.

Occlusive disease of the arterial system results in hypotension distal to the involved site; hence, the measurement of arterial pressure distal to the diseased vessel is an effective means of following the progression of the occlusive process. The measurement of systolic blood pressure is accomplished accurately by using the Doppler ultrasound technique, probably the one most important objective test of vascular measurement. This measurement can be taken both with the patient at rest and after the stress of exercise testing on a treadmill.

The plethysmograph and various isotopic studies can be used to measure total limb flow or regional blood flow and thereby assess the physiological results of arterial occlusion.

A pulse volume recorder measures oscillations superimposed on a constant pressure applied to the limbs in order to obtain the maximal possible amplitude of pulsation.

The reflex vasodilation test is a means of evaluating the possible usefulness of sympathectomy. The skin temperature and digital pulsations of the toes are measured in a controlled temperature laboratory before and after application of heat to the body of the patient. An increase in these measurements provides a rough estimate of the response to be expected from lumbar sympathectomy.

Invasive Vascular Examination

Contrast angiography offers the definitive means of visualizing the lumen of the arterial tree. Following the intra-arterial injection of a radiopaque medium, radiographs are taken at different intervals of time. The abdominal aorta, its main branches and the arteries of the feet can be examined by the injection of the contrast medium via the femoral artery. The percutaneous translumbar route of injection into the abdominal aorta is much less commonly used today than in the past.

Arteriography has gained significant importance with the increasing ability of the vascular surgeons to operate more distally in restoring arterial blood flow. Thus, the observation of the collateral circulation beyond a proximal occlusive site is an important feature in determining the ultimate efficacy of surgical intervention.

Treatment of Arterial Insufficiency

The treatment of the compromised arterial system in the leg and foot includes preventive measures. It is axiomatic that the patient must be educated in foot care, and this information must be communicated both orally and by written instructions. This information should include the following (but in greater detail):

1. Inspect (or have your family inspect) your feet daily for infection and lesions.

2. Wash your feet daily with a mild soap in lukewarm water.

3. Cut your toenails in the proper manner or have this performed by a podiatrist. Calluses and corns should be managed by a podiatrist.

4. Wear only proper fitting shoes.

5. Never apply a hot water bottle or other form of heat to the feet; never apply an antiseptic medication.

6. Never smoke tobacco.

The attending physician and podiatrist must function as a team, sharing the medical information available on any given patient. It is essential that both be aware of the vascular problem affecting the patient, its extent and those studies performed to evaluate the problem. They should both be knowledgeable as to the patient's systemic problems and medications prescribed. They must be alert to those conditions that diminish blood flow to the periphery such as congestive heart failure, and to problems of anemia and diminished oxygenation of peripheral tissue.

Both must realize the significance of careful surgical attention to calluses and corns. Overzealous removal of tissue may lead to infection and further compromise vascular flow. The prescription of appropriate footwear and orthotics is essential and this is of particular importance in the care of the diabetic patient with neuropathy. Unfortunately, it is not well appreciated among clinicians that neuropathic ulcers will fail to heal appropriately or will recur unless properly designed weight redistribution measures are prescribed. Such shoes and orthotics should protect pressure points in the insensitive diabetic foot.

Dermatophytosis may seriously affect an already compromised foot and lead to secondary bacterial infection and gangrene. If fungal lesions are few, treatment with one of the newer fungicidal preparations such as clotrimazole is in order. More involved fungal infection of the foot may be treated with a 1:4,000 solution of potassium permanganate as a foot bath.

Ulceration of the ischemic toe or foot is a serious condition, the implication of which must be made known to the patient and/or family if complete cooperation is expected. Treatment should include the following:

1. Bed rest initially is a prerequisite; weight bearing fosters nonhealing.

2. After the acute process responds to treatment, the patient may progress to a chair with the limbs dependent unless edema forms.

3. A foot cradle is desirable to prevent the bed covers from irritating the ulcer.

4. Analgesics should be dispensed as needed, the clinician exercising careful judgment.

5. A culture of the ulcer secretion with sensitivity studies is indicated. Since many ulcers have a mixed infection, a wide spectrum antibiotic in oral form is indicated; occasionally its intravenous use is more appropriate.

6. Local application of an antibiotic is infrequently helpful and may macerate adjacent viable skin.

7. The ulcer should be cleaned daily with hydrogen peroxide or povidone-iodine solution (Betadine) and dressed. Lamb's wool is used between the toes to protect the surrounding tissue from infection and to prevent pressure lesions.

8. Lukewarm Betadine compresses may be used to soften necrotic tissue for careful debridement. However, maceration of skin should be avoided.

9. Vasodilator drugs are not indicated in the treatment of occlusive vascular disease, including claudication or peripheral ulceration. They tend to lower systemic pressure which has been shown to increase collateral vascular resistance.

Surgical Treatment

Surgical candidates include patients with threatened limb loss who usually have the peripheral signs of ischemia, foot pain at rest, and may have nonhealing ulceration of the foot or frank gangrene; and patients with stationary arterial thrombosis who have debilitating claudication which affects their ability to work or interferes seriously with their lifestyle.

The procedures commonly used are femoropopliteal or femorotibial reconstruction using the reversed or autogenous saphenous vein. Less desirable is the use of a prosthetic graft in the former procedure. Operative risks and postoperative graft failures have diminished over the past several years. However, graft failure may recur and place the patient in jeopardy of a major amputation. In such cases, a second arterial reconstruction procedure may be successful. An axillofemoral Dacron bypass is occasionally performed when the risk of the standard procedure is high because of associated disease or in the presence of an infected graft.

Endarterectomy is less often used at present than in the past and is limited to segmental blocks in the superficial femoral and deep femoral arteries.

The place of lumbar sympathectomy in the treatment of chronic arteriosclerosis obliterans is controversial. It may play a role in the healing of small ulcers, although this is less applicable to diabetics since autosympathectomy is a common occurrence. There is general agreement that sympathectomy has no place in the treatment of intermittent claudication.

In recent years, recanalization of superficial femoral occlusions using a balloon catheter has been attempted. Only occlusions less than 10 cm. are treated because of low patency rates for longer recanalizations. After passage of the balloon catheter into the artery, the balloon is expanded sufficiently to compress the occluding material against the vessel wall.

Amputation is an unfortunate event that may become necessary when ischemia of a part results in incipient or frank gangrene. Since reconstructive surgery may effectively revascularize the foot or leg or limit the site of amputation, arteriography should be offered any patient who is a candidate for amputation. If reconstructive surgery is impossible or unsuccessful and amputation is inevitable, the patient must be prepared both emotionally and physically for this procedure.

Amputation of a toe or toes may be possible in those instances where digital arteries have been occluded in the diabetic foot, or by embolization, connective tissue disorders, or thromboangiitis obliterans. Occasionally, a transmetatarsal amputation of the foot is indicated in those cases where several toes are involved. In larger artery involvement, as in arteriosclerosis obliterans, a below-the-knee amputation is greatly to be preferred over an above-the-knee amputation since the immediate operative risk is less if the joint is preserved, and earlier ambulation and rehabilitation with a prosthesis are possible.

Acute Arterial Occlusion

Acute arterial occlusion represents the most profound emergency situation involving the arterial system of the lower legs, with the exception of acute arterial hemorrhage. The major causes are embolism, thrombosis and injury. Emboli may be of cardiac origin, primarily in rheumatic heart disease, usually mitral or aortic endocarditis, and frequently associated with atrial fibrillation or flutter. Other cardiac sources of emboli are the mural thrombi that occur on the wall of the left ventricle following an acute myocardial infarction, or prosthetic valves. Cholesterol emboli from the aorta may be dispersed peripherally and result in acute arterial occlusion, occasionally in the small digital arteries.

Sudden arterial occlusion may be the initial sign of arteriosclerosis obliterans, although a larger group of patients will have had symptoms of arterial insufficiency with the sudden worsening of symptoms presumably due to acutely superimposed arterial thrombosis. Trauma may produce acute occlusion such as external pressure on an artery.

Unusual muscular effort may result in the anterior tibial artery compartment syndrome. Less common causes include connective tissue diseases and blood dyscrasias.

While the greater number of acute occlusive phenomena in the legs will affect the superficial femoral and popliteal arteries, the three major vessels distal to the popliteal artery may also be acutely occluded.

Pain in the most distal part of the extremity is followed by numbness, coldness and tingling, these symptoms appearing quickly in 50% of cases and gradually over a period of one to several hours in the remainder. Significantly, pain is the initial symptom in only one-half the cases; hence, the diagnosis may be elusive if other symptoms occur prior to pain. The loss of cutaneous sensation is followed by the loss of muscular power of a variable degree dependent upon the suddenness and the extent of occlusion and the degree of collateral circulation.

The signs of acute arterial occlusion include pallor and mottling of the skin, the collapse of superficial veins, lowering of skin temperature, and the absence of pulsation in the areas involved. Neurological examination will reveal absent or diminished deep tendon reflexes, hyperesthesia or anesthesia, and a decrease or absence of muscle strength.

Emergency treatment is indicated, including initially elevating the head of the bed so that the limbs are dependent. The patient should be kept warm and the legs carefully protected by a soft, loose dressing. A foot cradle is useful in preventing the traumatic pressure of bed clothes on the ischemic limb. Heat of any type must not be applied to the limb. Opiates are essential for relief of pain and for their sedative effect. Vasodilators are of little value. Intravenous heparin therapy should commence immediately, as should treatment of any systemic disease that might be playing a role in the acute occlusive process. This includes cardiac arrhythmia, congestive heart failure, myocardial infarction and bacterial endocarditis. The age of the patient, his general vascular and systemic condition, and the results of medical therapy in the first few hours following occlusion will determine the need for embolectomy.

Thromboangiitis Obliterans (Buerger's Disease)

Thromboangiitis obliterans is a rare inflammatory and occlusive disorder affecting the small and medium-sized arteries and veins of the extremities. The diagnosis is less commonly made today, possibly because of more stringent criteria. The disease differs from arteriosclerosis obliterans in that it is ten times more common in males than females, occurs before the age of 40, involves the arteries of the upper extremities as well as the lower extremities, and is nearly always associated with cigarette smoking.

Claudication, most commonly occurring in the arch of the foot, but also in the calf, may be the initial symptom. Occasionally a cold, painful toe may inaugurate the disease process. Color changes occur as the disease progresses, and in advanced cases there is ulceration and gangrene of both fingers and toes. Absence of pulsations occurs in the pedal arteries and commonly in the radial and ulnar arteries. Acute thrombophlebitis in small and medium-sized veins may occur and is a clue to the diagnosis of thromboangiitis obliterans.

The occlusion of small arteries in this disorder appears to be episodic and is followed by the development of a collateral circulation of a degree sufficient enough to spare the part involved. If cigarette smoking should continue, further occlusive episodes occur and ultimately may lead to ulceration and gangrene.

Treatment includes a careful explanation to the patient of his disease state and of the role that cigarette smoking is playing. He must be advised to desist from using all forms of tobacco. Since avoidance of vasoconstriction is important, the patient should dress warmly and not expose himself to a cold environment. Vasodilating drugs are of little help and may actually shunt blood away from the ischemic area by dilating vessels elsewhere. Sympathectomy does have a role to play in those instances of moderate to serious arterial involvement short of extensive gangrene. The usual steps to protect the toes and feet from trauma must be carried out with the cooperation of an educated patient. Minor surgery on the digits and the care of ulcers should follow the precepts established in the treatment of those same conditions due to arteriosclerosis obliterans. Autoamputation of a digit may occur; in other instances, amputation of a toe or toes may be necessary and, uncommonly, a below-the-knee amputation may be indicated if disease has involved the dorsum of the foot.

Connective Tissue Diseases

Polyarteritis nodosa, systemic lupus erythematosus, rheumatoid arthritis and progressive systemic sclerosis infrequently cause an arteritis of a terminal digit and may progress to gangrene of a toe.

DISEASES OF VEINS

Acute Thrombophlebitis

It is appropriate to include acute deep thrombophlebitis in a discussion of vascular disorders of the feet, since the aftermath of the disorder, the postphlebitic leg, is frequently associated with stasis ulcers. These ulcers occur in the region of the ankle, just above or below the malleoli, more commonly the internal malleolus.

The three factors promoting venous thrombosis are the slowing of blood (stasis), intimal changes (nidus), and alterations in blood (hypercoagulability). While acute thrombophlebitis occurs frequently on an idiopathic basis, there are numerous conditions that predispose to this disorder, including trauma, the postoperative state, pregnancy, infectious disease, hematologic disorders, heart disease and neoplasms.

The thrombus most often forms in the deep veins of the calf muscles, although it may also form initially in the plantar, popliteal or the ileofemoral veins. Clinically, acute thrombophlebitis expresses itself as pain and tenderness in the calf in the case of involvement of the muscular veins of the calf. There may be slight enlargement of the calf itself. Homans' sign (calf pain following dorsiflexion of the foot) may or may not be present, and is not a pathognomic sign of acute thrombophlebitis since it may occur in muscle trauma, hematoma, myositis and irritation of sciatic roots.

Acute thrombosis of the popliteal and superficial femoral veins result in those symptoms and signs discussed in calf vein thrombosis as well as tenderness in the popliteal space, enlargement of the leg below the knee and edema of the distal tibia and ankle.

Involvement of the iliofemoral vein results in thigh pain, commonly lower leg pain, distended superficial veins, enlargement of the entire extremity and tenderness in the femoral canal.

While these are the classical presentations of acute thrombophlebitis, there are many instances in which a thrombus is present, particularly in the calf, with minimal-to-absent signs and symptoms. To facilitate the diagnosis, several noninvasive and invasive procedures are available. Perhaps most commonly used today is Doppler ultrasound, which approaches an accuracy of 80–95% when compared with deep vein phlebography. The thrombus can also be identified by isotope detection using radioactive labeled fibrinogen. When injected intravenously this isotope accumulates in the fibrin of a newly formed clot. There are serious disadvantages, however, including possible contaminated fibrinogen and unreliability of the test if other concentrations of fibrinogen are present. The most definitive diagnostic study is deep vein phlebography.

Once the diagnosis of acute thrombophlebitis is seriously considered or appropriately established, then immediate hospitalization is indicated. Treatment consists of bed rest, elevation of the leg, warm compresses applied to the limb, and intravenous heparinization. Recently, the use of agents that induce thrombolytic activity have been approved for clinical use. These include streptokinase and urokinase. Recommendations for their use include massive pulmonary emboli with or without shock, and extensive deep vein thrombosis where there is marked occlusion of the large veins of the lower or upper extremities with extension into the respective vena cavae. Many questions remain concerning the use of these drugs, which are used only in a hospital setting and only when the diagnosis has been as firmly established as possible.

Pulmonary Embolism

Pulmonary embolism is the more serious of the two prominent complications attributed to acute thrombophlebitis, the other being chronic venous insufficiency and the postphlebitic syndrome. Both pulmonary embolism and acute deep vein thrombosis may be unrecognized in more than one-half the cases in which they coexist. Thrombi in the lower extremities are said to be responsible for 60–80% of pulmonary embolisms.

Chronic Venous Insufficiency (Postphlebitic Syndrome)

Chronic venous insufficiency is the aftermath of iliofemoral thrombophlebitis and is the result of damage to the venous wall, incompetency of its valves, and partial-to-complete obstruction of its lumen. The stasis of venous blood flow leads to the transudation of protein-rich fluid through the vessel wall into the tissue spaces with chronic edema formation. The skin becomes pigmented and the tissues are subjected to low grade infection. Minor trauma may lead to ulceration.

Stasis dermatitis usually appears as weeping eczema with a covering of scaly, cornified material and surrounding inflammation. It may be accompanied by severe itching. Treatment consists of bed rest with the legs elevated and removal of the accumulated secretions and cornified superficial layers of skin. Lanolin or a steroid ointment may allay itching.

The prevention of stasis ulcer begins by attempts to control venous stasis. This is often achieved by the wearing of an elastic stocking fitted while the leg is edema free. The greatest care to prevent trauma should be exercised. Should an ulcer occur, bed rest and elevation of the leg may suffice to heal a small ulcer. Moist dressings of normal saline solution are helpful in healing, although caution must be exercised lest maceration of the surrounding skin occur. Infection is usually not a problem; hence, a systemic antibiotic is unnecessary except in very obvious infections, in which cases culture of the ulcer is indicated. The overzealous use of ointments and powders is to be avoided. Some clinicians will carefully use a fibrinolytic agent such as Elase in the ulcer site for debridement.

In the patient who is unable to be treated at bed rest because of his various duties and responsibilities, a nonelastic boot may be used in the treatment of the stasis ulcer. The Unna gelatin protein boot is applied to the extremity for 1–2 weeks, removed and reapplied until ulcer healing occurs. In those instances where a stasis ulcer does not heal and remains indolent, excision of the lesion followed by a split-thickness skin graft may be indicated.

LYMPH VESSELS

Acute Lymphangitis

Acute lymphangitis is inflammation of the lymphatic vessels as a result of bacterial spread from an infected or necrotic lesion, or a puncture wound of the skin. It is commonly due to beta hemolytic streptococci. Dermatophytosis between the toes is often an associated and antecedent feature, especially in those cases of acute lymphangitis involving the postphlebitic syndrome. Red streaks may be prominent and extend proximally from the infected area to tender and enlarged regional lymph nodes. Acute lymphangitis frequently begins with a chill and a fever ranging from 103° to 105°F.

Treatment consists of bed rest with elevation of the extremity. Procaine penicillin G is the antibiotic of choice when beta hemolytic streptococci are the offending organisms. In cases of staphylococcus infection, sodium oxacillin is frequently administered intravenously. However, it is appropriate to culture the secretions from the involved lesion, which frequently is in the foot. Since infection may enter the blood stream, blood cultures may also be indicated.

Lymphedema

Primary or idiopathic lymphedema may occur in childhood or in later life and is more common in females. One lower extremity is usually affected, but it may involve both legs. The edema, initially pitting, may be limited to the ankle and lower leg or extend to the thigh. Early in its development, edema will subside with elevation of the leg; later, as a fibroblastic reaction occurs in the subcutaneous tissue and the overlying skin becomes roughened, swelling becomes permanent and nonpitting. The skin is then subject to infection, cellulitis and ulceration.

Congenital lymphedema presents at birth. It may be hereditary and is called Milroy's disease. Secondary causes of lymphedema in the lower extremities include the spread of a neoplasm (carcinoma, sarcoma and Hodgkin's disease) to regional and distant lymph nodes with resulting interference in lymph flow and lymphedema formation.

In all cases of lymphedema, prophylactic care of the skin is important and includes a skin softener, the wearing of a fitted stocking if comfortably tolerated by the patient, and extreme care not to traumatize the leg. The judicious use of a diuretic may be helpful in limiting edema formation.

chapter 12

Podiatric Management of Vascular Complications

Edward L. Tarara, D.P.M.

Symptoms and signs in the feet, especially in elderly patients, can be clues to the presence of systemic diseases. When the foot is examined, the condition of the skin and the status of the circulation should be assessed, in addition to the mechanical function.

OCCLUSIVE ARTERIAL DISEASE

Arteriosclerosis obliterans is a diagnostic term used to describe a chronic occlusive arterial disease of the aorta and its major branches. The disease also involves the large and medium-sized arteries, especially those of the lower extremities. In the presence of diabetes mellitus, arteriosclerosis obliterans is more prevalent and more severe. The physical findings are those of occlusive arterial disease, decrease or absence of pulses in the extremity, pallor of the lower extremity on elevation, delay of venous filling time and dependent rubor directly related to the degree of ischemia.

The symptoms of arteriosclerosis obliterans result from ischemia of tissues supplied by the affected arteries. Symptoms may evolve gradually as a result of a slowly progressive obliteration of the arterial lumen or may appear abruptly as the result of an acute arterial occlusion. An acute occlusion may be the first clinical manifestation of the disease. If a relatively small portion of the arterial tree is occluded, the symptoms may be mild or totally unperceived. They may, however, progress in a series of episodes, with interven-

ing partial regression. Gradual progression is not inevitable; in many patients, the symptoms remain stable for years. Early in the course of the disease, even in mild cases, the affected extremity, and particularly the foot, may become excessively cold after brief exposure to a cold environment.

Intermittent claudication, often described as pain, aching, cramping, numbness or fatigue in certain muscles, develops only during exercise. Quick relief is obtained by rest without change of position. Intermittent claudication is almost always pathognomonic of occlusive arterial disease in the affected extremity. Although it is often unilateral initially, it may become bilateral at any time. During almost any stage of the disease, one leg may have more severe involvement than the other.

The distance that a patient is able to walk before distress develops depends on the extent and the severity of the arterial occlusion. It may be 10 yards or it may be a mile, but usually it is between half a block and two city blocks when the patient walks at an average pace on level ground. If a patient continues to walk after symptoms develop, the affected muscle frequently becomes spastic and produces a definite limp. Continued walking may then become impossible.

Pain while at rest signifies the presence of more severe ischemia of tissues and of a more advanced and severe type of occlusive arterial disease than does intermittent claudication alone. The digits, and perhaps the foot and lower part of the leg, are the initial sites of

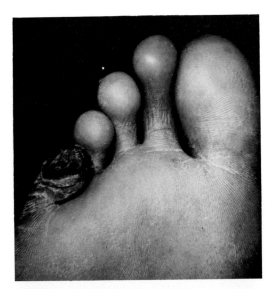

Fig. 12.1 Dry gangrene of fifth toe, arteriosclerosis.

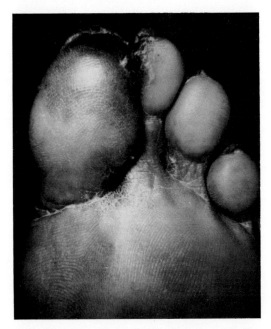

Fig. 12.2 Thrombosis and gangrene of hallux and second toe associated with pressure necrosis.

involvement. Occurring mainly during the night, it consists of a dull, moderately severe, persistent aching that may interfere with sleep. The patient may awaken and rub the affected area for hours in an attempt to relieve the pain.

When ulceration and gangrene are associated with arteriosclerosis obliterans, pain is usually moderate to severe. Hyposensitive patients and some diabetic patients with advanced neuropathy, however, may have minimal or no pain. Other patients may have severe pain that is difficult to control, even with opiates. The pain is persistent and, like pretrophic pain, is usually worse at night. It is often confined to the ulcerated or gangrenous region or just proximal to it.

Abnormal pallor on elevation and a delay in return of color and filling of superficial veins on dependency after elevation are pathognomonic of occlusive arterial disease, particularly if these findings differ in the two lower extremities. Both ulceration and gangrene usually appear first in the terminal portions of the digits, often around the nails or in a nail bed after an infection, and cause loosening and sloughing of the nail. In ischemic toes, pressure from shoes during ordinary walking can cause ulceration or gangrene. Ulceration of the foot or leg is usually the result of trauma, either mechanical or thermal, or some type of pyogenic infection of the skin.

DIFFERENTIAL DIAGNOSIS

The clinical differentiation of arteriosclerosis obliterans (ASO) from other vascular and nonvascular diseases is usually not difficult.

Thromboangiitis obliterans usually manifests itself under age 40 with the presence or history of superficial thrombophlebitis in nonvaricose veins and the presence of ischemic manifestation in the hands and fingers.

The presence of arterial calcification, diabetes mellitus or hyperlipidemia is strong evidence in favor of ASO. Any time there is impairment or absence of pulsation in the abdominal artery, femorals or popliteals, the lesion is almost always ASO. If bruits are heard over the major arteries in the lower extremities, ASO is most certainly the causative factor.

Arterial embolism is most commonly associated with heart disease and the embolus most commonly originates as an intracardiac thrombus. Occasionally an embolus may come from a mural thrombus in an atherosclerotic aorta or from an aortic, iliac, femoral or popliteal aneurysm. In these cases the thrombus is usually the result of advanced atherosclerosis and differentiating it from ASO may be difficult.

Raynaud's Disease. The differentiation of Raynaud's from ASO should present no difficulty. Raynaud's shows no evidence of occlusion of peripheral arteries, it develops in young women, mostly, and is bilateral. It has a tendency to involve the hands more than the feet with the characteristic color changes that occur in exposure to cold.

Livedo Reticularis. The cyanotic or mottled bluish discoloration of the skin of the extremities is bilateral and symmetrical. Pulsations are not impaired or absent in the posterior or tibial and popliteal arteries.

Ergotism. The pulsation of the major arteries in the lower extremities may be impaired or absent in patients with ergotism. The manifestations tend to be symmetrical and frequently a history of prolonged use of ergotamine or an ergot derivative is elicited. Discontinuation of the drug usually finds the symptoms of intermittent claudication disappearing and pulsation returning to normal.

Acute venous thrombosis or chronic venous insufficiency causes congestion and swelling of the leg. This is not present in ASO, unless gangrene of toes or the foot is seen. In acute venous thrombosis, pain usually is localized in the area of the large veins. In chronic venous insufficiency, pain, if it occurs, is associated with prolonged standing rather than walking.

The essential point of differentiation of ASO from venous problems is the absence of pulsation in posterior tibial and popliteal arteries in cases of ASO.

Most authors agree on the treatment of the ischemic limb; that is, to try to increase the blood supply either surgically or by building up collateral circulation through some of the following methods.

1. Avoidance of vasoconstriction by stoppage of all smoking.

2. In severe ischemia, warming the hospital or home room to 80°, and using boxes or cradles with controlled heat not to exceed 90°. In many instances this helps to relieve pain and improve circulation.

3. Raising the head of the bed is advocated by many authors, with heights from 6 to 16 inches to increase the hydrostatic perfusion pressure to the patient's feet. However, it is emphasized that the legs of a patient with ischemic disease must never be raised above heart level, even to disperse edema.

4. Exercise can be beneficial to help build up collateral circulations. Some authors advocate walking to the limit of the patient's tolerance three or four times a day. Others recommend the postural exercises (Buerger's exercises) and the Saunders oscillating bed.

5. The use of the Pavex boot and intermittent venous occlusion are only rarely suggested.

Foot problems in the elderly are the end result of a lifetime of disease residual, untreated deformities, trauma, abuse, lack of health education and lack of preventive measures in earlier years.

Physical Findings. Impaired pulsations, noted by palpation, are the most important and consistent physical finding in arteriosclerosis obliterans. Occasional patients have normal pulsations at rest, but during exercise the pulsations become impalpable.

The color of the skin is usually deep, dusky red on dependency, although a bluish discoloration may also be present. In severe cases marked pallor of one or more toes may be present.

A lower skin temperature of the foot or toes most affected can be detected upon simple palpation. A difference in temperature between the two feet is much more significant than equal coldness of both feet. There is loss of hair to the toes and dorsum of the foot, and occasionally we see loss of hair to the lower one-third of an affected extremity.

The skin, especially in the geriatric patient, becomes thin, shiny and almost parchment-like in consistency. Often one sees atrophy of the plantar fat padding beneath the metatarsal heads. Osteoporosis is frequently seen, especially in cases of advanced arteriosclerosis, particularly after long periods of rest in bed or lack of weight bearing to an extremity.

Prevention. Patient education plays an important part in the preventive therapy program: (1) teaching the patient how to care for his feet by daily hygienic care; (2) instruction in proper shoes and socks; (3) education as to the dangers of certain foot remedies that contain acids and other keratolytic agents; and (4) the dangers of home treatment with razor blades or cuticle scissors.

Many podiatrists routinely examine their patients with vascular insufficiency on a monthly or 6-week basis as a preventive therapy program. In this way the doctor can watch for any change in the vascularity of the lower extremity as well as observe any areas of the foot that may cause problems with infections or ulcerations. Most hospitals and clinics have printed brochures on foot care for their vascularly embarrassed patients. One of the most comprehensive and all-encompassing pamphlets is produced below.

You have a disease of the arteries of the legs. Certain parts of the arteries (blood vessels that carry blood to the legs) have become narrowed or obstructed, so that your legs and feet do not receive enough blood. Obstructions in the arteries are usually permanent and cannot be removed by medication. Sometimes, however, it is possible to bypass obstructed segments of arteries by means of surgery. Often the circulation can be improved by increasing the number and size of the collateral or "detour" arteries. This can be accomplished by time, treatment, and regular exercise.

Foot Care

It is extremely important to keep your feet as clean as possible. Wash your feet carefully and gently every day or every other day with mild soap and warm water and dry them carefully. *Never* use water warmer than 90°F; use a bath thermometer to check the temperature. *Rub the feet gently with a lanolin preparation* (or cocoa butter) *every day* to keep the skin as soft as possible. Rub the lanolin (for example, Lanolor) or cocoa butter thoroughly into the skin, but be sure that you do not leave an excess between the toes.

Exercise

Daily exercise usually helps to improve the circulation. We advise you to walk until your calf or thigh muscles hurt moderately; then stop, wait for the stress to subside, and walk again. Repeat this at least three to six times a day or as prescribed by your physician.

If discoloration of one or more toes, infection, or an open sore should appear, stop the exercise program and consult your physician promptly. Resume exercising only on your physician's advice.

PROBLEMS TO AVOID

Tobacco

Tobacco causes narrowing of the arteries which further reduces the blood flow to the legs, and it may also worsen the disease of the arteries; therefore, the use of tobacco is definitely harmful to you. *Never smoke or use tobacco in any form, not even a few cigarettes. This is extremely important.* The effect of one cigarette may last for 1 hour.

All Injuries

If the blood supply is poor, any small injury to the skin may result in serious infection, chronic ulcers or death of the skin (gangrene). Do all you can to avoid all types of injury to the feet and toes—scratches, cuts, cracks, blisters, burns or frostbite. When toenails need trimming, cut them straight across after soaking the foot in warm water and clean them carefully.

Toenails that are thickened or deformed and corns, calluses or bunions should *not* be cut or filed. If treatment is required, consult your podiatrist or have your physician refer you to a podiatrist; tell the podiatrist that the circulation in your feet is impaired. Removal of ingrown toenails and minor operations on the toes should *not* be done except in certain *rare* instances, and then only by a practitioner who is familiar with diseases of the blood vessels.

Redness and Irritation

If the feeling in the skin of your feet is impaired, as it often is in diabetic patients, look at and feel the skin of your entire foot daily to be sure that there is no area of redness or irritation. If you have any redness or injury, do not continue to walk but consult your physician and podiatrist *immediately.*

Ill-Fitting Footwear

Always wear comfortable shoes that do not bind or rub. In cold weather, wear soft woolen stockings and protect your feet from cold by wearing adequate outer footwear such as fleece-lined boots. *Feel the insides of new shoes or boots* with your hand to be sure that there are no prominent seams, rough spots or protruding nails that could injure your skin.

New shoes should be broken in gradually; wear them 1 hour on the first day and add 1 hour of wear each subsequent time. After each wearing, inspect your feet carefully for signs of irritation such as reddened areas. If these appear, do not wear the shoes until they have been adjusted and until you have consulted your practitioner.

Exposure to Cold and Heat

Avoid exposure of your feet to cold, because frostbite occurs more easily when the circulation is abnormal. *Never place a hot object,* such as a hot water bottle or electric heating pad, *on your feet,* no matter how cold they may become. Always test bath water with your hand to see that it is not too hot before stepping in.

Athlete's Foot

You may possibly have or may acquire "athlete's foot," which is an infection of the skin caused by a fungus. The fungus is frequently picked up at public shower baths, bathing beaches, hotels, and athletic clubs, particularly in warm weather. Athlete's foot causes the skin between the toes to become soft and to crack, or groups of small blisters may appear anywhere on the feet or the toes. Itching is common.

Careful treatment is important because athlete's foot may result in more serious ulceration and infection. Many of the available preparations are potent and may be harmful to your skin because of its poor circulation.

The following prevention program for patients with athlete's foot is recommended. If there is no break in the skin, (1) Keep your feet as dry as possible by changing your socks at least twice a day. (2) Use white, natural fiber socks or stockings (cotton or wool)—the synthetic fibers tend to allow heat and moisture to be retained within the sock. (3) Use a foot powder such as Desenex or Tinactin or, alternatively, some effective solution or ointment, such as tolnaftate (Tinactin) in a 1% solution or cream, which is available at the drugstore without a prescription. When blisters appear or weeping occurs, use other medications that may be obtained by prescription from your physician or podiatrist.

If there are cracks in the skin when you discover the athlete's foot, see your podiatrist or physician promptly. Likewise, if athlete's foot that seems minor does not respond to the foregoing treatment within a few days, consult your physician or podiatrist.

Strong Disinfectants and Other Medications

Do not use strong disinfectants, chemical compounds, ointments or corn cures. These may be harmless to feet that have a normal blood supply, but they may cause serious injury to feet that have an impaired blood supply. Do not use preparations containing iodine tincture, thimerosal (Merthiolate), carbolic acid, cresol or Lysol, carbolated petrolatum (Vaseline), or any other preparations for disinfectants or local treatment. *It is much better to leave the feet untreated than to take any chances.* If, in spite of care, a minor injury does occur, clean the part gently with soap and water and stay in bed for a few days. If the injury does not heal, call your physician or podiatrist.

No drugs given on a long-term basis have been found to improve the circulation significantly. Moreover, certain drugs given for other purposes, such as clonidine hydrochloride (Catapres) for hypertension or propranolol (Inderal) for hypertension or heart disease, under certain circumstances may actually *decrease* arterial blood flow to the limbs and digits and especially to the skin.

Several types of medication for headache, such as ergot-containing drugs and methysergide maleate (Sansert), even though taken in dosages indicated on the container, may also cause decreased circulation in the limbs. Consult your physician regarding any medication you use for headache or for any other chronic physical problem.

CARE OF CORN AND CALLUSES

A corn is a traumatic keratosis. Intermittent friction and pressure of a shoe, occurring with each step, produce irritation, especially on the dorsal aspect of the fifth toe. The site of the keratosis almost always overlies a bony prominence, condyle, joint or exostosis. The overlying epidermis reacts to the irritation and the normal rate of production of cells is accelerated. The cells become consolidated into a thick plate of horny tissue, much more homogeneous than the cornified layer it replaces and hence less subject to disintegration and desquamation. The typical corn is conical, with its base superficial and its apex impinging on the deeper structures. On radiologic examination a small, hypertrophied spur of bone may be found directly beneath the apex of the corn or a malalignment of the phalanges may be seen.

Shoes or stockings, or both, often are aggravating factors. In addition to the problems created by wearing a shoe of wrong size, wearing the wrong style or the wrong type of shoe for the occasion can create or exacerbate a painful corn or callus. The pointed shoe that impinges on the toe in the forward part or the so-called stretch stocking that "buckles" a toe contributes greatly to the intermittent friction and pressure developed with each step.

Occasionally, capillary loops are entrapped in the keratosis. This is usually the underlying reason for the thrombotic areas that do occur. An adventitious bursa may form between the keratosis and the bony protuberance. This may invite invasion by organisms. Sinuses leading into the bursa or even into the joint space can develop.

Treatment

Adequate care consists of dekeratinization of the compacted tissues with an end-edge scalpel or similar cutting instrument. Care should be taken not to cut too deeply, for an incision into the sanguineous tissues may fail to heal or may precipitate trophic changes leading to gangrene.

After the cornified layer has been removed, the next step is to attempt to inhibit the regrowth of the keratosis. One common and simple method is the placement of a U-shaped pad of felt directly behind the corn.

This eliminates or disperses frictional pressure on the region by distributing it over a wider area. Complementary appropriate foot care should be prescribed.

A callus may be described as a flat, amorphous mass of keratotic material usually found on the bottom of a foot under a bony protuberance. Intermittent pressure of the shoe and imbalance of a foot in walking are the usual causative factors. The callus is formed in much the same way that a corn is. However, because it covers a larger area it usually does not have the conical shape.

The important point in treating calluses is to alleviate areas of pressure with padding and protective devices. This can be accomplished with shoe inserts such as inlays. These may be rigid, semi-rigid, or soft—whatever structure that will reduce vascular demand by minimizing stress factors and increasing efficiency of the limb. The inlay may also help in increasing the length of walking time for patients who have severe intermittent claudication.

INGROWN TOENAIL

The common ingrown nail, although bothersome, usually is not dangerous to the average person. But to one whose arterial circulation is impaired, an ingrown nail is likely to become a serious problem because infection and gangrene may result.

Onychocryptosis is the term generally used to designate so-called ingrown or ingrowing toenails. Often, the only thing "cryptic" about the condition is what it really is. Many times, the nail plate has not "grown into" the nail lip and almost as often is not cryptotic. The problem may stem from the nail plate, the nail lip, or both—all lateral nail problems. This problem has a high prevalence among common foot complaints.

There are three basic types of lateral nail problems: (1) incurved nail, (2) onychocryptosis or ingrown nail, and (3) hypertrophic ungualabia. The patient may have one or a combination of two or more of these basic types when first seen, and the problem may be accompanied by paronychia with or without hypergranulation.

The *incurved nail*, or simple inverted nail, has a plate in which there is a sharp increase in the slight natural arc at the lateral border on one or both sides. The increased arcing may be congenital, may be a result of deforming pressures on the plate exerted subungually, extrinsically or both, or may be caused by interference with normal growth of the matrix from systemic factors or disease or from local disease or trauma. Not infrequently, a dorsally malformed terminal phalangeal tuft or a subungual osteoma or chondroma is responsible for the distorted plate. The symptoms of a simple incurved nail are usually tenderness, pain on walking, and pain (sometimes severe) on digital pressure.

Prophylactic care consists in trimming the nails properly; that is, cutting them straight across so that the corners of the plate are forward of the end of the groove in the nail lip. The stockings and shoes should be long enough to allow for the normal elongation of the foot on weight bearing.

Active treatment of the simple incurved nail consists of removing with a probe the cellular debris and callous tissue from the margin of the nail. The probe should not have a sharp edge because of the danger of injuring the nail bed when the border of the nail is elevated.

An *ingrown nail*, or onychocryptosis, although not as common as the incurved type, has much more harmful sequelae. The infected ingrown nail has granulation in the nail bed and groove and hypertrophy of the lip of the nail. As a result of the mutilation of the lateral border by improper trimming, a pointed shard or sliver frequently remains attached. As the nail plate grows forward, external pressures of footgear and function compress the soft labium against the sharp point, which then penetrates the skin.

Treatment consists of removing the shard or spicule of nail with a small straight-edge nail cutting forceps. Frequently the shard can be removed by an end-edge scalpel or onychotome directed backward to a point posterior to the base of the spicule or shard.

Warm ($32°$–$35°C$ [$90°$–$95°F$]) boric acid soaks should be instituted for 20–30 minutes every four hours. After these, dry sterile dressings should be applied to the area. A broad-spectrum antibiotic may be needed to combat the infection. Applying medicated powders or antibiotic ointments directly to the infected area is unsatisfactory in severe cases of arterial insufficiency. Rest in bed or hospitalization is recommended.

The third type of lateral nail problem, *hy-*

pertrophic ungualabium, was first described by DuVries. The lip of the nail is massively enlarged and often overrides a good portion of the nail plate. In extreme cases, both the lips and the anterior part of the toe cover much of the nail plate and leave only the central portion exposed. The hypertrophy almost always results from irritation of the epithelium of the nail groove by the lateral nail margin after repeated improper trimming of the nail. Sometimes, after avulsion of the nail plate for ingrown nail, the regrown nail is more or less covered by enlarged nail lips. Confining footwear compresses the lip against the nail border. The irritation and consequent inflammation establish a cycle leading to gradual hyperplasia of the lip and the groove, and eventually to permanent hypertrophy. Both the ingrown nail and the incurved nail eventually result in a hypertrophied lip if care is inadequate or nonexistent.

All three types of nail problems create difficulties because the border of the nail plate penetrates laterally into adjacent labium. Acute inflammation ensues, often followed by biogenic infection. If extensive pathologic change occurs in any of the three types of nail conditions, or if the condition is chronic and infection constantly recurs, surgical intervention is indicated.

Occasionally, as a result of trauma, we may see a thickened or onychogryphotic nail. Pressure on and irritation of a nail bed may sometimes cause a nail to become infected. Subungual ulcers, hidden beneath the gryphotic nail or a discolored or opaque nail, may cause great pain. Gentle removal of the nail by a skilled physician or podiatrist may relieve the pain and give the ulcer a chance to heal.

ULCERS AND GANGRENE

Many times, in spite of excellent care by the physician and podiatrist and the complete cooperation of the patient, and near-perfect foot hygiene, a corn, callus or ingrown nail will break down and become infected.

Treatment

The best way to prevent ulcers and gangrene is to protect the limb from trauma—physical, chemical or thermal. However, once ulceration occurs, one must treat it vigorously to try to stave off the ultimate gangrenous

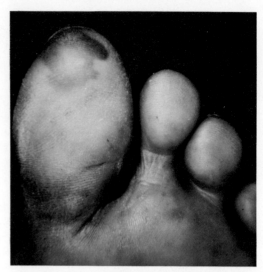

Fig. 12.3   Early spotty thrombosis of hallux.

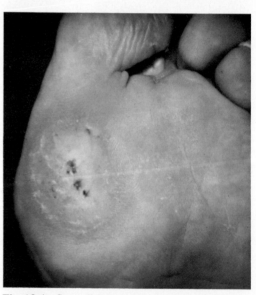

Fig. 12.4   Superficial ulceration, subkeratotic, arteriosclerotic.

process, and once an ulcer has healed measures must be taken to prevent recurrence.

Most authors agree that it is next to impossible to treat and heal any ulcer if the patient is ambulatory. Walking may facilitate the spread of any existing infection and extend the size of the lesion.

Management of ulceration or minor gangrene should include consideration of the following measures:

1. Protection from further trauma by wrap-

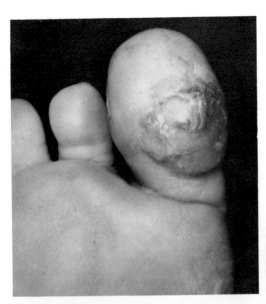

Fig. 12.5 Arteriosclerotic ulceration.

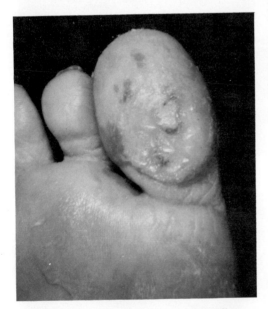

Fig. 12.6 Same as Fig. 12.5, early healing.

maceration that could delay or complicate healing.

4. Use of head-up position of bed to promote increased arterial blood flow.

5. Control of pain with adequate doses of any of the wide range of medications available.

6. Control of edema, if present.

7. Lubrication of the skin of the feet to prevent fissuring and dryness of the skin.

8. The use of thermostatically controlled

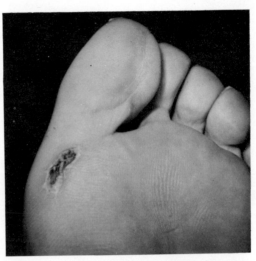

Fig. 12.7 Superficial gangrene from shoe pressure.

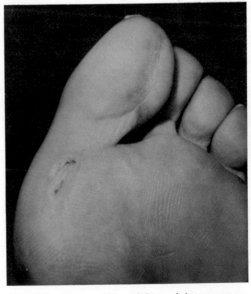

Fig. 12.8 Same as Fig. 12.7, resolving gangrene.

ping the limb loosely in cotton and the applying of wide gauze as an outside cover.

2. Local debridement with foot soaks, saturated boric solution or clean water, followed by dry dressings over the ulcerated area.

3. Culture of any discharge for antibiotic sensitivity.

Systemic antibiotics should be used, since the use of antibiotic ointments to the ulcer area could lead to local dermatitis and or environmental heat to help promote maximum blood flow in the skin.

After the ulceration has healed the prevention of recurrence of the ulceration is of utmost importance. Too often one sees a patient successfully treated in the hospital with good closure to the ulcer and good healing to the area only to have the patient return in 2–3 months with complete breakdown of the ulcer area with a more severe infection than the original problem.

Therefore, I feel it is mandatory to prescribe some measure to help prevent recurrence by use of an orthotic, shoe correction or special shoes for all patients with healed or healing ulcerations. The main purpose of any device or correction being to remove pressure and weight from the debilitated area when the patient ambulates.

For the patient with ulcerations on the top of the toes, it is imperative that they obtain shoes that give the toes enough room to prevent friction and irritation and recurrence of

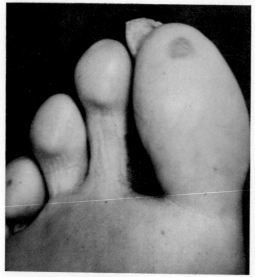

Fig. 12.9 Early bleb and thrombosis as a result of pressure in footwear from nail deformity.

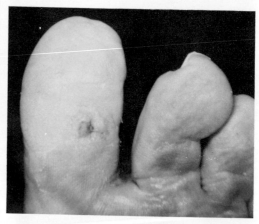

Fig. 12.11 Arteriosclerotic ulcer of hallux.

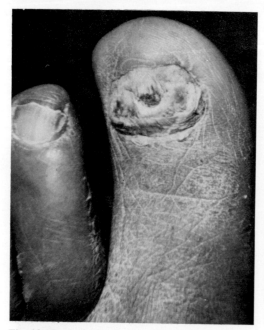

Fig. 12.10 Subungual ulceration and vascular insufficiency of toe and ulcer base.

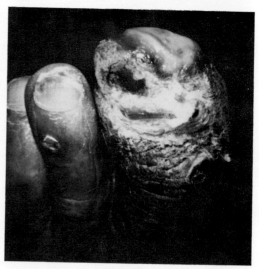

Fig. 12.12 Ulceration of hallux with hypergranulation tissue and secondary monilial infection.

the ulcer. The Inlay Depth Shoe[R] fills this need by providing extra depth across the toe box for adequate room.

Ulcers beneath the metatarsal heads, once they are healed, must be protected to prevent further breakdown and ulceration. Transverse metatarsal bars applied to the soles of the shoes have been of value to help relieve pressure on the healed ulcer.

Yale suggests the use of a ripple-soled shoe in which the ripples on the spongy outer sole beneath the ulcer are cut away to protect that area. Removing the pressure from the ulcerated area by the use of felt padding on the foot or an accommodative inlay has been helpful in preventing further breakdown in the ulcerated area.

Lately the molded (space) shoe has proved to be useful in these problem areas. An accurate mold is made of the feet, and allowances are made for the ulcerated area, so no pressure is put on that area. This special shoe protects any deformities of the feet, such as a bunion or hammer toes, because it is larger in the appropriate specific area and gives the foot more room. The molded shoe has also been very helpful in preventing further breakdown in ulcerated areas.

Plastazote and other polyurethanes can be placed inside shoes to act as cushions to protect the healed areas. These seem to work better than sponge rubber since they do not "bottom out" and retain their resiliency for longer periods of time.

SUMMARY

The care of the geriatric patient with vascular disease can be a never-ending fight to stave off the consequences of infections, ulcerations and gangrene. However, with the many advances in today's medicine, we are winning the battle many times and keeping the geriatric patient ambulatory.

chapter 13

Podiatric Management of the Diabetic Foot in the Elderly Patient

Arthur E. Helfand, D.P.M.

For the most part, dealing with foot problems in the elderly diabetic generally involves management of a mature-onset diabetic patient. However, it is perfectly feasible for us to consider dealing with patients who have been diabetic for many years and who may also present with concomitant systemic diseases. Most diabetic patients consider that there are some basic problems that they will be dealing with in relation to their lower extremities and, in particular, their feet. By the time they reach their senior years their concerns center on the loss of a limb, a serious infection, a period of hospitalization, a shorter life span and loss of ambulation and mobility, which would significantly remove their dignity and their independent activity. The primary concern in managing the diabetic foot in the elderly patient deals with the concept of prevention. Primary prevention to prevent foot problems from occurring; secondary prevention to identify foot problems at their earliest stages, and thereby prevent complications; and tertiary prevention by identifying the complications at a manageable stage and providing as much care as is feasible, consistent with the age of the patient and the progression of the disease. It should be noted, however, that no matter what steps are taken, it might be impossible to save an extremity or prevent a serious foot problem from occurring. However, early and periodic examination and close cooperation between all members of the team dealing with the patient's health care and his diabetes are major factors in establishing normal and good foot health for the elderly diabetic patient.

Diabetic foot care for the elderly cannot be separated from total patient care involving a team approach, including the physician, podiatrist, nurse, health educator, pharmacist, patient and his family. There is a great similarity in the management of the elderly diabetic foot and the patient with peripheral vascular insufficiency. Symptoms are similar and many diabetics present similar, multiple problems in a similar manner. The diabetic may also undergo some form of arthritic changes which causes the deformity that ultimately becomes an etiologic factor in the presence of diabetic ulcers. Patient management of the elderly diabetic must consider the usual needs of the patient in more than a biologic or physiologic sense. It must consider those intangibles and tangibles which might alter the patient, his way of life, and the methods and concepts of treatment. For the most part, diabetic patients in their senior years must be considered as patients with insensitive feet.

If one begins to look at the elderly diabetic as a total patient, we find that the individual is usually taking more than one drug at any given moment and may, in fact, demonstrate some drug sensitivity. The elderly diabetic is usually more susceptible to infection, not only because of the anatomic location of the foot itself and the diabetes, but also because of the associated avascularity, atrophy of tissue,

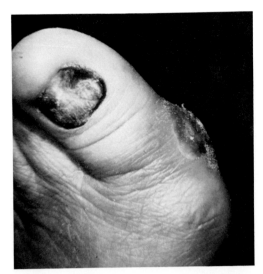

Fig. 13.1 Diabetic ulcer of hallux, associated with hallux valgus and repeated microtrauma.

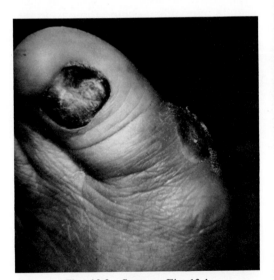

Fig. 13.2 Same as Fig. 13.1.

health status, thereby compounding the problems or complications. Aged diabetic patients are more prone to injury to the lower extremity with multiple complications due to neuropathic changes as an end result. They are more prone to immobility, impairment, disability, hospitalization and surgery following a minor foot infection. They are generally a greater risk for any type of therapy than a patient of the same age without diabetes mel-

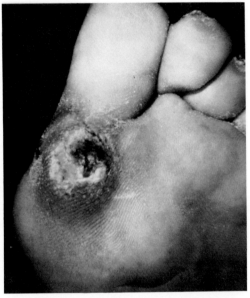

Fig. 13.3 Plantar view of Fig. 13.1.

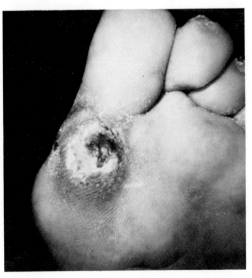

Fig. 13.4 Initial debridement of Fig. 13.1.

neuropathic changes, and the general lack of of concern for foot health that appears to be an endemic situation. The elderly diabetic tends to be concerned about life, as life in a sense to many elderly patients is in fact a terminal illness. They may have a lower threshold of emotional or physical stress, which in itself provides a limitation to ambulation. The elderly diabetic generally has more than one chronic disease and may be under treatment for multiple diseases at one time. However, it is also feasible for the poor, elderly diabetic to be unaware of his own

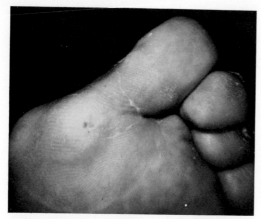

Fig. 13.5   Healing of Fig. 13.1.

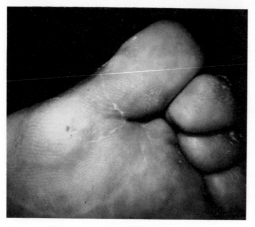

Fig. 13.6   Healing of Fig. 13.1.

litus and they present a general tissue state that does not heal well.

If we were to summarize diabetic foot pathology in the elderly patient we would think of the following general areas: paresthesia, sensory impairment, motor weakness, reflex loss, neurotropic arthropathy, absence of pedal pulses, atrophy of tissue, dermatophytosis, infections, dermopathy, onychopathy, angiopathy, ulceration, and gangrene.

The vascular symptoms in the elderly diabetic patient generally present some evidence of fatigue on ambulation and a general complaint of fatigue as a result of any activity. Pain may be a related factor due to the vascular insufficiency itself or may be neuropathic in origin. Pain may also be a result of arthritic or biomechanical changes in the foot and therefore must be differentiated significantly from the vascular evidence of dis-

ease. Coldness in the elderly diabetic generally represents localized avascularity to a specific segment of the foot or to the entire extremity. Heat, on the other hand, generally represents some infective or inflammatory process that is beginning or has been well organized. It should be noted that the patient may not complain of any symptoms whatsoever in the presence of infection if a neuropathy is well advanced. Patients may identify a bluish discoloration of the foot which should be a clear evidence of terminal vascular insufficiency to that segment of the extremity. Petechiae, when present, may also be related to a hematologic disorder, which may or may not be associated with diabetes itself. Numbness and tingling can be the end result of vascular insufficiency as well as neuropathy. Patients may complain of night cramps, which provide clear evidence of marked vascular insufficiency or may demonstrate intermittent claudication associated with localized muscular anoxia. Where claudication is present, patients generally can identify the distances they can ambulate prior to the onset of pain. The complaint of edema should also be noted in relation to its cardiorenal etiologic considerations. Phlebitis, when historically present, may be chronic in nature in the elderly patient and be another factor in the residual of edema. Patients may present with their initial symptom being dampness on hosiery, with the resultant identification of a diabetic ulcer. In a similar

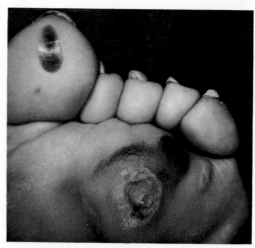

Fig. 13.7   Superficial gangrene, keratosis and deformity associated with continued microtrauma.

manner, the same general complaint of staining may be the initial symptom of a foot infection in the elderly diabetic patient. There should be some concern on the part of the practitioner in evaluating the elderly diabetic as to his previous or current activity or occupation, the use of alcohol and the use of tobacco.

The clinical findings in the elderly diabetic generally consist of color changes ranging from rubor to cyanosis, depending upon the vascular patency of the foot and the lower extremity. Temperature changes may similarly occur in relation to warmth to coldness. The condition of the skin is generally dry and scaly, due to xerosis and a lack of vascular supply to the lower extremity. Atrophy of the soft tissues will generally be pronounced and will be accentuated in the patient with an old arthritic foot problem. Patients who have utilized self-treatment for foot complaints by using self-prescribed rigid orthotics for long periods of time tend to demonstrate more atrophy than the average patient. The presence of infection is generally well demonstrated in the elderly diabetic patient during examination. Foot infections in the presence of vascular insufficiency should be viewed as a potential for amputation and should be dealt with in a guarded manner. All draining areas should receive a culture and sensitivity analysis to determine the appropriate antibiotics to be prescribed. Treatment, on the other hand, should consist of hospitalization where necessary, appropriate antibiotics through intravenous or oral methods, depending upon the severity and the patient, and a consistent review radiographically with bone scans to determine the presence of deep tissue infection and osteomyelitis.

Nail changes that occur in the elderly diabetic patient as a result of diabetes and vascular insufficiency generally can be termed diabetic onychopathy. The nail generally lacks a luster and usually presents some onychorrhexis. Thickening with onychauxis is feasible along with hypertrophy. The gradual thickening of the nail becomes a pressure area creating localized tissue ischemia when there is footwear incompatibility or neglect. The local pressure activity may produce some degree of ulcerative manifestation subungually. The presence of hemorrhage beneath the nail, in the absence of trauma, generally can be considered a complicating element of diabetic onychopathy. Treatment generally consists of periodic debridement of the hypertrophied structures and the use of an emollient on a regular basis to provide a degree of hydration and lubrication. Where there is footwear incompatibility, this needs to be corrected.

Edema, when present in the elderly diabetic patient, represents a clinical change that must be differentiated from localized and/or systemic etiology. Where cardiorenal pathology is present, the edema should be dealt with in an appropriate medical, diagnostic and therapeutic manner. Where the edema is a result of residual stasis, appropriate exercise and physical therapy may assist in reducing the edema, provided that it is not indurated and extremely well organized. Where swelling is associated with infection, appropriate antibiotics should be employed and the patient should be placed at bed rest or hospitalized if necessary. Edema may represent a serious complication in the diabetic elderly foot and should be carefully reviewed with the patient on a periodic basis. Blebs or small bullae, in the elderly diabetic patient, generally are the result of impending localized vascular insufficiency to specific areas. They may also be a residual of stress and trauma associated with tinea pedis, or idiopathic in nature. The treatment varies, based on the specific etiological factor. However, it is essential that trauma be avoided and, if drainage is attempted, that it be done under sterile conditions; a sterile needle and syringe probably are the best mechanisms for removing fluid from the bullae. As the blebs dry, they should not be debrided, as this represents a sterile area and merely needs to be protected from additional trauma. These lesions represent a potential for localized dry necrosis and can be managed on an ambulatory basis provided that the extension of the necrotic process is not extensive and does not become moist.

Varicosities present in the elderly diabetic represent a problem in relation to stasis and stasis ulceration as well as pruritus. Pruritus in the elderly diabetic can be managed with mild antihistamines, topical steroids, and the use of appropriate emollients to assist in the elimination of the effects of stasis and xerosis. When the eczematous area is moist and draining or an ulcer is present, an appropriate supportive dressing can be employed such as the Unna boot. Dextranomer can be used to help dry the wound. Topical enzymes may be used judiciously to assist in debridement. Treatment may also include the selective localized use of controlled ultrasound in water to assist debridement.

The diabetic ulcer associated with vascular insufficiency represents a somewhat different entity than the diabetic ulcer associated with neuropathic changes. For the most part, the ulcer associated with vascular insufficiency without neuropathy may present an extremely painful problem for the patient. The potential for gangrene and amputation is significantly greater. The ulcer generally appears dry but the potential for infection due to avascularity is significant. Radiographic examination of the part involved may demonstrate some osteolytic areas which may be the result of vascular insufficiency as well as osteomyelitis. Management of these ulcerations generally consists of some broad principles dealing with the appropriate antibiotics, removal of trauma from the area, attempts to provide as much revascularization to the part as is feasible, the use of whirlpool for local debridement, and anticipating that there will be a gangrenous area that will probably form in a dry manner. When this

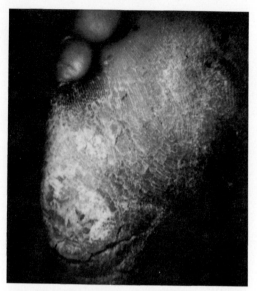

Fig. 13.9   Plantar view of Fig. 13.8.

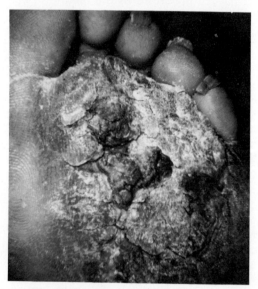

Fig. 13.10   Opposite foot of Fig. 13.8.

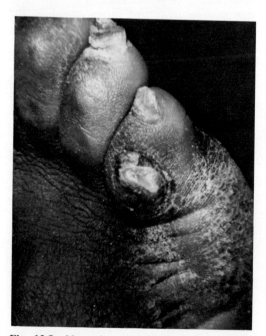

Fig. 13.8   Necrosis and ulceration with keratosis, deformity, xerosis and subcallosal hemorrhage.

dry eschar is present, unless there is severe infection involving the lower extremity, the eschar should remain in place with debridement not generally attempted. All attempts should be made to remove pressure from the area and to permit physical modalities to assist in the local revascularization of the area. If the ulcerated area progresses, gangrene will ensue with the ultimate determination of treatment depending upon the toxicity of the patient and the patency of the vascular system in the lower extremity. It should be noted that early consultation with vascular surgeons is appropriate to determine if bypass surgery in these cases would be of value. This should be done at the earliest possible moment.

When gangrene and necrosis are present as a result of vascular insufficiency in the diabetic patient, particularly without neuropathy, consideration must be given to the type, i.e., dry or moist, on the onset, its relation to trauma, its relationship to trophic changes and the presence or absence of infection. With infection present, a culture and sensitivity study should be taken and appropriate antibiotic therapy should be employed, along with bed rest and the use of mild compresses, such as saline or povidone-iodine, to keep the part irrigated. It is extremely important not to macerate the tissues which could well precipitate the development of moist gangrene from dry gangrene. If the area remains dry, and infection is not a predominant factor, the simplest treatment is to remove all pressure from the area, and attempt to revascularize the part within the feasible limits of physical modalities and other activities. It is extremely important to remember that bed rest probably is essential in these cases and hospitalization should be employed when control of the patient is inadequate. The early managing of these ulcerative processes can well prevent amputation in later stages, thereby reducing the total of social as well as health cost to society.

As a result of atrophy in the elderly diabetic patient one can anticipate a difference in limb symmetry. The usual consideration is a thinner limb, which represents a more guarded area for future ulceration, gangrene and amputation. Most elderly patients also have some residual of the arthritides. In these cases, there will be significant deformity present such as contracted and claw toes, hallux valgus and other related foot deformities. When this is accompanied by a marked absence of soft tissue, the osseous structures appear more prominent and serve as pressure points for the development of ulcerations and localized pressure necrosis.

The continuing examination and evaluation of the elderly diabetic patient should include the taking of the dorsalis pedis and posterior tibial pulses. Where these are inappropriately palpated, the popliteal and fem-

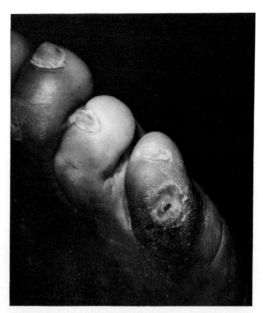

Fig. 13.11 Diabetic ulcer of fifth toe with heloma, rotational and contractural deformity.

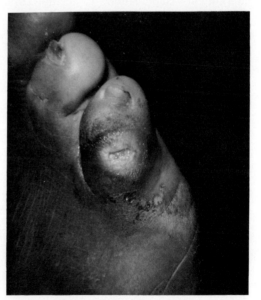

Fig. 13.12 Early healing of Fig. 13.11.

oral should be sought. The use of the plethysmograph, oscillometer, skin temperature studies, and Doppler flow studies will also assist in evaluating the vascular patency of the lower extremity. Other studies include the use of plantar ischemia, venous filling time and histamine reaction. Many times, a posterior tibial block may provide the best evidence of reflex vasodilatation to the area. Blood pressure should be carefully reviewed and the presence of hypertension may in fact produce pulsations which really do not affect the vascular competency of the particular extremity involved. Ophthalmoscopic studies can be part of the peripheral vascular evaluation of the elderly diabetic to help determine if the onychopathy, retinopathy, neuropathy and angiopathy are consistently present in the same patient. Radiographic examination of the elderly diabetic with vascular insufficiency will generally demonstrate some degree of calcification of the vessels and osteoporosis of the bones of the foot.

Other clinical findings associated with vascular insufficiency in the elderly diabetic patient include vasospasm demonstrating coldness, parethesia demonstrating organized impairment, rest pain indicating serious arterial impairment, weakness and muscular atrophy, which reduces the normal protective mechanisms of the foot itself, and a relationship of intermittent claudication to claudication time.

The diabetic patient with diabetic neuropathy and the presence of a neurotrophic ulcer represents a significant potential for amputation of the extremity, as the patient generally is unaware of pain, which is a primary guarding mechanism. The patient will demonstrate numbness and tingling of the ex-

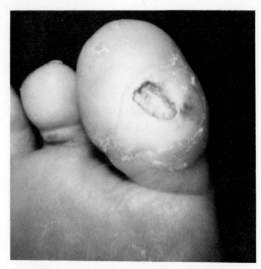

Fig. 13.14   Diabetic ulcer of hallux.

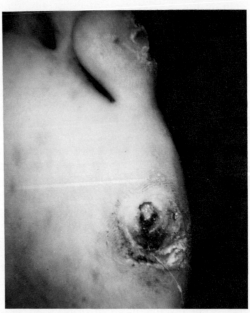

Fig. 13.15   Diabetic ulcer of head of fifth metatarsal, plantarly.

tremities with a varying degree of nocturnal cramps. There will be a loss or diminution of pain and temperature senses and a loss or diminution of vibratory senses. The deep tendon reflexes will generally be lost with it being most pronounced in the absence of the tendo achillis reflex. Anhydrosis and xerosis are generally accompanied by a dry scaly-like appearance of the foot. Where vascular impairment is most pronounced, there may even

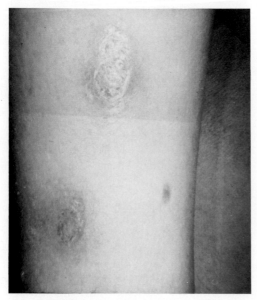

Fig. 13.13   Necrobiosis lipoidica diabeticorum.

be a hand-in-glove type of syndrome with the dryness serving as the line of demarcation. The entire lower extremity may demonstrate a waxy pallor. In these cases, hydration followed by lubrication needs to be done on a regular basis, after appropriate patient instruction.

There is usually a subsequent loss of the fat pad over the metatarsal head area. The absence of soft tissue in this area, together with pressure, generally produces a degree of hyperkeratosis as space replacement. Tendon contractures create clawed toes with further pressure on the prolapsed metatarsal area. Walking without adequate protection tends to produce localized pressure points followed by subcallosal hemorrhage due to the ischemia with ultimate breakdown to ulceration. It is extremely important that appropriate material be employed with footwear, such as orthotics, or as removable types of padding, to provide both weight dispersion and weight diffusion to prevent the pressure areas from becoming ulcerative residuals.

The extremities in the elderly patient with diabetic neuropathy may appear warm, as pulses in fact may be palpated. In the presence of hypertension, the chances for palpable pulses are even greater. When an ulcer is present, the classic neurotrophic ulcer appears as a thick callous overlying a dirty, yellowish ulcer with a fibrous, moist base, with a usual purulent discharge. A prime

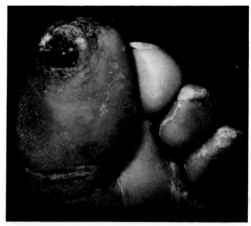

Fig. 13.17 Diabetic necrosis from pressure of tack in shoe.

concern in the management of this type of lesion is total avoidance of weight bearing to the part. With the presence of infection, appropriate antibiotics can be employed. With the presence of discharge, Dextranomer can be appropriately applied by the patient to help reduce the drainage. With the absence and removal of pressure from the area, ulcerations will generally heal. If they are permitted to persist for any period of time, osteomyelitis and the potential for infection and gangrene to be followed by amputation are significant.

The patient with diabetic neuropathy may present with peroneal involvement and a drop foot. Therefore, a careful foot orthopedic evaluation must be utilized on a bilateral basis to determine the degree of involvement so that some evidence of compensation can be utilized. The patient may also present with some tenderness over the calf muscles on palpation. There is generally a loss of position sense and associated arthropathy, or neuropathic bone disease may be present. Peripheral neuritis may be a clinical finding of diabetic neuropathy and may be the primary complaint of the patient. At the present time, no one specific treatment for the management of diabetic neuropathy in the foot has been advocated and a varied approach is needed for the patient. However, physical modalities do provide some relief of the symptoms and can be extended with the use of progressive resistive exercise techniques.

The presence of edema, which eliminates

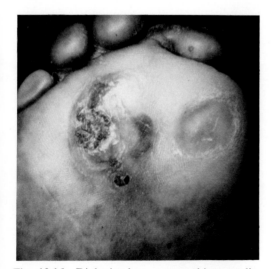

Fig. 13.16 Diabetic ulcer, neuropathic, past digital amputation. Note shifting of second toe.

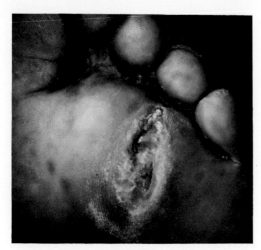

Fig. 13.18   Diabetic ulcer, neuropathic.

the local joint lines in the digits, accompanied by some gangrenous changes without pain, generally is a precursor to a toxic gangrene, which generally necessitates an amputation. The key considerations are early consultation and appropriate surgical management. It should be noted, however, that once amputation takes place, the potential for the opposite extremity to undergo a similar disease pattern in between 3 and 5 years must be considered and must, in fact, be communicated to the family to avoid future problems.

The radiographic findings in the elderly diabetic foot generally consist of the following demonstrable signs.

The trabecular patterns in the bones of the feet are thin. This is particularly noted in the digits in the metatarsals. There may be some clear evidence of decalcification along with arthropathy. Arthritis may be present with a destruction of the articular surface and osteoporosis may accompany the arthritic changes. Osteolytic formations may be present and the osteolytic areas may be the result of infection or a residual of an avascular activity. Frank evidence of deformity may be demonstrated. Such deformities may be related to trophic changes and the atrophy of soft tissue, causing contracture, or may be part of an arthritic process totally unrelated to the elderly diabetic's foot. However, the presence of these deformities represents a potential for ulceration and gangrene and should be viewed as a means of projecting a treatment plan for the elderly diabetic that will produce a reduc-

tion of pressure to these particular areas of deformity.

There are numerous changes that take place in the skin of the diabetic foot in the elderly patient. One of the most common of these is pruritus accompanied by scratching, followed by excoriation. The most common etiologic factor is excessive dryness and a xerotic or leather-like appearance of the foot and lower leg. It is related to the neurologic and vascular changes in the diabetic patient. Management can include the use of mild antihistamines such as 25 mm. of tripelennamine hydrochloride where the itching is severe. This should be used for a short period of time only if necessary. The use of emollients such as 20% urea cream and emollient lotion, preceded by a bath or hydration of the foot or extremity, can assist in maintaining a more normal appearance of the skin. Patients who are concomitantly being treated with physical modalities such as whirlpool and low voltage therapy to increase vascularization will also demonstrate marked improvement in the dryness and a relief of pruritus during the period of active treatment. The skin of the elderly diabetic's foot may also appear dehydrated. It will generally appear atrophic and shiny. Brownish pigmentation may also be present as a result of the deposition of hemosiderin. Where the atrophy and dehydration are marked, shin spots or pretibial diabetic lesions are common between the tibial tuberosity and the ankle. The presence of the pretibial lesions or diabetic shin spots generally represents a minute infarction of a small vessel and is a clear indicator of the

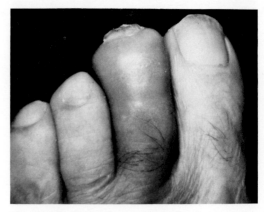

Fig. 13.19   Diabetic osteomyelitis of second toe.

severe friability of the vascular system in the lower extremity. It should also be noted that these lesions tend to heal by scar formation and are in fact very slow to heal. All efforts need to made to provide proper patient instructions and to utilize hydrating and lubricating techniques to maintain the normal integrity of the skin tone.

Cutaneous infections are more common in the elderly diabetic than in the nondiabetic patient and represent a serious potential for severe complications in the elderly diabetic, the potential for gangrene and the loss of the limb. If one would begin to view foot infections in the elderly diabetic as a potential for amputation, many of the serious sequelae of bacterial infection could be eliminated. Bacterial infections may appear as localized abscesses, superficial infections, cellulitis, lymphangitis, or lymphadenitis, and may progress to gangrene. In the presence of a bacterial infection, a culture and sensitivity analysis would provide some tangible evidence as to the appropriate antibiotic that would be most effective. However, clinical judgment would warrant the institution of oral antibiotic therapy at the onset of the cutaneous infection. Many times, however, because of the neuropathic changes in the elderly diabetic patient, the individual does not seek

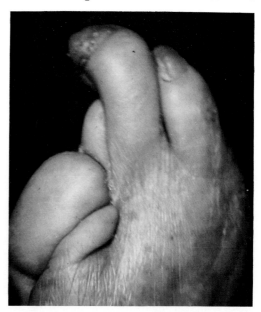

Fig. 13.21   Opposite foot of Fig. 13.20.

care until the infection is well organized and swelling is significant. In the presence of vascular insufficiency, hospitalization should be considered so that appropriate antibiotics may be accompanied by bed rest and all of the supportive measures. These measures would include the use of warm compresses, intravenous antibiotics, and supportive drugs for pain. As the edema decreases, ambulation should be encouraged and discharge planning should include appropriate patient education. There should be a significant review of the patient's history and his social activities to determine the etiologic factors that precipitated a bacterial infection in the elderly diabetic patient. Many times there is a shoe-related trauma as a result of inadequate footwear which may be due to an economic problem rather than a medical problem. Where feasible, the patient's family should be closely tied to the total management of the infected elderly diabetic.

Fungal infections of the skin (dermatophytosis) are also common in the elderly diabetic patient. They may appear as chronic intertriginous scaly lesions, an acute vascicular eruption, or a chronic hyperkeratotic type of tinea. For the most part the etiologic factors include *Trichophyton rubrum*, *T mentagrophytes* and *Monilia*. For a monilial infection, appropriate

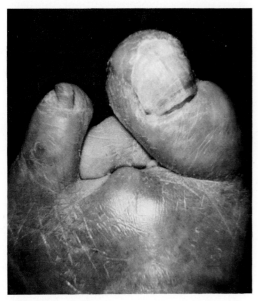

Fig. 13.20   Postdigital amputations for diabetic gangrene.

topical nystatin therapy generally provides adequate resolution of the problem. Where the organisms are of the *trichophyton* variety the appropriate choice of therapy depends upon the clinical manifestation of the disease. Where the infection is moist and draining, the consideration of secondary bacterial infections must be considered. Appropriate antibiotics as well as antifungal therapy are needed at the onset. Mild aluminum acetate soaks or compresses will assist in relieving some of the inflammatory changes and help produce a drying affect. Appropriate antibiotics would control the bacterial infection. Topical clotrimazole solution generally has proven the best initial step in the management of these superficial mycotic infections. Where the area is chronic and scaly, particularly in the intertriginous areas, clotrimazole solution again has proven to be a most satisfactory topical medication; it should be accompanied by an antifungal foot powder to assist in drying. Where the tineal involvement is chronic and hyperkeratotic, the use of ointments generally proves to be more successful than the use of solutions and/creams. For marked hyperkeratosis with inflammatory reactions, iodochlorhydroxyquin and hydrocortisone creams tend to be an initial approach to therapy to help reduce the inflammatory process and decrease some of the areas of hyperkeratosis. The patient can then be changed to a cream such as clotrimazole to provide for a sustaining antifungal effect. Although systemic antifungal drugs are indicated in some cases, careful observation of the patient is required. Because of the fact that many elderly patients are already on various types of drugs for other systemic diseases, the topical approach may prove to be the best initial direction for the management of superficial fungal infections.

The skin of the elderly diabetic generally presents some degree of tissue ischemia, which may vary in color from cyanosis to rubor. Pallor may also exist as an initial finding. There is usually a loss of hair on the digits, proceeding up the leg to the tibial tuberosity. This also provides significant demonstrable evidence of the vascular supply to the lower extremity. These trophic changes demonstrate the avascularity and, in effect, provide some degree of demarcation as to the superficial blood loss. Patients generally have decreased sensation in the skin itself and there are changes relating to a loss of the ability to distinguish between hot and cold. Elderly diabetic patients generally present with a lack of sweating and, where excessive hyperhydrosis is present, appropriate diagnostic activity should be initiated to rule out the presence of a superficial fungal infection.

Diabetic patients may also demonstrate necrobiosis lipoidica diabeticorum, which is generally pathognomonic of diabetes. A yellow discoloration may also be seen over the smaller joints of the foot associated with carotenosis. Idiopathic bullae may also be present which many times are the predisposing clinical signs of early necrosis and gangrene.

Elderly diabetic patient may also demonstrate some changes in relation to drug reaction which would include urticaria, erythema multiforme and photosensitivity.

Fissures or cracks in the skin are also common in the elderly diabetic patient, particularly in the areas of the heels. This is due primarily to a gradual atrophy of the soft tissue, repeated microtrauma, avascularity, and a lack of lubrication in the skin itself. The impingement factors related to footwear must also be considered. Once a heel fissure breaks the epidermal continuity, the resultant delayed healing time is similar in effect to a decubitus ulcer. Many approaches for therapy have been advocated, but our approach generally has been to control any bacterial infection that may be present. Local tissue stimulants such as compound tincture of benzoin can be utilized if the denuded area is clean. Efforts must be made to reduce local trauma to the heel area. This can be accomplished by the use of a Styrofoam heel cup, a plastic heel cup, or a plaster of Paris splint, molded to the heel and worn in an appropriate shoe. These measures generally provide an initial approach to healing. Physical modalities such as whirlpool and low voltage therapy can be used to increase the local vascular supply to the denuded area. Judicious topical enzymes can be used to remove some of the necrotic tissue that may be present, but care should be taken to utilize such preparations on a sporadic basis providing 2 or 3 days of contact followed by 2 or 3 days of absence. This mechanism provides better control over the destruction of tissue. Surgical debridement generally is avoided, as these areas are usually free of infection and the introduction of a surgical technique may in fact precipitate an infected or early necrotic process. Once the areas are healed, some protection should be continued in the shoe to prevent continued trauma and pulling on the skin of the heels. The Styrofoam or plastic

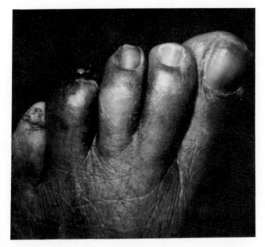

Fig. 13.22   Osteomyelitis and ulcer of fourth toe with necrosis.

heel cup generally has proven to be the best approach to this and the final determination is based on patient tolerance and patient response.

Nail changes that occur in the diabetic patient are those generally associated with vascular insufficiency, and represent a diabetic onychopathy. They include onychorrhexis, onycholysis, dryness, onychophosis, onychauxis, onychogryphosis, and with trauma, onychia. Trauma also provides a precipitating factor for onychomadesis, and the possibility of a subungual ulcer.

Diabetic ulceration in the elderly patient generally takes two forms: one form is associated with vascular impairment and the other with diabetic neuropathy. In each case, there are generally some primary etiologic factors and some significant principles in relation to treatment. In the elderly patient most diabetic ulcers that are associated with vascular insufficiency without neuropathy are related to a spontaneous infarction of a superficial vessel. The area generally becomes hemorrhagic, and necrosis and gangrene are rapid. Generally speaking, the type of gangrenous area present is dry and many times

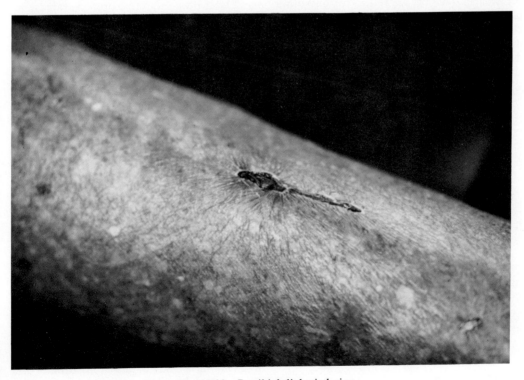

Fig.. 13.23   Pretibial diabetic lesion.

is very superficial. Repeated microtrauma from the presence of external activities may prove to be the precipitating factor. These include mechanical factors such as new or poorly fitting footwear, home treatment and self-inflicted surgical attempts, physical trauma, and the mechanical activity of neglected hyperkeratotic lesions. The formal factors relating to trauma include the inappropriate use of electric heating pads, hot foot baths, hot water bottles, heat lamps, or the prolonged exposure to cold and moisture. The chemical factors relating to local trauma include strong topical agents and antiseptics and the inappropriate use of over-the-counter corn cure products which permit the invasion of bacteria and the second degree chemical burn to occur, thereby producing a break in the integument and the initial phases of ulceration.

Adding to these areas of activity, repeated microtrauma is magnified by the presence of neglected hyperkeratotic lesions, bony prominences, especially those associated with arthritic changes, and heat-reflecting substances from footwear such as rubber and nylon. It should be noted that footwear for the elderly diabetic, as well as for any other individual, should be viewed as an article of clothing and should be changed and modified to the particular activity for which it was designed.

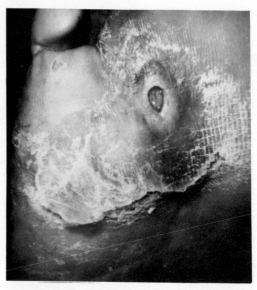

Fig. 13.25   Neurotrophic ulcer and early necrosis.

It must be recognized that the primary etiologic factor in the development of the vast majority of diabetic ulcers in the geriatric patient, exclusive of those that are precipitated by a pure infarctive process, represents a repeated local microtrauma and generally a chain of events. It generally begins with some disturbance of local foot mechanics either as the residual of some biomechanical change that has taken place over the years, a change in gait, or in fact the incompatibility of the foot to adjust to either the daily activities of the patient, footwear, or the residuals of deformity related to one of the arthritic processes. In areas where there is continued friction and trauma, hyperkeratosis begins to form as a protective mechanism and space replacement.

With further trauma and continued disturbances in local foot mechanics, the hyperkeratosis, which in effect is a hyperplasia, continues to magnify and becomes an additional traumatic factor. With continued trauma, there is a softening of the subaollosal epidermis and dermis with local hemorrhage appearing beneath the hyperkeratotic tissue. The related ischemia and hemorrhagic areas begin to develop bacterial growth and present, generally, an invasive infection. Poor hygiene, shoe trauma, or incompatibility and the use of self-treatment generally enhances the spread of the infection and produces re-

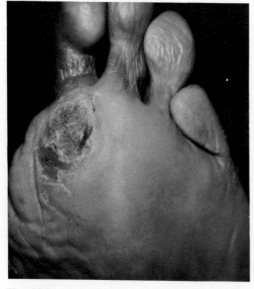

Fig. 13.24   Keratosis and ulceration as a result of weight transfer; postamputation of partial first ray.

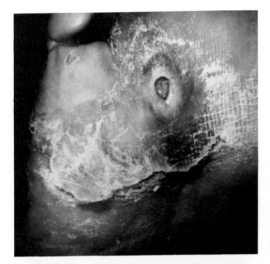

Fig. 13.26 Predebridement of Fig. 13.25.

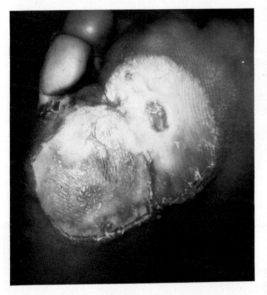

Fig. 13.27 Postdebridement of Fig. 13.25.

occur when the infected area is significant enough to reduce both arterial and venous blood flow to the area, thereby creating local death of the part.

The general principles in the management of the diabetic ulcer consist of means to decrease the local trauma. These include absolute bed rest and, for the most part, hospitalization as most elderly patients are unable to

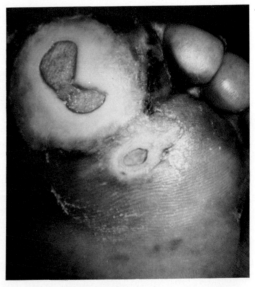

Fig. 13.28 Neurotrophic keratosis and early necrosis of Fig. 13.25.

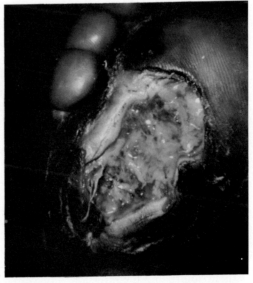

Fig. 13.29 Moist gangrene of Fig. 13.25, preamputation.

peated trauma which continues to embarrass the local area. With neuropathy there is less ischemia. but the invasive type of infection is generally present. The area then ulcerates with hyperkeratosis surrounding the ulcer. There is a tendency for the ulceration to attempt to heal by the hyperkeratotic areas progressing from the margins of the ulcer to the central portion. There is no healing of the base. Once covered with hyperkeratosis, the ulcer no longer drains and the chain of events begins again, with a developing invasive type of infection. Gangrene and necrosis generally

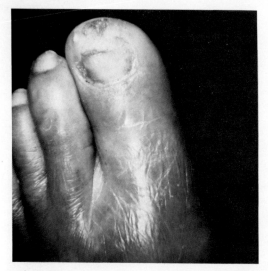

Fig. 13.30   Osteomyelitis and ulceration of hallux.

provide appropriate care for themselves in their usual surroundings. There is also some concern pertaining to compliance on the part of the elderly, and a short period of hospitalization to appropriately manage both the ulcerative area and the diabetes mellitus generally is the most economical factor in preventing large expenditures of funds for the rehabilitation of an amputated patient. Local trauma can also be reduced by changes in footwear, the use of surgical shoes, the use of orthotics to minimize pressure to localized areas, and Plastazote shoes.

The infection needs to be controlled. Antibiotic sensitivity tests should be done and the appropriate medication prescribed. Generally speaking, large doses of antibiotics are essential and the method of use would depend on the patient, his vascular supply, and the clinician's judgment. There should be no trauma to the foot itself and an appropriate foot cradle may be used when the patient is in bed.

Radiographic studies should be employed to determine the absence of osteomyelitis and arteriography completed to clearly review the potential for more definitive care by the vascular surgeon. Tepid saline compresses may be used to wash the area, and the use of povidone-iodine as a compress and soak assists in controlling the infection. Topical enzymes may be used judiciously to help remove some of the necrotic tissues. Our experience indicates that the use of the enzymes should be carried out for 2 or 3 days and then suspended for 2 or 3 days to permit the proper evaluation of the enzymatic process. If the area is significantly draining, a product such as Dextranomer can be employed to help remove some of the draining from the lesion.

Attempts can be made to increase the vascular supply to the area by avoiding prolonged elevation, reducing edema, and using of physical modalities such as whirlpool, low voltage therapy and exercise. The use of peripheral vasodilators has become somewhat questionable, but there is evidence in some patients that these drugs do provide some local increase in the vascular supply to an ulcerated area.

Once the infection is under control and there is no frank evidence of bone involvement, the local debridement can be completed under appropriate conditions. Debridement of the majority of diabetic ulcers in the elderly patients generally does not require any form of anesthesia. All of the hyperkeratotic tissue should be removed, within the appropriate judgment of the clinician.

In the presence of deep infection, incision and drainage are required if the antibiotics do not reduce the infective process. Once debridement has been completed, and the patient begins to become ambulatory, the use of a surgical shoe or Plastazote sandal to permit ambulation is advisable. This reduces the degree of ambulation that a patient can accomplish and, in addition, permits the use of significant dressings to reduce local trauma. It has been our experience to permit patients to become actively involved in the treatment of their diabetic ulcers, and we believe that dressing changes two or three times a day help prevent infection and permit the patient to recognize changes that occur that might be detrimental to the ulcerative process. As healing begins to take place, there is a need for periodic debridement of the hyperkeratotic tissue. There is no set period of time that can be identified, as the treatment regime for each individual patient must be tailored to his condition and to his activity status. Once the patient is ambulatory and no longer confined to bed either at home or in the hospital, ambulatory care can be completed and maintained through the healing process. It is not unreasonable to see patients go for long periods of time with an extremely slow healing ulcer or an ulcer that may resist healing altogether. However, as long as there is no threat to life and the patient does not become toxic, treatment should be carried out on an ambulatory basis.

Once the lesion has healed and is satisfactorily dried, the next step involves appropriate patient education and those means to prevent the ulcer from recurring. Skin care becomes essential and the use of emollients on a continuing basis is important. Changes in footwear need to be considered and the use of appropriate orthotics employed. One of the prime considerations that one must recognize in the diabetic with ulceration in later years is that the ulceration will probably recur. If the lesion is present in the area of the metatarsal head, there is usually an atrophy of soft tissue. Appropriate materials can be used in the form of dense polyurethane foam in removable types of orthotics to diffuse pressure from the area and disperse pressure from the ulcerative site. Where deformities exist such as contracted digits, the use of moldable silicone orthotics, tube foam, lamb's wool and, if necessary, removal of the toe box of the shoe may prove to be an appropriate means of treatment.

When the infected process has progressed to present osteomyelitis, significant gangrene, necrosis and toxicity, amputation of part of the foot—a below-the-knee or above-the-knee amputation—must be considered. Arteriography and peripheral vascular scans should precede this activity and a team decision should be made in relation to surgical care of the patient.

Shoe modification may also include wedges, bars or specially constructed shoes that will permit the clinician to remove weight bearing from the infected area. Surgical shoes or plastazote shoes will also help reduce pressure to the foot.

One of the most significant activities in dealing with the elderly diabetic patient is to counteract the fear of amputation. Most elderly patients are aware of someone who has lost an extremity as a result of gangrene. This fear itself can be a deterrent to ambulation and management.

Giving the elderly patient hope and making him recognize that his or her problem can be managed and that he or she can remain an active member of society and maintain his dignity is a significant catalyst in helping the patient begin the process of rehabilitation. Team care in the management of the elderly diabetic is perhaps more essential than in almost any other condition involving the foot of the geriatric patient. The team must include all of the professionals involved in care, as well as the patient and his family.

chapter 14

Physical Therapy for Elderly Patients with Foot Conditions

Joseph Bruno, P.T.

The philosophy of rehabilitation is almost as important as the rehabilitation procedures. Regardless of the degree of severity of the disability, regardless of the ultimate prognosis, or whether it may be terminal, there is always something that can be done to offer the patient 5 minutes, 5 hours, 5 days or more of comfort either physically or emotionally.

The approach by physical therapy to geriatric management should be basically the same as for any disease, but should be modified to accommodate to the physiology of the aging patient.

Although the chronic degenerative diseases become the major problems with the aged, it should be remembered that acute disease can also attack the aged. The treatment of the chronically ill patient is primarily symptomatic because most diseases are of a chronic nature and irreversible at this time. The biologic aspects of disease, as well as the concomitant psychologic and social sequelae, and the holistic approach must be considered. The practitioner must aid the patient in the discovery and use of reserve potentials to help him attain the highest possible emotional and functional level. He, the practitioner, can always lend a willing ear to the patient or to the patient's family, because frequently the psychological and emotional disturbances overshadow the physical disability which may be present.

The process of evaluation should include physical, psychological and sociological factors. Realistic goals should be set, both on a short and long range basis. A flexible physical therapy plan is formulated and instituted. It should be periodically reassessed and appropriate changes in treatment made as the patient's condition changes. Medicare by law requires the referring physician to reevaluate the patient at least every 30 days.

At the time of interview, if possible, have another member of the family present to verify the patient's statements or add to the patient's statement anything that he may have forgotten. This also applies in prescribing a home treatment program, which also provides the patient and the patient's family with better rapport.

Aside from the regular diagnostic methods of the x-rays, laboratory studies, etc., special examinations should be included such as range of motion, muscle testing, and activities of daily living (ADL).

Range of motion examination is of primary importance and generally should be done actively and passively. If the patient cannot actively move a part, the disability may be neuromuscular or musculoskeletal. Usually passive motion is greater than active motion.

For the sake of standardization, the terminology and the method of measuring and recording joint motion should be based upon the principles advocated by the American Academy of Orthopedic Surgeons. The neutral zone method as described by Cave and Roberts in 1936 is used.

In this method, all motions of a joint are measured from defined zero starting positions rather than 180°.

The motion of the extremity being examined should be compared to that of the opposite extremity, if possible. In the event that the opposite extremity is also lost or affected, then the motion should be compared to the "average motion" of a person of similar age, sex and physical stature.

Limitation of joint motion may be complete, as in ankylosis, or it may be due to pain (physiologic splinting) and this should be recorded as such. For example: "Active motion dorsiflexion of left foot is 0–3° (pain—physiologic splinting)."

The use of the goniometer is preferable, but the angle of motion can sometimes be estimated by an experienced person without the use of a goniometer.

Lower extremity measurements should include:

Length: measure from anterior superior spine to the internal malleolus.

Circumference of thigh: measure from 5 inches above the adductor tubercle.

Circumference of calf: measure from 5 inches below the adductor tubercle.

Circumference of foot: measure from the distal and proximal ends of the metatarsals.

Average Range of Joint Motion: Lower Extremity

Hip

Flexion—113°
Extension—28° (hip and spine)
Abduction—48°
Adduction—31°
Rotation in flexion
   Internal—45°
   External—45°
Rotation in extension
   Internal—35°
   External—48°
Abduction in 90° of flexion: 45–60° depending upon age

Knee—Straight Leg Raising 70–90°

Flexion—134°
Extension—0°
Hyperextension—10°

Ankle

Plantar flexion—48°
Dorsiflexion—18°
Hind foot—subtalar
   Inversion—5°
   Eversion—5°

Forefoot

Inversion—33°
Eversion—18°

Toes

Great toe: flexion distal joint—60°; proximal joint—30°; extension-distal joint—0°; proximal joint—63°.

Second to fifth toes: flexion distal—0–55°; middle—0–38°; proximal—35°; extension-proximal joint—0–40°.

MANUAL MUSCLE TESTING

The technique of manual muscle testing as advocated by Dr. Robert W. Lovett, professor of orthopedic surgery at Harvard University, and his staff should be the method of choice for muscle examination. This technique is recommended for the sake of standardization because it is by far the most widely used method in the world today and will facilitate communication both within and outside the profession.

The grading system is based upon:

1. Evidence of a muscle contraction or the absence of a muscle contraction.
2. Range of motion (ROM), with gravity eliminated or against gravity, whether the ROM is complete (full grade) or incomplete (minus grade).
3. The amount of resistance that can be given at the completion of the range of motion (break test).

The following grades according to Lovett and his associate and according to the numerical system used by the Polio Foundation are as follows:

Normal = N = 5 = complete range of motion against gravity with "normal" resistance.

Good = G = 4 = complete range of motion against gravity with resistance less than normal.

Fair = F = 3 = complete range of motion against gravity.

Poor = P = 2 = complete range of motion with gravity eliminated.

Trace = T = 1 = contraction of muscle which is either visible or palpable, but is not strong enough to cause motion.

Zero = O = No evidence of contraction.

S or SS = spasm or severe spasm.

C or CC = contracture or severe contracture.

An asterisk may be placed next to the muscle in spasm or contracted to denote that range of motion is limited.

The test position for any muscle to be examined is usually the primary action of that particular muscle and is usually the best motion for exercising a specific muscle.

Some of the advantages of muscle testing are:

1. Acts as a common base for communication with all medical practitioners, and it becomes a "soft tissue x-ray."
2. Aids in diagnosis of neuromuscular diseases.
3. Aids in assessment of peripheral nerve injuries.
4. Aids in determining segmental nerve involvement, e.g., a disc, tumor, etc.
5. Aids in treatment by:
   a. Providing greater understanding of the *Why* of poor foot or body mechanics.
   b. Providing a better evaluation for orthotic devices.
   c. Prescribing a more comprehensive exercise program, including the type—passive exercises, active assistive exercises, voluntary active exercises or active resistive exercises.
   d. Establishing a ready reference if reconstructive surgery is contemplated (with tendon transplants, muscle usually loses a grade).
6. Becomes a record of progression or regression of muscle power by periodic retesting.

This method of testing is best utilized for lower motor neuron conditions. It is not designed for upper motor neuron conditions. It also must be borne in mind that it is a subjective test.

ACTIVITIES OF DAILY LIVING (ADL)

The primary goal of rehabilitation is to restore function to the patient within his capabilities to enable him to care for himself with minimal outside assistance.

In order to assess a patient's ability to perform activities of daily living it becomes necessary to have the patient demonstrate his capabilities rather than accept his statements. These activities should be recorded on the patient's chart or on an available chart with a checklist. Special emphasis should be on walking activities, whether independent or with the use of aids such as crutches, walkerette, cane, orthotic device, or prosthesis, and whether he can do level walking, stair climbing, etc.

The practitioner who knows normal gait patterns, although the lower extremity plays the most important conspicuous role in locomotion, must also observe other body segments such as the pelvis, trunk, upper extremities, neck and head, as they also play an important role in normal human gait.

Pathological gait is any variation from the normal human gait. It is usually asymetric, excessive, arrhythmic, antalgic, podalgic, etc. With the analysis of the pattern of locomotion, you will recognize hemiplegic gait, drop foot gait, ataxic gait, painful back gait, painful foot gait, etc.

Special note should be made here of Petren's gait. It is a gait similar to Parkinson's, the inability to initiate semi-automatic motor activity—the patient's feet seem glued to the floor and he then glides them across the floor inch by inch. There is no gross motor or sensory deficiency evident when the patient is in bed or sitting.

Therapeutic programs should be scheduled according to priorities of goals. The patient and his family should be part of the rehabilitation team; they should be instructed in how to prevent contractures and atrophy. The reasons for each element of the therapy should be explained to the patient and his family.

THERAPEUTIC PROGRAMS

Special consideration must be given to the treatment of the geriatric patient with the various physical therapy modalities.

Thermotherapy

The use of heat and cold is more in the realm of an art than a science in the practice of medicine. Every form of externally applied heat will increase the surface temperature and affect the skin as well as the deeper tissues. Heat in any form should be applied with caution to the extremities of the geriatric patient, because of the multiple deficiencies such as neuropathic, vascular and skeletal deficiencies, hypotonia of muscle and atrophy of skin.

Whirlpool

The application of heat to a part which is motionless and dependent, as is commonly done when a patient is placed in the average arm or leg whirlpool, is definitely contrary to good physiologic and scientific judgment. The heat produces increased pooling of blood, and without the pumping effect of muscular activity, will result in increased edema, which may further complicate the original problem.

Kinetic whirlpool is the combining of exercises of the foot and ankle while in the whirlpool to aid the circulation and overcome the gravitational effects of the dependent position.

Special care should be exercised so that the patient's limb does not rest on the edge of the seat or on the rim of the tub; or that rolled up slacks or pants, do not cause constriction of the circulation.

Avoid direct activity of the jet, especially upon excoriated or devitalized skin. Water temperature should be 93–102°F depending upon the general physical condition of the patient and the condition being treated.

Treatment time: 10–20 minutes.

Frequency: daily to once a week.

Kinetic low profile or full body immersion whirlpool. Water temperature should be 93–97°F depending upon the general physical condition of the patient and the condition being treated.

Hot Packs or Compresses

Hot packs or compresses are applied locally for periods of 10 minutes to 1 hour; time is dictated by the condition to be treated and the practitioner's judgment. Added caution should be exercised because of the weight of the compresses, which could result in local ischemia and increase the danger of burning.

This same principle applies to home treatment, especially with electric heating pads. Patients may fall asleep with the appliance

on (even if it is on low intensity), increasing the duration of the heating, thereby increasing the danger of burning.

Treatment time: 10–30 minutes.

Frequency: once or twice daily.

Contrast Baths

These consist of the alternate immersion of feet and legs in containers of hot and cold water. The hot water should be at 102–105°F and the cold water at 65–75°F. Start with hot water for 4 minutes, then cold for 1 minute. Repeat four times, ending with hot water. This process acts as a blood vessel exercise, causing the vessels to contract and relax, thereby increasing blood flow.

Treatment time: 20 minutes.

Frequency: daily, three times a week; twice a week.

Paraffin Baths

This is another method for applying heat and is especially useful in arthritis of the hands and feet. The skin generally feels soft and more pliable following a treatment. The paraffin mixture consists of seven parts paraffin and one part mineral oil so that the melting point becomes about 126°. Special caution should be exercised in the presence of neuropathy and severe peripheral vascular disease.

Treatment time: 10–20 minutes.

Frequency: daily; three times a week; once a week.

Infrared

In treating the lower extremities, especially the foot and leg, a simple and safe device is a radiant light baker 18–24 inches long and governed by a three-way switch of low, medium and high intensity. Usually the intensity would be on medium, and in the case of vascular insufficiency low intensity can be used. The baker can be placed over the abdomen for reflex heating. When the radiant light baker is utilized, the patient receives a diffusion of heat over a large area. When irradiation by a lamp is used, and if the lamp is placed close to the part being treated, there is danger of burning. If the lamp is placed at too great a distance from the patient, the infrared rays are ineffective.

Infrared is generally combined with other physical therapy modalities or procedures such as massage, low voltage current, ultrasound, exercise, etc. The advantage of infrared is that it does not touch or cover the skin; therefore it can be monitored easily and generally does not cause any discomfort of touching or of weight.

Treatment time: 10–30 minutes.

Frequency: once or twice daily.

Deep Heat

There are three types of deep heat presently used: short wave diathermy, microwave diathermy and ultrasound.

With short wave and microwave diathermy the patient should experience a mild sensation of heat. Special care must be exercised with the aged, because dosage is determined by the patient's sensation, which is generally impaired. If the patient is confused and or disorientated these modalities should not be used.

Treatment time: 15–30 minutes.

Frequency: daily; three times a week; twice a week.

Ultrasound

The sonation may be applied either paravertebrally, locally or both. If both are to be used at the same treatment session, the paravertebral application should precede the local.

Dosage is usually prescribed in watts per square centimeter of the transducer. Care should be exercised so that the intensity used during treatment does not cause pain or produce uncomfortable heating. The clinician should be aware of the reflection of sound waves as they strike bone (30–35% reflection) and join together with the sound waves being applied. Overdosage can cause a flaccid paralysis. If the patient's sensation is intact, this rarely happens.

Ultrasound being one of the most potent agents used in physical therapy, the understanding of the physiology, biophysics and technique of application is a prerequisite for safe application. Some of the techniques used are: direct contact, underwater, continuous, pulsed, phonophoresis, and combined ultrasound and electrical stimulation simultaneously.

Treatment time: 3–10 minutes per area, depending on area of body.

Frequency: daily; three times a week; once a week.

Cryotherapy

Cryotherapy is the use of ice, ice bags, cold compresses, ethyl chloride and fluoromethane sprays.

Cryotherapy is usually used following acute trauma (including surgery) the first 1–3 days. When heat is not effective in relieving pain and muscle spasm, cold would be indicated for patients with acute lumbar sacral pain, spasm and acute sciatic radiation due to trauma or the arthritides. The treatment would be indicated for those patients who do not respond to the more conventional approaches to treatment. Ice (frozen in 5-ounce cups) is applied to the affected areas with the same technique as is used with the transducer of ultrasound: small overlapping circular movements until the ice is melted. This is then directly followed by direct contact continuous ultrasound to the same area.

Ultraviolet rays

This treatment is bactericidal, bacteriostatic and fungicidal. It is also used for stimulation of tissue repair, especially in infections, such as indolent ulcers. It is also used in pruritus and for counterirritation.

The usual precautions should be exercised regarding the hypersensitivity of blondes, blue eyed patients and the aged. Also, certain substances increase sensitivity: (1) Fluorescent materials—eosin, methylene blue, tryptoflavin and quinine. (2) The endocrines—insulin, thyroxin, adrenalin and Pituitrin. (3) Drugs—tetracyclines, sulfas, chlorpromazines, barbiturates. Ultraviolet rays are prescribed in erythema doses which cause reactions in the skin that are classified as follows: suberythema dose, first degree erythema dose, second degree erythema dose, and third degree erythema dose. The method used for determining the erythema dose for your ultraviolet lamp is the sleeve test. This test should be done periodically, because the lamp does deteriorate with time and use. Wood's filter over the ultraviolet lamp is used for the detection of ringworm by fluorescence.

Goeckerman's technique is used for psoriasis. Coal tar should be applied to the lesions before the application of ultraviolet rays in order to intensify the reaction.

Massage

Special care should be exercised with the geriatric patient because of the dryness of the skin, the hypotonicity of the muscles and the sensitivity to pressure. Massage should not be painful. It has either sedative or stimulating effects. It does not increase muscle strength or reduce deposits of fat.

Massage is generally used in conjunction with other physical therapy modalities, especially following the application of heat, after exercises. When attempting to reduce edema in the foot and leg the limb should be elevated in order to utilize gravity to aid in circulation. The proximal positions of the lower extremity should be massaged first, in order to make room for the excess fluid from the distal portions. The massage movement of frictions, which is synonymous with digital kneading, is very useful in stretching adhesions, loosening of superficial scars, and breaking up myositic and fibrositic deposits.

Counterirritation

Counterirritation increases the blood supply to the tissues in and around the areas being treated. To produce counterirritation, ointments, (imadyl unction, methyl salicylate, etc., massage, and second and third degree erythema doses of ultraviolet ray could be used. Suction cups are more commonly used in Europe, and as recently as in May 1979 we saw them used in the Peoples Republic of China, along with acupuncture with electricity.

Counterirritation has been used for centuries and is still effective for the relief of pain, loosening of postoperative adhesions, myositis, lumbago, lumbosacral sprain, strain and arthritis.

Low Voltage and Low Frequency Currents

Low voltage and low frequency currents consist of three basic types: direct (galvanic), alternating (sinusoidal), and faradic. Medical galvanism is a direct current which produces electrochemical effects without contraction of muscle. It is employed when the polar effects are desired, such as:

Positive (+)	Negative (−)
Acid	Alkaline
Sedative	Irritative
Vasoconstriction	Vasodilation
Hardens tissue	Liquifies tissue
Repels positive ions	Repels negative ions
Mild thermal effect	Mild thermal effect

Other indications are: to reduce pain, reduce swelling, soften scar tissue, increase local circulation (using labile technique), aid in nerve regeneration and iontophoresis,

Iontophoresis (Table 14.1) is the introduction of drugs into the body by the galvanic current. The law of magnetism prevails: like poles repel, unlike poles attract. The technique is based upon the fact that the ions to be introduced through the intact skin will be repelled into the body. For instance, to introduce histamine into the body (histamine ionizes positively) the positive pole is used; to introduce iodine (iodine ionizes negatively) the negative pole is used. The ointment or solution should be 2% or less. Indications or contraindications for iontophoresis are dependent upon the effect of the drug: histamine for vasodilation; contraindication is cardiac asthma (can induce an attack); copper as a fungicide; chloride as a softening agent; magnesium as an astringent; procaine hydrochloride as an analgesic, etc. Treatment time is 5–30 minutes for iontophoresis and an average of 20 minutes for medical galvanism. Dosage formula for iontophoresis or stabile medical galvanism, especially for the geriatric patient, should be one-half to one (0.5–1 MA) milliampere per square inch of the smallest surface electrode. ALL OTHER STANDARD PRECAUTIONS SHOULD BE OBSERVED.

Surgical galvanism, by the use of the negative pole (liquifies tissue when dosage formula is exceeded), is effective for the destruction of certain skin lesions and the removal of unwanted hair (electrolysis).

Interrupted galvanic current is used to contract denervated muscle until reinnervation occurs, provided prognosis for regeneration is good.

Slow sinusoidal current can also stimulate denervated muscle directly if the frequency is 25 hertz or less. Theoretically the slow sine

Table 14.1.

Iontophoresis

Ion	Source	Polarity	Physiology	Indications
Chloride	Sodium chloride	Negative	Sclerolytic	Scars, adhesions
Copper	Copper sulfate	Positive	Caustic, antiseptic, astringent	Fungus infections, indolent and varicose ulcers, bromidrosis
Histamine	Imadyl	Positive	Vasodilator, analgesic	Myositis, myofasciitis, fibrositis, intermittent claudication, phlebitis, peripheral vascular disease, arthritic conditions, rheumatism, varicose ulcers
Iodine	Iodex	Negative	Sclerolytic, antiseptic, analgesic	Myositis, myofasciitis, fibrositis, tendonitis, arthritis
Magnesium	MgSO$_4$	Positive	Anti-inflammatory analgesic	Neuritis, osteoarthritis, rheumatoid arthritis, bromidrosis
Mecholyl	Acetylcholine	Positive	Vasodilation, analgesic	Peripheral vascular disease, intermittent claudication, varicose ulcers, phlebitis, TAO, neuritis, rheumatism, arthritis (same as histamine)
Procaine	2% in alcohol or ointment	Positive	Vasodilation, analgesic	Neuritis, bursitis, gout

wave should have no ionic or polar effects, but in practice it does. Use the same precautions as when using the galvanic current.

Faradic current is an induced current, whose impulse lasts only about 1 millisecond, which is too rapid to stimulate denervated muscle.

Table 14.2 lists electrodiagnostic tests that can be done with an office apparatus having galvanic and faradic currents.

Galvanic Tetanus Ratio Test (GTR)

It was long believed that a muscle contracts only on the "make" or "break" of the galvanic current and that, during the intermittent flow of the current, the muscle relaxes. It has been shown that, depending upon the state of the muscle and the use of sufficient current intensity, both the normal and denervated muscle may sustain a continuous or tetanic contraction throughout the duration of the direct current flow.

Innervated muscle requires little current to contract it; much current to tetanize it. But, when a muscle is denervated, it requires relatively less current to contract it, but the same or slightly more than threshold (rheobase) current to tetanize it.

Technique:
1. Determine twitch rheobase. Record MA.
2. Increase milliamperes (MA) until there is a sustained contraction (tetany). Record MA.

Nerve Status	Galvanic Tetanus Ratio
Normal	3.5 to 6.5 times rheobase
Denervated	1.0 to 1.5
Regenerated	1.0 to 20.0 then back to normal

Table 14.2.

Reaction to Degeneration Test (RD Test)

		Faradic	Galvanic
Normal reaction	Nerve	Tetanic contraction	Brisk single contraction
	Muscle	Tetanic contraction	Brisk single contraction
Partial RD	Nerve	Diminished response	Diminished response
	Muscle	Diminished response	Sluggish response (vermiform)
Full RD	Nerve	No response	No response
	Muscle	No response	Sluggish response (vermiform)
Absolute RD	Nerve	No response	No response
	Muscle	No response	No response
Prognosis:	No RD	2–4 weeks	
	Partial RD	6–12 weeks	
	Full RD	6–12 months	
	Absolute RD	no return	

Hysterical Paralysis. Stimulation with a tetanizing current is the simplest test. This will cause a contraction of the muscle, which will exclude the diagnosis of a peripheral nerve pathology. If, with *a good history*, there is no evidence of an organic nerve lesion and the distribution of the "paralysis" is doubtful, hysterical paralysis should be suspected.

Myotonic Reaction. A tetanizing current, when applied to a muscle, will elicit a contraction which will persist even after the stimulus has been removed, sometimes for as long as 20 seconds. Patients with myotonia congenita (Thomsen's disease) and other forms of myotonia will exhibit this reaction.

Myesthenic Reaction (Jolly Test). Usually the muscle of choice is the orbicularis oculi. (This is the muscle which usually shows weakness first.) A tetanizing current is used over the motor point at the rate of 100–200 interruptions per minute. At first the muscle will contract normally; but within 30 seconds or less, the amplitude of the contraction will begin to diminish and finally stop. If contractions continue for 8 minutes, the test is considered negative.

Applications in Operating Room

1. Identification of Motor Nerves by electrical stimulation (faradic current) is useful for traumatic injuries where interference by complete or partial sectioning of a nerve is affected (stabbing, gunshot wound, etc.). This can be tested during surgery for continuity from above or below the site of injury. Dosage: 0.5 MA at 0.3 seconds or shorter duration.

2. Curare Levels. Curare acts on the motor end plates and prevents efferent stimuli from reaching and contracting muscle. A stimulus greater than threshold is determined before the administration of the curare. This current is introduced at intervals. If the contractions are normal the curare level is low; if the contractions cannot be elicited electrically, the curare has reached a paralyzing level.

3. Tendon Transplants. Surgeons can, with a nonpolarizing tetanizing current, check the proper length.

Principles of Clinical Application

Physiologists have stated that all forms of voluntary muscular contractions are tetanic in nature. The brain cells do not send out a single stimulus, but successive volleys of impulses.

Physiologists have stated that stimulation active exercise (SAE) will produce the same chemical and physical phenomena connected with normal muscular work. When a muscle cannot or does not contract voluntarily or reflexively, it tends to revert to a noncontractable connective tissue type. This can be reversible in most cases, especially when it is possible to have a muscle contract again, whether by SAE or by voluntary active exercise. SAE could be defined as electrical stimulation of nerve or muscle or both by an electrical current which will cause a contraction of muscle followed by a period of relaxation. This can be accomplished with the use of an interrupted current, surged current or a pulsed current of slow or medium rate.

In the clinical application of electrical stimulation to normally innervated muscle, the ideal current would be one that is most comfortable and causes the least amount of ionic concentration.

Electrodynamic or electrokinetic currents will usually motivate the patient to exercise the part even when it is too sore to touch or massage. It can stimulate an individual muscle or a group of muscles, depending upon the desired effect. The method of application is by transcutaneous electrical nerve stimulation: (1) sensory or (2) motor effects.

The placement of electrodes should be based upon anatomical and physiological principles. There are many sites and methods of application which are determined by the etiology and the effect desired. Bearing the preceding statements in mind, the following basic four techniques have evolved, using a two circuit, low volt generator with independent volume controls for each circuit.

Technique 1–anatomical. This technique is used for stimulation active exercise of a specific muscle or for exercising a group of muscles that produce a specific motion. To produce dorsiflexion of foot at ankle place electrode over anterior tibial group of muscles (red circuit). To produce plantar flexion of foot at ankle place electrodes over plantar flexor group of muscles (black circuit). To exercise isometrically, energize both circuits at the same time, adjusting current to counteract each other (using a surge or slow-to-medium pulse rate). To exercise isotonically, use selector switch on reciprocal or alternating; this will then energize only one circuit at a time. Depending upon electrode placement and motion desired, this can activate or stimulate other muscles or groups, such as lumbricales and interrossei for hammer toe or abductor hallucis longus for hallux valgus.

This technique could also be used preoperatively and postoperatively to prevent adhesions and fibrosis. It can also be used for muscle reeducation by providing the patient with a visual image, and kinesthetic information about the muscle, tendon and joint involved, and also provide mental awareness.

Technique 2—Vascular. The objective of this technique is to increase circulation by the contraction and relaxation of the greatest number of muscle fibers at one time by electrical stimulation. Each muscle fiber will act as an accessory heart or pump. Any current that can cause a period of contraction, followed by a period of relaxation, could be used to increase circulation to the part.

With innervated muscle, an alternating nonionizing current such as interrupted rapid sinusoidal, surging rapid sinusoidal, interrupted faradic or surging faradic, etc., would be the currents of choice. A strong continuous tetanizing current should not be used, because it would cause the muscle stimulated to remain in a continuous state of contraction (spasm) which would inhibit circulation.

The placement of electrodes should be in areas in which the greatest number of muscle fibers can be stimulated at one time. This could be over the nerve trunk supplying a muscle or a group of muscles.

This technique is used to influence the peripheral vascular deficiencies of arterial, venous and lymphatic origin.

Without vascular disease, the following are some of the factors that could influence the circulation adversely.

1. Flaccid paralysis
2. Spastic paralysis
3. Disuse—hypokinesis
4. Shortening of muscle
5. Contracture
6. Scar tissue
7. Fibrosis
8. Fibrous ankylosis
9. Bony ankylosis
10. Pain
11. Chronic low grade spasm
12. Stress and anxiety
13. Trauma
14. Surgery
15. *Anything that affects contraction and relaxation of muscles.*

All or most of the above factors could be found in the aged patient. Vascular disease affects the lower extremities mostly because of the distance the blood must travel to the heart and because of the added effect of gravity on the return flow to the heart. The need for increased contraction and relaxation of muscle is apparent to prevent stasis.

If a patient cannot or will not engage in enough ambulatory activity, the use of SAE, alternate contraction and relaxation, would be indicated. Stimulation active exercise puts less demand on circulation than does ambulation. The element of fatigue is also decreased when using electrical stimulation.

Many geriatric patients utilize only the number of motor units absolutely necessary for function. By utilizing electrical stimulation you may be able to make patients aware of unused motor units that do not make up their usual habit patterns.

Technique 3—Sensory. This technique is used for pain, muscle spasm and neuropathies. The currents of choice are continuous tetany, 3/4 pulse rate or any other current that may break up the cycle of spasm or cycle of pain. The technique to be selected will be dependent upon the etiology, symptoms, location and character of pain. The placement of electrodes is varied; the method of choice falls upon the clinician as a result of his findings. In the treatment of pain, the electrodes may be placed over the point of greatest pain, segmental nerve supply, dermatomes, acupuncture points, trigger points or any other neuroanatomical or physiological sites.

The earlier use of the electrical currents for the relief of pain was the reduction or alleviation of muscle spasm through fatigue or the utilization of Sherrington's law of reciprocal innervation. The former was accomplished by applying electrodes over the muscles in spasm until they fatigue or by placing electrodes over antagonists of the muscles in spasm. The usual treatment time is 20 minutes. In recent years, with the advent of the transcutaneous electrical nerve stimulator (TENS) units, renewed interest has developed in pain relief. One theory, called the gate theory, presumes that the impulse from afferents, when activated, would close the gate and thus not permit smaller diameter afferent fibers to transmit pain information to a conscious level. Another theory states that electrical stimulation may liberate endogenous endorphins and enkephalins, which are morphine-like substances which have an inhibitory action.

To use technique 3 for neuropathies, place electrodes over areas involved, usually the plantar and dorsal areas of the feet. Turn selector switch to "automatic setting" on the low volt generator which will give 1 minute of tetanizing current, 1 minute of a surging current and 1 minute of a pulsating current, in cycles, for 20 minutes of treatment time. The patient should also be instructed to "bombard the sensorium" by rubbing or touching the affected parts with different types of stimuli; the hands, woolen cloth, cotton cloth, leather, warm, cold, etc. The results will be pleasant to both the clinician and the patient.

Technique 4—Psychosomatic. The psychosomatic effect of electrotherapy will and does invade and become a part of the other techniques, as it is present in all forms of therapy.

Technique 1—anatomical—aids in motivating the patient.

Technique 2—vascular—aids in relieving anxiety, which will directly affect the circulation.

Technique 3—sensory—relieves pain and anxiety, thereby also relieving associated muscle spasm.

Technique 4—psychosomatic—there is no definite pattern of application of electrodes based upon anatomic or physiologic principles used, but it is important to use strong suggestions.

The exception is hysterical motor paralysis. The paralysis is treated by placing the electrodes over the affected muscles and strongly urging the patient to try the motion as the clinician synchronizes the intensity of the current (manually) to cause the paralyzed muscles to move in unison with the patient's effort. Many times it becomes very gratifying to see an "immediate cure."

EXERCISE

The clinician must give specificity to his prescription for exercise. He must be knowledgeable about the wide range of effects that exercises are capable of producing and how to select the specific exercise for the specific condition.

Examples of effects of exercises for specific objectives are:

1. Exercises to mobilize joints
2. Exercises to reeducate muscle
3. Exercises to improve coordination

4. Exercises to improve or develop strength
5. Exercises to increase endurance
6. Exercises to increase circulation
7. Exercises to prevent fibrosis—inter- and intrafascicular
8. Exercises to reduce edema
9. Exercises to reduce painful period
10. Exercises to prevent thrombophlebitis
11. Exercises to improve respiratory system
12. Exercises for relaxation
13. Exercises that are calorie consuming for the diabetic
14. Exercises to prevent atrophy of spirit

An exercise program can be "tailored" to practically all patients. Hans Selvye, an authority on stress, states that by exercising intelligently, a man can train his heart to resist attacks that otherwise might kill him. It does not matter that he has been training with calisthenics and is later attacked not by physical stress but by emotional stress; cross resistance will help his heart withstand the attack in any case.

Hypokinesia

Hypokinesia or disuse syndromes can be and many times are more catastrophic than the primary disabilities. Regardless of the primary disability, whether it be a stroke, acute arthritis, fractured hip, etc., preventive treatment should be instituted almost immediately. If not, then some of the secondary complications of atrophy, contractures, decubiti, demineralization, hypostatic pneumonia, kidney stones, infections and even death can occur.

The involvement could be general, such as in acute generalized rheumatoid arthritis, or it may be local, such as immobilization in a leg cast, necessitating inactivity. The more the inactivity, the more the susceptibility to secondary complications. It is of primary importance that the range of motion be maintained and that contracture be prevented. If motion is free, strength can always be increased, but if contracture develops, it becomes extremely difficult to restore range of motion, even with the restoration of normal strength.

Davis' Law (Functional Adaptation of Soft Tissue)

At this point it is helpful to remember the Davis law of functional adaptation of soft tissue. Ligaments or any soft tissues put under even a moderate degree of unremitting tension will elongate by the addition of new material.

Conversely, when ligaments or other soft tissues remain in an uninterrupted, loose or lax state, they will gradually shorten as the affected material is removed, until they maintain the same relation to the bony structure with which they are united that they did before their shortening. If Davis' law persists for any length of time, Wolff's law can take effect.

Wolff's Law (Functional Adaptation of Bone)

Every change in the form and position of the bones or their function is followed by certain definite changes in their internal architecture and equally definite secondary changes in their external conformation. These changes are in accordance with mathematical laws.

The use of various physical therapy modalities in the treatment of disabilities and diseases, when properly applied, has been very beneficial. Unfortunately, however, too much dependence is often placed on the therapeutic benefits supposedly received from the application of phyiscal therapy modalities and not enough personal effort is made to assist the joint in regaining movement.

The emphasis should be placed upon *motivation*. Voluntary effort and active exercise are the chief stimulants for the restoration of motion.

Exercise programs should have reachable goals, with the patient and his family part of the rehabilitation team. They should be instructed in how to prevent contractures, how to prevent atrophy, and that when a part is put through the full range of motion (active or passive) each day, they will not lose that motion.

A variety of deformities can be caused by faulty posture, wear and tear, stress, strain, trauma, degeneration, inflammation, infection, malnutrition, metabolic, neurologic or endocrine disturbances. A general exercise program, in conjunction with specific corrective exercises directed at a specific disability, should be instituted.

Therapeutic programs should be scheduled according to priorities and goals and structured so they can be modified as the condition of the patient changes.

Each exercise program should employ the simplest forms of exercise which will produce the greatest therapeutic benefit to the body. In researching the literature, even up to the present time, exercises for weakness and pronation of the feet have included such devastating and frustrating exercises as rolling a rubber ball between the soles of the feet and grasping marbles with the toes. Some children would have difficulty doing these exercises; imagine a geriatric patient attempting them!!

Weight bearing is the fundamental function of the lower extremity. The hip, therefore, is subservient to the foot. When alterations in the thigh or hip occur, the mechanism of the leg and foot will be affected. The clinician should be aware of rotational defects, shortening or lengthening defects which may alter the gait pattern, and foot mechanics.

Considerations in Formulating Exercise Program

1. Think of muscle function in terms of agonists and antagonists.
2. With imbalance, generally muscles that are contracted or in spasm are the agonists and those that are stretched, the antagonists.
3. The objectives of the treatment program would be:
   a. To stretch the contracted muscles.
   b. To shorten the stretched muscles.

These objectives can be accomplished by:
1. Manual or mechanical stretching (agonists).
2. Stretching exercises (agonists).
3. Orthotic devices (supportive).
4. Muscle strengthening exercises (antagonists).

Heel Cord Stretching Manual

Grasp os calcis by hand and use forearm in conjunction with hand and forcefully dorsiflex foot at the ankle (especially for children and CVA patients or where balance or coordination is a problem).

Exercise 1

1. Patient should remove shoes, then:
2. Stand at arm's length from wall, feet slightly apart and in-toed.

3. Lean toward wall, keeping body straight.
4. Heels must remain on the floor.

Exercise 2

1. Patient should remove shoes, then:
2. Stand at arm's length from wall, feet in-toed.
3. Place ⅛ inch, ¼ inch, ½ inch, etc., under metatarsal heads of feet.
4. Lean toward wall, keeping body straight.
5. Heels must remain on the floor.

Exercise 3

1. Patient should remove shoes and stand on the bottom step, facing down. Then:
2. Place one foot on the landing.
3. Place other foot on step.
4. Foot on step will be the one being stretched (this will be the rear foot) (intoed).
5. Heel on step must be down.
6. Be sure that the patient holds on to stair rail.

Exercise 4

1. Have patient remove shoes.
2. Have patient hold onto table, etc., for balance.
3. Instruct patient to partially squat (20°–40°).
4. Be sure that patient's heels are down and intoed.
5. Incline patient's trunk forward.
6. Care should be exercised with the geriatric patient.

Peroneal Stretching

1. Sitting, cross one leg over the other. Grasp forefoot and strongly invert, adduct and dorsiflex to the count of 1001 to 1005, audibly, using sets of five.
2. Teach the patient to walk in an adducted position, with toes flexed in the shoes.

Muscle Strengthening Exercise for Anterior Tibial Muscle

With the patient sitting, apply 2½-pound weight over forefoot, having patient dorsiflex and invert, hold and count 1001, 1002, 1003, 1004 and 1005, audibly using sets of five. Increase weight progressively as tolerated.

Muscle Strengthening Exercise for Posterior Tibial Muscle

With the patient standing, have him hold for balance and raise body on toes (intoed position).

Exercise for Lumbricales and Interossei Muscles

1. Patient should remove shoes and stockings, then:
2. Stand with an intoe position which will align the metatarsophalangeal joints with the edge of a step, stool or board.
3. Curve toes over edge, maintaining this position for 5 seconds (1001 to 1005).
4. Relax.
5. Repeat above three sets of five.

Exercise for Hip

Flexion: with the patient sitting, place 2½-pound weight over his ankle; have patient bring knee to chest.

Extension: with patient in prone position, extend thigh backward, keeping knee straight.

Abduction: with patient lying on his side, raise leg up; with patient supine, bring leg out to the side.

Rotation—lateral: with patient sitting, bring foot behind other foot.

Rotation—medial: with patient sitting, keep knees together, separate feet outward.

Exercises for the Knee

This exercse will increase strength and improve circulation in the entire lower extremity. With patient sitting, place 2½-pound weight over dorsum of foot, and have patient extend leg; hold and count 1001, 1002, 1003, 1004 and 1005. Increase weight slowly and progressively as tolerated. To enhance muscular contraction of the quadriceps, have patient dorsiflex foot at the same time.

With a patient who cannot exercise one leg at the knee, it would be advisable to have him exercise the uninvolved leg, thereby aiding the affected limb by cross-education.

To Strengthen Hamstrings

With patient in prone position, apply 2½-pound weight around ankle and have patient flex leg at knee.

With patient standing, and holding onto table or other fixed object, flex leg at knee.

Teach patient to *think* exercise as well as do exercise. Ultimately we should—as Dr. A. E. Helfand stated—"Keep Them Walking," whether it is with people assistance, assistive devices, or, ideally, independently walking.

The psychology of the disabled is a very important factor, because the contraction of muscles properly and coordinately is under the control of the will. The conditioned reflex or habit must be taught the patient who must do conditioning or restorative exercises over and over again until he can move all parts, especially the affected parts, without conscious effort.

Therapeutic exercises are rarely contraindicated in the ambulatory patient. Caution should be employed in the presence of cardiac disease. Each case must be considered individually. The type of exercise will be dependent upon the site and the nature of the condition and with the age and general health of the patient. Most exercise programs should be begun gently and increased gradually.

The pathology or condition will dictate the type of exercise possible, such as passive, active assistive, voluntary active or active resistive. Whenever it is possible, it has been our experience that a progressive resistive exercise program has proven best because of the following:

1. Cerebration is required when performing resistive exercises, thereby not only exercisng the muscle but also the brain.

2. It is a more controlled exercise. The patient must consciously extend the leg, and then consciously let the leg flex, utilizing both concentric contraction upon extension and eccentric contraction when allowing the leg to flex.

3. Dr. Thomas DeLorme and others found that active exercises against resistance, within limits of pain, proved more effective in restoring motion and hypertrophy than did passive or active nonresistive exercises.

4. Strength once developed with resistive exercises is more difficult to lose and generally can be maintained with minimal effort.

5. In normally innervated individuals, unilateral resistive exercises cause contralateral increase in strength and endurance. This suggests that the nature of the motor nervous system is such that the whole body is responding even when only part of the body appears to be doing the work. It also suggests that both sides of the body should be exercised in

order to secure the most rapid return to normal or nearest normal neuromuscular function.

6. Dr. Frances A. Hellebrandt, a physiologist, emphasized that a person must exert maximal effort in order to achieve the minimal rate of increase in function. She also stated that great caution should be exercised with maximal heavy resistive exercises to the aged, because of Valsalva phenomenon.

7. Our technique consists of teaching progressive resistive exercises with a minimal weight of 1½ or 2½ pounds and slowly progressing with increases of weights and repetitions. Usually a set consists of five repetitions. On occassion, this could be reduced to two repetitions if necessary. Each set is done four times a day, arranging the time to coincide with a normal daily function, such as before breakfast, before lunch, before dinner, and before going to bed. By doing the exercises before meals, the cardiovascular system is not embarrassed by working to supply blood for digestion and exercise at the same time. In doing the exercises, when the patient has lifted the weight to the extent of this motion, have him count 1001, 1002, 1003, 1004 and 1005 audibly, which aids both cerebration and minimizes the Valsalva phenomena by "letting air out." We also caution patients to monitor their respirations: "If you are breathing too hard, or think that you are tired, stop and rest longer between repetitions." When the patient has progressed to two and ultimately three sets, he should rest between sets 3 to 5 minutes. Finally, increase weight resistance and return to one set again.

8. Signs of overdosage are increased pain that lasting for over 12 hours, and decreased strength or range of motion.

9. For vascular insufficiencies, increase repetitions and lessen weights.

10. *Motivation* is the key to successful exercise programs.

Following are guidelines for a successful exercise program:

1. The patient should be informed of the objectives of the exercise program and its importance.
2. The patient should be instructed in how to perform the specific exercises, with minute detail, including positions, alternate positions, and improvisations if necessary.
3. The patient should be taught no more than two exercises at one visit and be able to do the exercises properly in the office or clinic.
4. Goals should be frequently modified in the rehabilitation of the older patient. This applies to the time allowed for specific gains as well as to final objectives.
5. The patient's performance of the exercises should be reevaluated upon each subsequent visit. At this time, the clinician can review the complete program using verbal encouragement, telling them how good they are, at times how bad they are, and give them "hell" if necessary. Make necessary corrections, if indicated, or increase the number of exercises.
6. Have patients write, using their terminology, a description of the exercises taught. Most printouts are too difficult to interpret.

Contraindications and/or Precautions

Heat

1. Tendency to hemorrhage
2. Hyperpyrexia
3. Decompenssated cardiovascular disease
4. Sensory deficit, including anesthesia (local)
5. Severe peripheral vascular disease
6. Prolonged heating may cause demineralization of bone

Diathermies, In Addition to Heat

1. Metallic implants
2. Over malignant tumors
3. Vascular disease—reflex heating may be used
4. Patients who are not fully alert or are disoriented

Ultrasound, In addition to Heat

1. Over malignant tumors
2. Acute infections (local application)
3. Vascular disease—may be used paravertebrally
4. It is theoretically possible that the circuitry in pacemakers might pick up electrical impulses from radar stations, microwave ovens or ultrasound. With the newer pacemakers it almost never happens. Today's pacemakers, which supply precisely timed electrical impulses

to the heart muscles to keep it beating in proper time, are now built inside titanium shields that almost always protect the circuitry from external emanations.

Massage

1. Acute inflammation (abscesses, etc.)
2. Tumors, malignant
3. Aneurysm
4. Diseases of the skin
5. TB joints
6. Hyperpyrexia
7. Acute thrombophlebitis
8. Acute neuritis

Ultraviolet

1. Hyperpyrexia
2. Malignancies of the skin
3. Albino
4. Neurodermatitis
5. Drugs—tetracyclines, sulfas, barbiturates, insulin, thyroxine, adrenalin, etc.
6. Diabetes—precaution

Exercise

1. Hyperpyrexia
2. Acute inflammation
3. Acute infection
4. Acute thrombophlebitis

Cold (non-ambulatory)

1. Hypersensitivity to cold
2. Impaired sensation—could cause frostbite

Intermittent Vascular Occlusion

1. Acute infection
2. Acute thrombophlebitis
3. Threat of embolism
4. Open lesions
5. Sensitive tissues
6. Hyperpyrexia

Procedures

Vascular

Physical therapy procedures for influencing vascular deficiencies of arterial, venous, capillary and lymphatic origin have been used according to the earliest written records in the practice of medicine. Some of the physical measures used in the past and at present have included:

1. Rest
2. Heat—direct and indirect—as compresses, Hydrocolator, hot packs, whirlpool, carbon dioxide baths, infrared, (radiant light baker, light cradle) diathermies, short wave and microwave, which are used only for reflex heating, and ultrasound for paravertebral sonation.
3. Cold—cold compresses and ice packs.
4. Heat and cold—contrast bath.
5. Mechano-therapy-massage — pressure suction boot, vasopneumatic compression, intermittent venous occlusion, oscillating bed or chair, elastic garments, venous gradient supports, Unna paste boot, postural therapy, and the use of protective devices, lamb's wool, sheepskin, orthotic devices, special shoes.
6. Ultraviolet radiation—first degree erythema for stimulation reaction, second degree erythema for stimulation and bactericidal reaction to open lesions.
7. Electrotherapy—iontophoresis, using vasodilating drugs, histamine, mecholyl, electrical stimulation as stimulation active exercise (S.A.E.) using a non-ionizing current, such as interrupted faradic or interrupted rapid sinusoidal currents, etc.
8. Exercise—Beurger, Beurger-Allen, walking, passive, active assistive, voluntary active, progressive resistant exercises (PRE), stimulation active exercise (SAE) endurance (submaximal resistance with increasing number of repetitions), general conditioning exercises, including exercises to improve respiration.

The objective of physical therapy in vascular insufficiency is to increase or stimulate the flow of blood through the area and avoid circulatory stasis as well as to increase the nutrition and tissue drainage. Some of the causes that can be helped by physical therapy are:

1. Edema, whether due to trauma or poor muscle tone, especially of the legs and abdomen, making the fascia lax, promoting venous congestion.
2. Fibrosis or adhesions, whether interfascicular or intrafascicular.
3. Hemodynamic mechanisms that are usually associated with the more cata-

strophic types of conditions necessitating prolonged bed rest such as in the case of the quadraplegic, hemiplegic or rheumatoid arthritic. We should also look for this same phenomenon when a lower extremity has been immobilized in a cast for a long time.

4. Muscle spasm, whether due to pain, stress or anxiety.
5. Inactivity.

The natural stimulus to circulation is active movement. The most important modality of physical therapy is a supervised, controlled, active exercise program for vascular insufficiency. Exercise will increase arterial, venous, lymphatic and capillary flow. It will make patent capillaries that are not patent and produce new capillaries.

In contrast, inactivity causes lymphatic and venous stasis. Every time a muscle contracts it releases metabolites, causing dilatation of arteries and capillaries, resulting in increased oxygen and nutrition, and waste removal from that part. Edema, if not removed, will tend to organize into fibrous tissue, making the area hard and indurated. If the edema is due to trauma, it tends to organize more quickly and diminishes the "pumping effect" of muscular contractions, thereby, reducing function and activity. This demands quick response of treatment; the sooner treatment is instituted the better.

The strength of muscular contraction depends upon the number of motor units stimulated; the greater the number of motor units stimulated, the greater the therapeutic effect.

Where one segment of a limb is unable to move, active movements of other segments will help maintain the circulation. If active movement is lost, passive exercises are necessary, or the use of the interrupted direct current. The duration of the stimulus of this current is sufficient to stimulate the muscle directly if denervation has occurred. When using this current, observe all safety rules that apply to the galvanic current.

The clinician must always be aware of the effect of emotional disturbance on the well-being of the geriatric patient. With mental depression, the patient's symptoms may increase, including disturbance of the gastrointestinal tract, generalized weakness, skin disorders, tension, pain and anxiety. The latter—pain, tension and anxiety and their associated muscle spasms—will decrease the circulation by mechanical pressure of muscular contraction. Just as circulation is generally improved when a patient sleeps, so will the circulation improve upon the relaxation of muscle spasm with relief of pain, stress and anxiety.

Physical therapy with the use of modalities and especially exercises generally acts as a motivating and viable approach to a visible and measurable degree of improvement. The aged patient must be reassured that he is doing well now as compared to before, that he can walk three blocks now, compared to one block.

The Bruno-Helfand technique utilizes most of the elements necessary in the management of vascular insufficiency by:

1. Producing movement, either with the resistant exercises or without the patient's cooperation by electrical stimulation in the form of SAE or both.
2. The application of the radiant light baker, whirlpool and SAE, aiding in relieving pain and associated spasm.
3. Emotional stress and anxiety are usually relieved. Satisfying the psyche when the patient can see and feel that something is being done relieves his emotional stress and anxiety. The patient also will have the opportunity to discuss his problems while treatment is being applied.
4. The patient becomes part of the rehabilitation team by implementing at home or in the hospital the progressive resistant exercise program and limb posturing technique, if indicated.

Bruno-Helfand Technique and Methodology

The current of choice should be a non-ionizing one, causing a period of contraction followed by a period of relaxation.

Placement of the electrodes, using a two-circuit electrical stimulator with individual intensity controls, is as follows. Black circuit: place the electrodes of one circuit on the anterior thighs. Red circuit: place the electrodes of the other circuit in the popliteal areas.

The object of placing the electrodes on the anterior thighs and the popliteal areas is to contract the greatest amount of muscle fibers

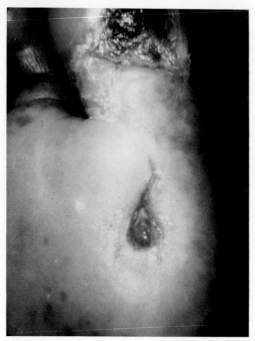

Fig. 14.1 Dry gangrene—pretreatment, vascular etiology.

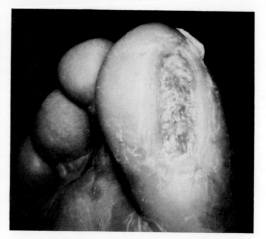

Fig. 14.3 Healing of Fig. 14.1.

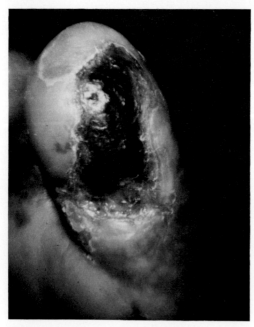

Fig. 14.2 Early treatment phase of Fig. 14.1.

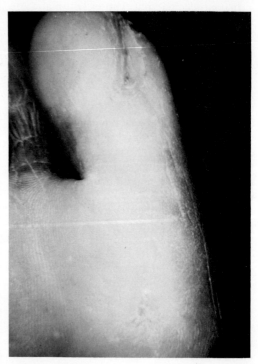

Fig. 14.4 Healing of Fig. 14.1.

in the lower extremities at one time, aiding the circulation. The black circuit over the anterior thighs will cause the large bulk of muscles to contract. The red circuit in the popliteal areas will stimulate the sciatic nerve before and after it divides, contracting the hamstring muscles, portion of the adductor magnus, and all of the muscles below the knee. Concurrently, a radiant light baker, (24 inches in length) is placed over the lower extremities at a medium or low intensity. A good rule of thumb is to apply heat more proximally in direct ratio to the severity of

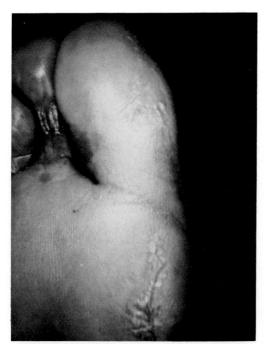

Fig. 14.5   Healing of Fig. 14.1, 1 year later.

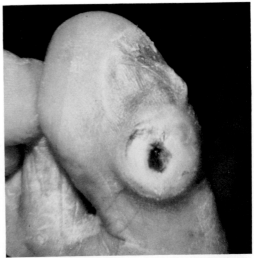

Fig. 14.7   Initial debridement pretreatment, diabetic etiology.

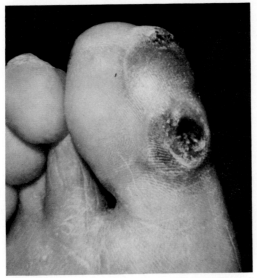

Fig. 14.6   Diabetic ulcer, bulla, hemorrhage and deformity.

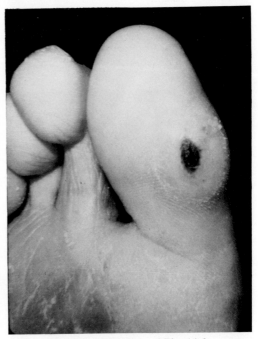

Fig. 14.8   Healing of Fig. 14.6.

the vascular deficiency. If gangrene is threatened, the heat should be used only reflexively. Indirect heating is generally safe and results in reflex vasodilation of the lower extremities. Caution should always be exercised when using heat in any form, because with a poor transportation system, what is normally mild heat becomes a more vigorous heat. When edema is present, a modification of the above technique could be used. The methodology is the same as above except for the use of a short or full leg air splint to provide external counter pressure.

The approach is physiologic. The air splint takes the place of the skin and fascia that

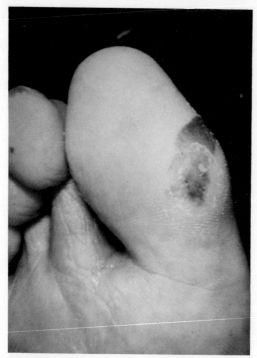

Fig. 14.9   Additional hemorrhage of Fig. 14.6.

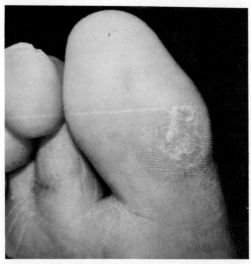

Fig. 14.10   Healing of Fig. 14.6, 1 year later.

have become stretched because of the edema, as well as the lax fascia, as a result of the hypotonic condition of the muscles. Upon each impulse, electricity causes the muscle to contract, pushing against the splint, thereby propelling the fluid cephalically.

A low profile whirlpool (bathtub size) in which the patient sits fulfills the physiologic law of not needing to fight gravity of the dependent position. In the presence of an ulcer, it is used not only for its beneficial effect on the circulation, but also for the purpose of debridement. This is also a kinetic whirlpool in which the patient exercises the lower extremity by flexing and extending at the hip, knee, ankle and toes. This will act as an additional pump for the body's transportation system. Duration of treatment is usually 20 minutes. Temperature of the water may vary with the severity of the vascular insufficiency; the worse the deficiency, the lower the temperature, 93–98°. This procedure is used at the Pennsylvania College of Podiatric Medicine and at the James C. Giuffré Medical Center.

In conclusion, the patient is instructed in a modified progressive resistant exercise program "tailored" to the patient and his condition. Sitting on the treatment table, the patient is asked to extend his leg against a recorded resistance (1 pound, 2 pounds, 5 pounds, etc.) which is attached to his forefoot. When the leg is in full extension, the patient counts audibly 1001, 1002, 1003, 1004 and 1005. To say "1001" takes approximately 1 second, to think it takes much less time. The purpose of speaking 1001 is not only that it takes a second to say, but more importantly, especially with the geriatric patient, that it aids in preventing the Valsalva phenomenon.

The home exercise program is prescribed initially as one set of five repetitions, to be done before breakfast, before lunch, before dinner and before going to bed. Upon subsequent visits, the clinician should have the patient do the exercises in his office, commenting on the performance, increasing the weight resistance, or increasing the number of repetitions. This will demonstrate to the patient the clinician's sincere interest in the importance of the exercise program. Frequency of treatment is 3 times a week. As the patient improves, the frequency can be reduced until the patient can be maintained on a progressive resistance exercise program (PRE).

Trauma Involving the Lower Extremities

In the treatment of trauma, correct body alignment for the erect position is essential, because of the direct pressure of the joints of the lower extremities on one another. Therefore, not only must the involved joint be treated, but also the integrity of the adjacent joints must be protected.

Weight bearing is the fundamental function of the lower extremity; the hip and knee are therefore subservient to the foot. Alterations which occur in the hip, thigh or knee may also be manifest in the foot.

Treatment should be aimed at reducing or preventing the sequela of trauma, such as pain, edema, atrophy, fibrosis, contractures, ankylosis and paralysis. The goal of the treatment is to lessen or minimize further damage due to inactivity imposed upon the patient because of immobilization. The earlier treatment is begun, the better the possible results. Keep the patient ambulatory, if necessary, using assistive devices such as walkers, walkerette, crutches or canes. The method used will be dictated by the condition or the amount of pain.

Usually the treatment for pain is given in order to prepare the patient for the most important part of his treatment: a program of supervised active exercises. Heat, cold, electrical stimulation (stimulation active exercise) or the analgesic current (TENS), massage, ultrasound, and whirlpool are some of the modalities used to prepare the patient for an exercise program. One technique that was found to be successful was to use the low volt generator, using an analgesic current, attached to an electrode over the area of pain; this procedure enables the patient to do more strenuous exercise. We have also used a TENS unit in the same manner with similar results.

"Edema is glue" said Watson-Jones. He also noted that not only immobilization but also functional inactivity produces joint stiffness and adhesions. The degree of atrophy will be dependent upon the length of immobilization and inactivity. There will also be decreased muscle strength.

Being aware of the benefits of cross-education, one should institute muscle strengthening exercises to the adjacent joints and to the unaffected extremity. The unaffected extremity must do all or most of the weight bearing, particularly in fractures or reconstructive surgery.

Strong resistive isometric exercises of the muscles within the cast or splint can be performed safely. Tendonitis, synovitis, fascicular, intrafascicular and intramuscular fibrosis can be prevented by producing motion which affects the muscles and their tendons within the sheath.

Adhesions are one of the most important factors that may affect joint motion and may, if not attacked quickly, produce permanent disability. Aside from the surgical and forced manipulation under anesthesia there are also two conservative approaches: (1) massage, using, basically, friction or digital kneading over scar tissues or other fibrotic or consolidated structures, and (2) passive (stretching) and active resistive exercises. It would be also proper to utilize heat in the form of hot packs, whirlpool, ultrasound, etc., preceding massage or exercises to aid in relieving pain and breaking up of fibrosis by softening scar tissue. The exercises, especially progressive resistive type, not only increase blood supply to the part but also mechanically stretch the affected parts.

If "alienation" occurs because of a physiologic or mental block, the patient cannot activate muscles to produce motion voluntarily. Whether due to fear or pain, the patient cannot be motivated. We have found the following technique to be highly successful. Cut windows in the cast in order to apply electrodes from a low volt generator to stimulate the muscles to move, either as SAE or for muscle reeducation. Following cast removal, we have also used this technique of stimulation active exercise and voluntary active exercise together, using electrical stimulation as a "pacer" for voluntary active exercises.

Paralysis may occur if there is pressure placed upon a nerve, either from the trauma itself or as a result of pressure from splints or plaster on the peroneal nerve, causing a drop foot. A drop foot brace, passive exercise, electrical stimulation and muscle reeducation should be used until function returns, when tests so indicate.

Contracture and ankylosis may occur in any joint of the lower extremity. Residual stiffness may become permanent in the hip, knee, ankle or foot. The plantar fascia and the intrinsics are especially prone to contract after fractures. Other factors that may be involved in permanent disabilities are: an improper exercise program, lack of cooperation, voluntary or involuntary malalignment and joint damage, infection, permanent nerve damage, rheumatic fibrositis or arthritis and myositis ossificans.

There may be many manifestations presented to the clinician if conditions are not ideally corrected. Foot pain with subsequent disability is a common complication of lower extremity fractures. Flexion deformities of the hip or knee will give a shortening effect to the affected lower extremity, resulting in an excessive type gait with increased trauma to the foot, or rotational defects. The feet should be examined for imbalances, callosities, traumatic arthritis, blistering, and possible subsequent infections. If the patient is a diabetic, the above may become magnified due to the added lack of vascular supply, causing an ulcer which may develop necrosis and gangrene, and endanger life itself.

Surgery and Geriatrics

Most physical therapy procedures should be instituted in parallel with surgery. In fact, most times it is advisable to instruct patients in an exercise program before surgery, thereby implanting a posthypnotic suggestion, facilitating postoperative motion as desired. It has the added advantage of not hurting, making the patient willing to listen and learn.

We must set up goals for each procedure, postoperatively.

1. To relieve pain—the use of analgesic inducing modalities such as cold, heat, massage, transcutaneous electrical nerve stimulation and exercise are prescribed as tolerated.

2. To reduce swelling—casting, splinting, bandaging and exercises are used. The exercise program could be voluntary active, and/or stimulation active and limb posturing.

3. To prevent adhesions—a graduated exercise program should be instituted, as early as 1 day postoperatively. The exercises would be isotonic or isometric, or both, depending upon whether the part is in a cast. These could be done either voluntary actively or stimulation actively. Following surgery it is not unusual for a patient's muscles to become "alienated" due to pain, fear of having pain, or apprehension resulting in mental block. SAE will provide the patient with a visual image, mental awareness and kinesthetic information from the muscles, tendons and

joints involved, thereby aiding in the return of his ability to perform voluntary active exercise.

Function of uninvolved parts of the lower extremities must be maintained. Exercise programs should be aimed at the knee and hip to maintain proper alignment of the complete lower extremity.

Early ambulation should be instituted, usually on the first postoperative day. If crutches or walkerette are to be used, the patient should be instructed and supervised for both level walking and stair climbing.

The three point crutch gait is the easiest and safest crutch gait to use for nonweight bearing on one lower extremity. As healing progresses, the patient is instructed in partial to full weight bearing crutch gaits.

Bunionectomy

Mobilize the limb as early as possible without jeopardizing healing. Relieve pain before exercises, by using whirlpool, heat, massage, electrical stimulation, etc. The exercise program should be aimed at restoring function of the toes and foot and, finally, comfortable ambulation. The following exercise is designed to improve or restore plantar flexion and dorsiflexion of the toes.

1. Stand on a step, board or book with metatarsal heads in line with the edge.
2. Curl toes down and maintain them in the flexed position for the audible count of 1001, 1002, 1003, 1004 and 1005.
3. Relax for at least the count of 1001 to 1005; the patient may take more time if needed.
4. Extend toes and maintain for an audible count of 1001 to 1005.
5. Relax as in step 3.

This exercise may be augmented, when the surgeon feels that it is feasible, with toe raise. Frequency: three sets of five repetitions, before breakfast, lunch, dinner and before bedtime. If function is not restored in the great toe both plantarly and dorsally, a podalgic gait will result.

Arthritis

Whether arthritis is caused by trauma, inflammation, poor posture, strain, stress, infection, degeneration, congenital abnormalities, metabolic, neurologic or endocrine disturbances, physical therapy treatment should be instituted both during and after the diagnostic procedures and parallel to medical treatment.

The objectives of physical therapy are to relieve pain, maintain or improve range of motion, maintain or improve maximum muscle power in muscles about the affected joints and to prevent deformity.

The basic approach to treatment is rest by splinting or casting, and controlled exercise. Cold is used in some acute forms of arthritis, but heat in various forms is more commonly used. Treatments include heated tub baths, whirlpool, contrast baths, hot compresses, paraffin, ultrasound, diathermy or radiant light baking. Other forms of physical therapy used have been iontophoresis, phonophoresis, light massage and electrical stimulation using both the sensory effects (TENS) the kinetic currents (SAE) and active and passive exercises as tolerated. While the patient is immobilized in splints or casts, he should be taught to do isometric exercises in an attempt to maintain muscle strength and also benefit from the concomitant effects of muscle contraction. The treatment of arthritis is for the relief of pain and spasm in preparation for a therapeutic exercise program. Exercise is the key to the treatment of arthritis. It is imperative that the joint mobility be maintained at least passively. Muscle strength can always be improved, but if joint motion is lost, even with normal muscle strength joint motion may not be regained. If it is possible to actively or passively put a joint through its full range of motion at least once a day, full joint mobility will be maintained, preventing capsular and tendinous tightening.

In the convalescent and chronic stages, a graduated exercise program to combat prolonged bed rest, maintain or restore range of motion and prevent muscle atrophy should be initiated.

The proper balance between rest and exercise, though difficult to achieve, should be tried. If, following exercise or other physical activity, there is resultant pain and stiffness persisting without gradual remission over a 12-hour period or longer, the tolerance of the joint was probably exceeded and the activity to such a degree should be decreased. Use heat or cold, rest and passive motion to the joint as a palliative measure.

Correct body alignment for the erect position is essential because of the direct effect of the joints of the lower extremities on each other. If the knee develops a flexion contracture, the hip and ankle will attempt to compensate by flexing at the hip and plantar flexing at the ankle.

If the patient is in severe pain, or if there is a significant residual articular damage, then aids to ambulation such as crutches, canes, braces and molded shoes should be used to increase the stability of the joint or protect it from further damage.

Early ambulation should be instituted if possible and, if crutch walking is indicated, the proper crutch gait should be taught and supervised. For example, if both feet are painful, the crutch gait of choice would be four point alternate gait.

Some self-help devices:
1. Firm mattress
2. Rubber shoelaces
3. Zippered shoes
4. Velcro fasteners
5. Long handled shoe horns
6. Device for putting on socks or stockings
7. Adapted chairs and toilet seats
8. Wall bars for tub or toilet
9. Wheelchairs with special attachments
10. Crutches, with modifications, such as platform type, canes with large hand grip, etc.
11. Special large hand grip for forks, spoons, knives, combination knife and fork, etc.

Geriatric Hemiplegic Patient

1. Inspect the uninvolved extremity for range of motion and strength and prescribe an exercise program to counteract disuse syndrome.
2. Inspect the hemiplegic lower extremity; examine for range of motion, both active and passive, at the hip, knee, foot and ankle.
3. Prevent secondary contractures; most common contractures result from external rotation of the hip, hip and knee flexion, equinus and varus.
4. Look for any local manifestations on the foot because of the altered gait pattern.
5. Prescribe a proper fitting shoe and drop foot brace, if indicated.

6. Institute neurophysiologic approaches to the therapeutic exercise program.
7. Reassure the family that most hemiplegic patients respond better when they are incorporated into "regular family life."
8. Maintain the patient at maximum functional level and continue professional supervision for as long as he has some residual disability. This program may continue for the remainder of the patient's life. It is intended primarily to prevent contractures and other possible complications, which can be insidious and sometimes catastrophic. Maintaining function is beneficial to the psyche as well.
9. Look for possible preexisting disabilities such as arthritis, old fractures, peripheral vascular disease, diabetes, osteoporosis, or simple corn. A painful corn can and has delayed ambulation of the hemiplegic as well as the podiatric patient.

Crutch Gaits

There are a number of standard crutch gaits. The most suitable crutch gait for the geriatric patient should be a slow and safe gait. The patient should be instructed to keep his crutches in front of him and to take small steps.

The patient's condition will dictate the type of gait most suitable for him. When a patient's condition dictates nonweight bearing on one lower extremity, postoperatively, because of fractures, casts, etc., then the following crutch gait is indicated.

Three Point Alternate Crutch Gait

Crutch, foot sequence:
1. Right crutch
2. Left crutch
3. Lift or shuffle unaffected foot.

This is a safe gait because there are always two points on the floor. Many times if the patient's balance is very good, he will automatically do a swing through crutch gait. When a patient's condition dictates partial weight bearing on one lower extremity, because of a fracture, postoperative weakness or paralysis, the following crutch gait would be indicated.

Three Point Simultaneous Crutch Gait

Crutch, foot sequence:
1. Both crutches and affected extremity
2. Stronger or unaffected extremity

The amount of weight placed on the affected extremity can be varied depending upon the amount of weight placed on the hand grips of the crutches.

When a patient's condition dictates partial weight bearing on one side and then the other, such as trauma, arthritis or weakness bilaterally, the following crutch gait would be indicated.

Four Point Alternate Crutch Gait

Crutch, foot sequence:
1. Right crutch
2. Left foot
3. Left crutch
4. Right foot

This crutch gait is a very safe gait because there are always three points of support on the floor.

Measuring Crutches

1. Crutch length is measured from just below the axilla to 4 inches lateral to the foot.
2. To measure for position of hand grip, elbow should be flexed 30°.
3. There should be a space of two fingers between the axilla and the axillary bar of the crutches.

Measuring Cane or Walkerette

A cane or walkerette is measured from the floor to the greater trochanter. If there is contracture or ankylosis of the elbow, one should measure from the wrist to the floor. The cane is used on the opposite side of the affected part, except when the upper limb is affected.

Cane gait

Cane, Foot Sequence:
1. Advance cane, on unaffected side and affected foot simultaneously.
2. Advance unaffected foot in front of affected foot.

Walkerette

Place the walkerette in front of the patient, leading with the weaker extremity, if any, and follow with the other extremity, placing one foot in front of the other. Avoid canes or walkerettes with wheels for the geriatric patient, because they require greater coordination.

Safeguards when the patient is at home on crutches:

1. Stairs: remember that the good extremity goes up (to heaven) and the bad extremity goes down (to hell).
2. If the cast is too heavy or if the patient is weak, elevate the shoe (on unaffected side) high enough that it can clear the floor.
3. Remove small rugs, toys, lamp cords, clothing, etc., from the area the crutch walker is using.
4. Avoid water and oil spills in the home or street.
5. Do not walk in dark rooms, turn on bright lights.
6. When the patient is about to sit on a chair, be sure he can feel the edge of the chair against the back of his leg.

Prescribing Physical Therapy

Just as much care should be given to the prescription of physical therapy as an internist gives when prescribing a specific drug or combination of drugs. Because it is very difficult to assess the patient's tolerance for a physical therapy modality, especially exercise, it is best to prescribe as follows:

1. Diagnosis (Figs. 14.11 and 14.12).
2. Precautions: diabetes, heart disease, hypertension, blindness, loss of hearing, with fractures—full, partial or non-weight bearing.
3. Goals: decrease pain, decrease swelling, increase ROM, increase strength, gait training.
4. Identify the part or parts to be treated.
5. Frequency of treatment: daily, 3 times a week, twice a week for 1, 2, 3 or 4 weeks.
6. Schedule a return date of referring practitioner within 30 days.

DIAGNOSTIC CATEGORIES AND SOME SUGGESTED MODALITIES

Many different methods have been described in this chapter; some can be used alone, and others may be used in combination. The choice of method depends on a variety of factors, the two most important being the age of the patient and the site and extent of the lesion. The details of the treatment will depend upon understanding the significant factors of the physiologic, pathologic and psychologic aspects of each case.

Abscess

1. Hot compresses—Hydrocolator packs, etc.
2. Infrared
3. Ultraviolet rays—local and general (for associated debilitation if indicated)
4. Whirlpool—povidone-iodine
5. Diathermy—microwave, short wave
6. Ultrasound
7. Controlled ROM exercises

Adhesions and Scars

1. Exercise—(stretching) passive and active resistive
2. Electrical stimulation (SAE)
3. Massage (especially digital kneading)
4. Ultrasound
5. NaCl iontophoresis
6. Diathermy
7. Infrared
8. Whirlpool
9. Hot compresses

Amputation

1. Preprosthetic training
2. Shrinking of stump
   a. Bandaging
   b. Stump shrinker
3. Range of motion
   a. ROM exercises
   b. Muscle strengthening exercises
4. Exercises after healing—intensification of step 3.
   a. Massage to prevent adhesions of skin to bone which would result in breakdown of skin with concomitant complications of infections, inability to ambulate, ulcers, etc.
5. Pain
   a. TENS
   b. Electrical stimulation
   c. Heat
   d. Cold
   e. Ultrasound
   f. Massage

JAMES C. GIUFFRÉ MEDICAL CENTER

REQUEST FOR PHYSICAL THERAPY CONSULTATION

Name _____ _____ _____ Age _____ Sex _____
              (last)   (first)   (middle)

Address _____

Referred By: _____ Frequency _____ Date _____

Diagnosis: _____
_____

Precautions _____

Goals _____
_____
_____

Physical Therapy Plan: _____
_____
_____

Date	PHYSICAL THERAPY PROGRESS NOTES

Fig. 14.11   Request form for physical therapy consultation—outpatient.

Arteriosclerosis Obliterans

1. Bruno-Helfand technique
   a. Electrical stimulation (SAE)
   b. Radiant light baker (RLB)
   c. Exercises (PRE)
   d. Whirlpool (kinetic)
2. Iontophoresis: histamine, mecholyl, (vasodilating drugs that ionize)
3. Intermittent venous occlusions (Jobst)
4. Contrast bath

Arthritis

1. Exercise—active and passive, as indicated
2. Warm compresses

JAMES C. GIUFFRÉ MEDICAL CENTER
Girard Avenue at Eighth Street
Philadelphia, Pennsylvania 19122

PHYSICAL THERAPY DEPARTMENT

NAME _____ RACE _____ AGE _____ SEX ____ RM # _____
    (last)   (first)   (middle)

ADDRESS _____ REFERRED BY: _____

DIAGNOSIS (on admission) _____ ADM. DATE: _____

DIAGNOSIS (parts to be treated by Physical Therapy) _____

PRECAUTIONS (diabetes, cardio-vascular, weight-bearing, surgery, etc.) _____

PHYSICAL THERAPY PRESCRIPTION (express in terms of goals) _____

CONSULTATION FOR PHYSICAL THERAPY PLAN (by Physical Therapist) _____

APPROVED BY REFERRING PHYSICIAN: _____

(Referring physician's signature)

COMMENTS, CHANGES, ETC: _____

Fig. 14.12 Request form for physical therapy consultation—inpatient.

3. Electrical stimulation (SAE and TENS)
4. Whirlpool (kinetic)
5. Infrared (RLB)
6. Massage
7. Paraffin
8. Ultrasound (phonophoresis)
9. Iontophoresis (histamine, iodine, etc.)
10. Acute—cold compresses, ice

Atrophy

1. Exercise—passive, active assistive, voluntary active, active resistive
2. Electrical stimulation (SAE)
3. Massage

Buerger's Disease

1. Bruno-Helfand technique
   a. Electrical stimulation

b. RLB
c. PRE
d. Whirlpool (kinetic)
2. Intermittent venous occlusions (Jobst)

Burns

1. Whirlpool (povidone-iodine) (kinetic)
2. Exercises—active (and passive, as indicated)
3. Ultraviolet ray

Bursitis

1. Ultrasound
2. Ice (acute)
3. Rest
4. ROM (once daily, passively)
5. Iontophoresis (procaine, iodine)
6. Infrared
7. Exercises—following acute phase
8. Paraffin
9. Diathermy
10. Massage
11. Electrical stimulation
12. Whirlpool

Callosities—Corns

1. Correct faulty shoe or poor foot mechanics
2. Orthotic device, if indicated
3. Exercises to implement function of device
4. Pain
   a. Whirlpool
   b. TENS
   c. Warm compresses
   d. Infrared
   e. Electrical stimulation

Causalgia

1. TENS
2. Exercises—as tolerated
3. Cold compresses
4. Electrical stimulation (SAE)
5. Limb posturing

Cellulitis

1. Warm compresses (continuous, if possible)
2. Infrared
3. Whirlpool (povidone-iodine)
4. Passive motion gently to maintain range of motion

Cerebral Palsy

1. Should be treated for any local manifestations podiatrically
2. Neurophysiologic approaches to therapeutic exercises, such as facilitation techniques, etc.
3. Any method you have had with any degree of success

Chilblains

1. Whirlpool—cool (kinetic) (90–93°)
2. Electrical stimulation (SAE)
3. Intermittent venous occlusion
4. Exercise

Contraction of Gastrocsoleus Complex

1. Heat—preceding exercises
2. Stretching exercise
3. Muscle strengthening exercises to dorsoflexors (antagonists)
4. Electrical stimulation (SAE)
5. Night splint

Contractures

1. Warm compresses
2. Infrared
3. Whirlpool (kinetic)
4. Paraffin
5. Diathermy
6. Ultrasound
7. Massage
8. Electrical stimulation (SAE)
9. Exercises
   a. Passive for stretching and increasing ROM
   b. Voluntary active to strengthen both antagonists and agonists to break up intrafascicular and interfascicular fibrositis

Contusions

1. Acute—cold
   a. Compresses
   b. Ice
2. Exercises
3. Whirlpool (kinetic)
4. Warm compresses
5. Infrared
6. Massage
7. Paraffin
8. Diathermy
9. Ultrasound

Decubitus

Usually heels and lateral malleoli
1. Whirlpool (povidone-iodine) (kinetic)
2. Electrical stimulation (SAE or vascular technique)
3. Ultraviolet
4. Exercises
5. Limb posturing

Disc Etiology Cramps

1. Electrical stimulation—lumbosacral area, leg and foot
2. Infrared
3. Exercises for low back

Dupuytren's Contracture

1. Ultrasound
2. Stretching exercises
3. Strengthening exercises to antagonists (PRE)
4. Iontophoresis (NaCl)
5. Massage
6. Warm compresses
7. Infrared

Eczema

1. UVR (Ultra violet ray)
2. Medicated baths

Epidermophytosis—Athlete's Foot

1. $CuSO_4$ iontophoresis
2. Ultraviolet ray
3. Good foot hygiene and shoe hygiene

Felon

1. Warm compresses
2. Whirlpool (povidone-iodine)
3. Ultraviolet ray
4. Maintain range of motion

Fibromyositis

1. Ultrasound
2. Massage (digital)
3. Exercise (active and passive)
4. Paraffin
5. Infrared
6. Hot compresses
7. Whirlpool (kinetic)
8. Diathermy
9. Electrical stimulation (SAE)

Frostbite: Immersion Foot, Trench Foot

1. Whirlpool 90–93° (kinetic)
2. Exercise while in whirlpool as well as out
3. Intermittent venous occlusions
4. Electrical stimulation (SAE or vascular)
5. Contrast bath

Fractures

1. Exercises—passive, active assistive, voluntary active and active resistive, isometric in cast
2. Whirlpool (kinetic)
3. Electrical stimulation (SAE)
4. Infrared (RLB)
5. Hot compresses
6. Paraffin
7. Intermittent venous occlusions
8. Massage

Furuncle

1. Hot compresses
2. Infrared
3. Diathermy
4. Whirlpool
5. Ultraviolet ray

Gangrene

1. Whirlpool (povidone-iodine) 93–95°
2. Reflex heating—abdomen and low back
3. Electrical stimulation (SAE)
4. Exercise—mild
5. Ultrasound—paravertebrally
6. Iontophoresis (procaine)
7. Massage—not acute

Hallux Valgus

1. Orthotic device
2. Ultrasound to painful area
3. Whirlpool (kinetic)
4. Electrical stimulation
5. Exercise

Hematoma

1. Acute—cold
2. Hot compresses
3. Whirlpool (kinetic)
4. Infrared
5. Ultrasound—not acute
6. Massage
7. Exercises—not acute
8. Electrical stimulation—not acute

Herpetic Neuritis

1. TENS
2. Ultrasound
3. Galvanism
4. Cold
5. Ultraviolet ray
6. Electrical stimulation (analgesic currents, such as TENS)

Hyperhidrosis

1. $CuSO_4$ iontophoresis (+)
2. $MgSO_4$ iontophoresis (+)
3. Foot and shoe hygiene

Intermittent Claudication

1. Bruno-Helfand technique
   a. Electrical stimulation
   b. Radiant light baker
   c. Progressive resistant exercise
   d. Whirlpool (kinetic)
2. Iontophoresis
3. Intermittent venous occlusion
4. Therapeutic walking
5. Diathermy—reflex heating

Joint Stiffness

1. Mobilization techniques
2. Exercise
3. Whirlpool (kinetic)
4. Massage
5. Hot compresses
6. Infrared
7. Ultrasound
8. Electrical stimulation

Ligament and Fascial Strain

1. Kinetic whirlpool (foot, toe and ankle exercises, done while in whirlpool)
2. Ultrasound—acute—low intensity
3. Massage
4. Orthotic device and exercise
5. Electrical stimulation

Metatarsalgia

1. Electrical stimulation
2. Massage
3. Exercise
4. Whirlpool
5. Ultrasound
6. Orthotic device and exercise

Morton's Neuroma

Following surgery—residual symptoms, usually due to physiologic splinting causing fibrosis and secondary contracture of muscles of the foot and ankle, especially the intrinsics.

1. Electrical stimulation
2. Infrared
3. Exercise—active and passive
4. Whirlpool (kinetic)
5. Ultrasound

Multiple Sclerosis

1. Should be treated for any local manifestation podiatrically
2. Neurophysiologic approach to therapeutic exercises

Muscle Cramps

Due to other than vascular disease, such as fatigue, trauma

1. Whirlpool
2. Rest
3. Electrical stimulation
4. massage
5. Exercises to improve endurance

Muscle Spasms

1. Electrical stimulation
2. Infrared (RLB)
3. Exercises
4. Massage
5. Diathermy
6. Cold
   a. Ice massage
   b. Compresses
   c. Ethyl chloride spray—do not frost skin
   d. Fluoromethane
7. Whirlpool (kinetic)

Muscular Dystrophy

1. Should be treated for any local manifestation podiatrically
2. Exercise

Myalgia

1. Whirlpool (kinetic)
2. Infrared
3. Hot compresses
4. Massage
5. Ultrasound

6. Diathermy
7. Exercise
8. Paraffin
9. Electrical stimulation
10. Iontophoresis
11. Cold

Myositis

1. Compresses
2. Infrared
3. Whirlpool (kinetic)
4. Cold compresses
5. Ultrasound
6. Diathermy
7. Massage (digital kneading)
8. Electrical stimulation
9. Exercises
10. Iontophoresis

Myositis Ossificans

1. Ultrasound
2. Diathermy
3. Exercises to maintain or increase ROM

Neuralgia

1. TENS
2. Cold
3. Warm compresses
4. Infrared
5. Massage
6. Ultrasound
7. Electrical stimulation
8. Controlled exercise

Neuritic Pain in Scar Tissue

1. Digital kneading
2. Ice massage
3. Stretching exercises and PRE to antagonists
4. Ultrasound
5. NaCl iontophoresis (negative pole active)
6. TENS
7. Electrical stimulation

Nevus

1. Electrodessication
2. Electrocoagulation
3. Surgical galvanism (negative pole)
4. CO_2 snow

Osteomyelitis

1. Whirlpool (povidone-iodine)
2. Ultraviolet ray
3. Controlled exercise

Paresis or Paralysis

1. Infrared
2. Whirlpool and hydrogymnastics
3. Electrical stimulation
4. Exercises
   a. Passive—maintain ROM
   b. Active assistive
   c. Voluntary active
   d. Active resistive
5. Massage

Paronychia

1. Whirlpool (povidone—iodine)
2. Ultraviolet ray
3. Hot compresses
4. Good foot hygiene

Periostitis

1. Whirlpool
2. Warm compresses
3. Diathermy
4. Ultrasound
5. Cold
6. Controlled exercises

Peripheral Nerve Lesion

1. Warm compresses
2. Infrared
3. Whirlpool
4. Massage
5. Electrical stimulation
6. Exercises
7. Bracing

Peripheral Vascular Disease

1. Bruno-Helfand technique
   a. Electrical stimulation
   b. RLB
   c. Exercise as tolerated
   d. Whirlpool—low profile, if available
2. Short wave diathermy—reflex heating to lower back and pelvis
3. Ultrasound—paravertebrally
4. Intermittent venous occlusions
5. Iontophoresis

Phlebitis

1. Warm compresses
2. Infrared
3. Whirlpool
4. Controlled exercise if patient is ambulatory

Plantar Fasciitis

1. Electrical stimulation
2. Ultrasound
3. Whirlpool (kinetic)
4. Rest
5. Exercises when feasible
6. Paraffin
7. Cold
8. Massage

Plantar Wart

1. Ultrasound
2. Electrosurgery

Poliomyelitis (Anterior)

1. Kenny hot packs
2. Bracing when indicated
3. Exercises—muscle reeducation

Pruritus

1. Ultraviolet ray
2. Medicated baths

Psoriasis

1. Goeckerman's   technique—ultraviolet ray

Raynaud's

1. Bruno-Helfand technique
   a. Electrical stimulation
   b. RLB
   c. Exercises—PRE—therapeutic walking
   d. Whirlpool (kinetic)
2. Iontophoresis
3. Intermittent venous occlusions

Scars

Same as adhesions

Scleroderma

1. Bruno-Helfand technique
   a. Electrical stimulation
   b. RLB
   c. Exercise as tolerated, PRE

2. Iontophoresis
3. Intermittent venous occlusions

Sensitivity of Soles of Feet

Following prolonged bed rest or immobilization in plaster.
1. Prevention by exercise in bed or in cast
2. Stimulation active exercises by electrical stimulation
3. Check for secondary contracture of gastrocsoleus complex, stretching exercises, ROM exercises as tolerated
4. Whirlpool (kinetic)

Sprain

1. Ice—acute
2. Immobilization, casting, strapping
3. Isometric exercises in cast or when joint motion causes pain
4. Whirlpool (kinetic)
5. Ultrasound
6. Hot compresses
7. Infrared
8. Paraffin
9. Diathermy
10. Massage
11. Iontophoresis
12. Isotonic exercises (PRE)
13. Electrical stimulation

Strain

1. Immobilization, cast, strapping
2. Isometric exercises in cast
3. Whirlpool (kinetic)
4. Ultrasound
5. Electrical stimulation
6. Ice—acute
7. Hot compresses
8. Infrared
9. Paraffin
10. Diathermy
11. Massage
12. Iontophoresis
13. Isotonic exercises (PRE)

Stump

See Amputation

Sudeck's Atrophy

1. Electrical stimulation, SAE
2. Whirlpool—cool (92–94°) (kinetic)
3. Exercises as tolerated

Swelling—Depending upon Etiology

1. Limb posture
2. Bruno-Helfand technique
   a. Electrical stimulation
   b. RLB
   c. Exercises—PRE
   d. Whirlpool (low profile—kinetic)
3. Massage
4. Intermittent venous occlusions
5. Paraffin

Synovitis

1. Ultrasound (phonophoresis)
2. Hot compresses
3. Whirlpool
4. Infrared (RLB)
5. Paraffin
6. Exercises
7. Electrical stimulation
8. Cold

Tendon Repair or Transplant

1. Ice—first 24 hours
2. Electrical stimulation (SAE)—mild
3. Isometric exercises
4. Isotonic exercises
5. Whirlpool (kinetic)
6. Infrared

Tenosynovitis

1. Ultrasound—phonophoresis
2. Electrical stimulation (TENS)
3. Immobilization cast, strapping
4. Ice (acute)
5. Hot compresses
6. Whirlpool
7. Infrared
8. Iontophoresis

Thrombophlebitis

If bedridden:
1. Warm compresses
2. Infrared
3. Iontophoresis
If ambulatory:
1. Warm compresses
2. Infrared (RLB)
3. Iontophoresis
4. Electrical stimulation
5. Exercises as tolerated
6. Whirlpool

Trigger Points

1. Electrical stimulation
2. Ice
3. Ultrasound
4. Ethyl chloride spray
5. Fluoromethane

Ulcers

1. Bruno-Helfand technique
   a. Electrical stimulation
   b. RLB (radiant light baker)
   c. Exercise, PRE
   d. Whirlpool, (low profile—kinetic)
2. Ultraviolet
3. Ultrasound (under water to ulcer) or paravertebrally
4. Iontophoresis
5. Intermittent venous occlusions
6. Diathermy, reflex heating
7. Infrared, RLB

Vascular Deficiencies

1. Intermittent claudication, etc.
2. Bruno-Helfand technique
   a. Electrical stimulation
   b. RLB
   c. PRE
   d. Whirlpool (kinetic)
3. Iontophoresis
4. Intermittent venous occlusions
5. Diathermy (reflex heating)
6. Ultrasound—paravertebrally

Verruca Vulgaris Plantaris

1. Electrodessication
2. Electrocoagulation
3. Surgical galvanism (negative)
4. Ultrasound

CONCLUSION

All patients, especially the geriatric patient, should be treated with reverence and dignity.

Treat the patient as a whole person. Do not use the patient's first name, it can be demeaning. Many dislike being called "Mother," "Dad," etc.

Treat the patient with compassion, he or she will know you care.

Treat the patient by making him a part of your rehabilitation team, telling him how important he is in his own recovery. And finally, when your patient is in pain, and is troubled, BE THERE, LISTEN, AND TOUCH.

chapter 15

Pharmacologic Considerations for Elderly Patients[a]

Bruce I. Weiner, Pharm. D., D.P.M.

Today's practitioner sees a spectrum of pathological conditions in his day-to-day practice. Often overlooked, however, is the range of patients treated. Traditionally, we have thought of only three age groups of patients and have limited therapeutics to age only. We must recognize that there is a fourth age category of the geriatric or senior and that there are many more criteria for therapeutics than age alone.

In this chapter, I will attempt to discuss many of the areas traditionally overlooked by many practitioners, primary care and specialists alike. We will be looking at the nutrition of the geriatric patient, many of the drug interactions seen in this group and how this class of patient should be viewed so as not to expect the causes and effects seen in others.

The initial source for patient information about symptoms, medications taken, and drug reactions is the patient himself. Patients and, more specifically, geriatric patients may be using more than one physician, numerous specialists, and more than one source for obtaining their medications.

We must be aware of these facts when taking an initial history. This aspect is as important as our physical examination and cannot be minimized. A family practitioner may have prescribed Dyazide[b] for a patient's hypertension. This same patient sees another practitioner for stasis dermatitis. As part of the treatment regimen he may wish to use a diuretic to decrease the edema. He asks the patient if she is taking any "water pills." She replies that she is not. The thiazide component in the Dyazide may be missed because of this confusion about the drug's indications. This is an example of problems that can be minimized if we always obtain a complete drug history, and stay familiar with the latest changes in the area of pharmaceutics.

THERAPEUTIC CONSIDERATIONS

Often, the geriatric patient seen for a foot problem is taking more than one medication. This consideration alone is important when one thinks of adding an additional pharmacologic agent. Interactions between drugs are commonplace and entire texts have been devoted to this subject alone. Many of the more frequently seen problems will be discussed in this chapter. Interactions, as will also be discussed, can be in the form of potentiation, where one drug can increase the activity of another. Some drugs are antagonists to one another, and the effect may be decreased

---

[a] Drugs mentioned by the author are done so for discussion purposes and with regard to current practice and policies. It should not be inferred that lists are complete, or discussions inclusive. For that information refer to appropriate reference texts. Doses mentioned are only for comparison and depict the normal adult dose in use today. For complete information refer to appropriate references.

[b] Dyazide—trademark of Smith Kline & French Laboratories.

when given concomitantly. These effects can be minor or absolute, where one drug would totally inactivate the action of another. As mentioned, in geriatric medicine multiple daily doses of drugs are commonplace and it behooves the practitioner to know all there is about this area of pharmacologic interaction, for the possibility exists for not only inactivation of drugs, but for lethal iatrogenic combinations.

There is more than one excellent text in this area and some have monthly revisions. The federal government is also trying a method of collecting data in this area from practitioners, but is encountering some problems. Lastly, never minimize a patient's comments related to drug therapy. An individual even in his lay state still is the best source of information about the occurrences within his body. To negate a patient's concern is analogous to ignoring a clinical finding of yours, and in today's world of medical-legal practice these cannot be minimized.

Nutrition

Nutrition, though traditionally thought by many, to be an extension of nursing care, should be included in the realm of pharmacology. There are many investigations that are concerned about diet and nutrients and their effect on drugs and drug therapy.

Proper nutrition has been referenced as far back as Hippocrates, the father of medicine (460–370 B.C.), who is said to have considered the diet as a very important part of a patient's therapeutic regimen. There must be a proper balance of proteins, carbohydrates and lipids. The geriatric patient is able to store essential factors less efficiently than younger adults and the need here is very important. The older patient frequently demonstrates vitamin and other essential element deficiencies than can not only prevent normal responses to medications and healing but create distinct pathologic states on their own.

Vitamins were originally thought of as nutrients but are better classified as separate entities when given in separate dose regimens. The vitamin class can be divided into lipid soluble and water soluble groups. Neither can be totally synthesized in the body. Vitamins A, D, E and K are lipid soluble and as such can be stored by the body for later use. Vitamins C and B complex are water soluble and cannot be stored.

Lipid Soluble Group

Vitamin A (usual adult dosage—50,000 IU daily) contributes to the maintenance of normal skin appearance and a deficiency of this vitamin results in a hard, keratinized skin that is prone to infection. An excess of the vitamin can cause skin peeling and flaking and some vague pains in the long bones of the body. The availability of this drug in a water soluble form relates to its transport media not to its in vivo effect.

Vitamin D (usual adult dosage—50,000 IU daily) is essential for the maintenance of normal bony states and blood levels of the bony constituents. A decrease in this vitamin results in an impairment of bone, mineralizations and even pathologic fractures, while an abundance can result in increased calcification of the bones and soft tissues.

Vitamin E (usual adult dosage—400 IU daily). This vitamin's needs have not been completely understood to date, but it seems to act at many different organ system levels. A significant decrease in this vitamin experimentally may cause hemolytic anemia in the young, while an overabundance may retard bony growth in the young.

Vitamin K (usual dosage—5 mg. daily) is essential in the normal coagulation of blood and alterations in vitamin K level can be predicted. A decrease will decrease the blood's coagulation ability, and an increase above normal can cause hemolytic anemia and jaundice, as well as toxicity to red blood cell membranes.

It should be repeated at this juncture that these lipid soluble vitamins can be stored so that a cumulative overdose is possible even after the drugs are discontinued and, further, that high doses of this group are even more dangerous than the water soluble variety. This condition has been termed hypervitaminosis.

Water Soluble Group

The normal adult usage of ascorbic acid is 500 mg. daily).

Ascorbic acid (vitamin C) is needed for the maintenance of normal skin and wound healing as well as for the maintenance of blood vessel strength and functions. A deficiency of this vitamin has been classically described by many and termed scurvy. One finds a generalized weakness, inflamed joints, diseases of the gums and teeth, delayed wound healing and muscle cramping.

Because it is easily flushed from the body overdoses of vitamin C are difficult to see but with the advent of megavitamin therapy kidney stones and false positive glucose tolerance tests have been reported.

Vitamin B_1—thiamine (normal adult dosage—100 mg. daily) is essential, as are most of the "B" group in maintenance of normal neural function, especially the peripheral nerves. A classic description of thiamine deficiency is seen with beriberi, and accompanied by nausea, disorderly thinking, edema of the lower extremities or paralysis of the lower extremities, termed the "dry" type as seen with chronic alcoholics.

Vitamin B_2—riboflavin (normal adult dosage 25 mg. daily). A patient with this deficiency can exhibit a cheilosis around the mouth edges and glossitis of the tongue, as well as a dry scaly skin.

Vitamin B_3—niacin (nicotinic acid) (normal adult dosage 100 mg. daily). This vitamin is also essential and a marked deficiency has been described as pellagra that exhibits the 3Ds: dermatitis, diarrhea and dementia. An excess amount acts as a peripheral superficial vasodilator with the resultant flushing of the skin.

Vitamin B_5—pantothenic acid (normal adult dosage—100 mg. daily as calcium pantothenate). A decrease of B_5 can cause leg cramps and hand/foot paresthesia.

Vitamin B_6—pyridoxine (normal adult dosage—50 mg. daily). A deficit of this vitamin can cause dermatitis, weakness and neuritis.

Vitamin B_9—folic acid (normal adult dosage—1 mg. daily) deficiency is exhibited as megaloblastic anemia; some growth retardations are seen with inadequate amounts.

Vitamin B_{12}—cyanocobalamin (normal adult dosage—25 mcg. daily) deficiency is exhibited as megaloblastic pernicious anemia.

Vitamin H—biotin (normal adult dosage—300 mcg.). A deficit can cause dermatitis and muscle pain.

Minerals

Potassium (normal adult usage—25 mEq. daily) is generally used as the chloride salt. This mineral is generally deficient in the elderly. Potassium is found in citrus fruits and milk. These foods are not popular with the aged. Diuretics and diarrhea may cause potassium loss.

Calcium (normal adult usage—650 mg. daily) as a salt is essential in bone metabolism. With a decrease frequently osteoporosis is seen, but it is difficult to relate calcium levels to osteoporosis. The elderly are not in the sun as often as younger groups (vitamin D factor) and do not consume as much milk, which may account for the pathology seen in this age group.

Zinc—as the sulfate (normal adult usage—660 mg. daily) has been discussed in the literature relative to wound and tissue healing. Impure zinc oxide (calamine) is reported in the literature as early as 1550 B.C. and in people with delayed wound healing. Studies are trying to correlate decreased zinc levels with this disorder.

Alcoholics exhibit low zinc levels, but once again the etiology may be difficult to ascertain. Hospitalized patients exhibit low zinc levels which are probably a major factor in tissue repair and prolonged hospital stays.

We find that food habits may be among the firmest of our lifestyle habits. Immigrants rapidly change their clothes and language, but not foods. This finding may serve to preserve vitamin deficient diets among family members. It should also be noted at this juncture that all medications, including vitamins, are best prescribed on a mg./kg. basis. The normal doses listed are for generic comparison.

Geriatric Pathology Practice Techniques

Initially we might ask why are geriatrics any different from the general adult population? They are older but does that matter so much? Probably not. However, the question does raise many others. How does the geriatric patient differ from the general adult population in his response to therapy? Concerning nutrients, the geriatric may have a poor appetite because he has fewer teeth, so his food selections are fewer. His smell and taste sensations are lessened and he may have less coordination, making it more difficult to hold and use eating utensils.

Certain drugs may interfere with nutrients and cause problems with the elderly such as:

1. Steroids with vitamin A, C, D, B_6 and zinc

2. Tetracyclines with vitamin C, K and zinc
3. Chloral hydrate with vitamin B$_6$ and zinc

The senior individual is more likely to develop infections than is his younger counterpart and the antibiotics used and abused are constantly being compromised by new strains of resistant organisms, especially in the hospital environment. A patient's lower extremity is constantly showered with bacteria and so the risk of infection is usually greater at that site. This age group may experience more exposure to corticosteroids, which increases the risk of infection due to the immunosuppressive activity of the drug. Use of alternate day therapy may reduce some of the effects generally seen with this class of drugs. Several recent studies have shown that more than 50% of the elderly do not take drugs as prescribed, obviously accounting for varied responses.

It would be better if the practitioner used written prescription instructions over oral ones. Instructing patients to use a calendar helps, as does a suggestion to put their daily regimen of "pills" in a separate vial so there is no doubt whether or not they have taken them. The practitioner writing medications for older people should follow this format.

1. Use the drug that is most suitable for the condition.
2. Write directions that are clear and concise.
3. Determine that no sensitivity exists.
4. Determine that no drug interaction exists.
5. Determine the product's pharmaceutical elegance.
6. Be aware of patient compliance.
7. Be astute enough to recognize patient responses.

Many older people have misconceptions about medications and unfortunately so do some practitioners. Later in this chapter we will be discussing many over-the-counter preparations and we will attempt to clarify that area of misconception. The following are the most common fallacies.

1. *Generics are cheaper than brand names.*
   This is not universal. The cost to the consumer is governed by supply and demand. The patient may have to take more of the medication because it has a lower bioavailability. Also, the pharmacist can often dispense any brand he chooses and may not pass the direct savings on, as his reason for dispensing a certain brand may not be directly linked to that specific brand. The prescriber, and sometimes the pharmacist, is unaware of the actual manufacturer of the drug, only the distributor of the generic. The doctor's best course of action is to deal with a reputable pharmacy that is concerned with the product and service he is providing, not merely the sale!
2. *The government controls all drug production, so all chemical equivalents are the same.*
   The FDA is still not capable of policing the drugs produced here. Many generic drugs distributed here are bulk manufactured in other countries. The seller need not list the manufacturer's country of origin.
3. *Generics are as good therapeutically as the same branded product.*
   Each manufacturer has an identity, good or bad. This relates to personnel, equipment, quality control, origin of material, etc.

Brand name companys do all of the research on new drugs for the future.

Before discussing foot related geriatric medications, it is probably best to further discuss the specifics of the geriatric patient that might further compromise our ability to treat them. We have already spoken of the geriatric patient not taking his medicine as prescribed, but what other factors are hidden from practitioners at first glance?

Aging has been a concern since the time of the ancient Egyptians, who used to use rejuvenating elixirs, but it has only been rather recently that a lot of attention has been directed toward the elderly. The FDA has not required special labeling for the geriatric on drugs, yet many agents exhibit long term toxic effects obviously more important to these people. They have generally less renal and liver function which closes the gap between therapeutic doses and toxic doses. They are increasingly sensitive to drugs and they may exhibit altered or unexpected responses. Aging tissues exhibit decreased blood flow for fibrosis. The geriatric psyche must also be considered. The older patient (senior) may perceive symptoms differently. Cerebral insufficiency may prevent him from remembering how a problem began. We can summarize the drug modifying effects into six areas for clarity.

1. *Age*—reduced physiological efficiency, less hepatic, cardiovascular and renal function, less oral absorption, a higher incidence of pathologic diseases.
2. *Body size*—dosage should be done by weight, not age group. Is a 90-pound person going to need as much drug as a 225-pound person?
   In addition, in old age, muscle/fat ratio changes, thus affecting drug response.
3. *Genetic factors*—drug allergies—abnormal immunological response to drugs, or an idiosyncratic drug reaction, abnormal metabolic response to drugs.
4. *Temporary condition*—meals, emotional stability, fatigue and residual drug effects.
5. *Pathological conditions*—vomiting/diarrhea decreases absorption; gastric ulcers and liver dysfunction can preclude use of certain drugs.
6. *Tolerance and tachyphylaxis*—rapid tolerance to drugs.

The above should serve as an example of how complex the senior is to treat. The presence of the senior's multiple pathologic states has necessitated use of many drugs together. The incidence of adverse drug reaction with one to five drugs is 18.6% and with six or more is 81.4%.

These drug interactions and reactions can be minimized if we list and recognize some aspects of their occurrence.

1. Inadequate professional knowledge.
2. Patient physiological characteristics as mentioned earlier—size.
3. Patient behavioral characteristics—vitamins and over-the-counter preparations.
4. Patient dietary habits.
5. Environmental pollutants.
6. Pharmacologic or drug effect factors.
7. Pharmaceutic factors such as dosage forms and generics.
8. Diagnostic lab procedures.

Also the keeping, maintenance and use of accurate records can go a long way toward helping the practitioner in his quest to minimize these problems.

Drug Therapy

First, we must recognize what the senior perceives as a drug. Frequently the mention of aspirin is not included and, as we are aware, all over-the-counter products are drugs and should be listed as such, for many of them can interact with legend drugs that may be ordered. Interactions will be discussed in the drug classes.

Medications for foot problems can be divided into 3 categories for clarity of discussion: (1) Topical agents (both over-the-counter and prescription), (2) injectable agents, and (3) systemic agents (both over-the-counter and prescription), the last having the highest potential liability for the patient.

Topical Over-the-counter Preparations (for the Geriatric Foot)

A barrage of products has been and continues to be applied to the foot, most of which are intended for the relief of pain. The external analgesics act as counterirritants that provide warmth and irritation to the skin in attempt to crowd out the pain sensation. The psychological implication of "doing something" cannot be minimized in the drug's effectiveness. Methyl salicylate, camphor, menthol mixtures, turpentine oil, thymol and capsicum have all been used. Liniments are generally oils or water in oil emulsions, or alcoholic solutions of soap to help the spreading or massaging ability.

There are gel preparations that warm and lotions that are made to dry the skin. Ointments will allow increased percutaneous absorption while balms are generally aromatic petroleum combinations. These preparations have some effectiveness locally on chronic types of arthritic aches and stiffness but are very temporary in their duration of action. They also may pose a problem in the patient with decreased sensation or broken skin.

Anti-infectives are another common area for self-medication and can cause significant problems. Alcohol has a very short lived effect on the skin of about 1–2 minutes and is not universally effective in its spectrum of action. Of course, we are still looking for that agent!

A popular newer agent is the tamed form of iodine or povidine, which is very effective and has an affinity for the skin so that its effect may last longer than some of the others.

It has a relatively low index of reaction and is used in foot ulcerations for its astringent and drying effects. It can, however, like many of the metallic compounds, inactivate topical enzymes frequently used in ulcer sites. Historically, mercurials have been used topically by the public but their effectiveness is also short lived. Also, they are rather harsh on open areas. Ammonium compounds such as Zephiran[c] were very popular, but actually Zephiran is a very poor antibacterial agent and is inactivated by many agents and even tissue debris.

Stains are extremely effective as antibacterial/antifungal agents. Gentian violet and scarlet red and others also are astringents which makes them very effective as an agent to use interdigitally, but their major drawback is that they stain and are very messy and they obscure the field in which they are used. Topical creams and ointments with antibiotic properties are excellent agents to prescribe for the older person because of their high index of effectiveness. Neosporin[d] combines three antibiotics, namely neomycin, bacitracin and polymyxin B in an ointment or cream base. We must note that the ointment formulation is an occlusive one and the geriatric patient probably would do best not to use it interdigitally. Topical ointments and antifungals have always been popular with older patients and so there are shelves of products in the drugstore to choose from.

The most popular and probably one of the most effective antifungal agents today is tolnaftate. It was originally a legend item but the governmental agencies reclassified it because of its safety in use. It is available as a cream, liquid and powder, and the practitioner has an excellent product at his disposal and one that can save the older patient some money.

Dry skin is a frequent visitor and generally the approach is to moisturize, soften and lubricate the area. Products to avoid are those that occlude, stain, have a greasy feel to them or that can actually coat the skin and prevent moisture from entering the skin.

The agent of choice is Carmol 20.[e] This is a 20% urea cream that should be applied after washing or soaking the feet. It is also available as a 10% lotion for milder cases. Zinc oxide ointment is a good protectant for weeping lesions and may actually facilitate the healing process. At all costs avoid corn/callous removers. Most of them contain salicyclic acid, acetic acid or zinc chloride. They are irritating, very caustic and corrosive. The geriatric may have trouble seeing his foot. He has decreased coordination to apply to the exact area and generalized decreased sensation; both of these factors are precursors to a burn, infection, ulceration and, occasionally, an amputation. Many over-the-counter preparations were introduced when controls were rather lax and because of grandfather clauses are protected today. The alternative to these products is a competent practitioner.

Topical Prescription Items

Though technically an over-the-counter preparation, Domeboro[f] soaks are almost exclusively written for by prescription. As a dissolving tablet or powder, it is an excellent astringent with some antibiotic and antifungal properties. Used on foot ulcerations, open fissures or after nail surgery, it shortens the period of drainage and may actually promote healing.

Anti-infectives are commonly prescribed and the nonocclusive agent of choice is Neosporin-G cream.[d] It differs from the over-the-counter preparation in that it is in a cream vehicle and has the addition of gramicidin. It can be used interdigitally which is an additional advantage.

Hexachlorophene, a cumulative topical antibiotic, has gone to legend status and, because of its supposed percutaneous systemic toxicity, has all but fallen into disuse. It is mentioned here only as a historical note for its previous vast popularity.

Halotex[g] and Lotrimin[h] are very effective antifungal agents. Available as creams and liquids they empirically work very well against the common tinea seen infecting the feet. Lotrimin also is effective against candida infections sometimes seen on the foot. Topical steroids are very useful for inflammatory conditions. The more potent steroids such as

---

[c] Zephiran—trademark of Winthrop Laboratories.
[d] Neosporin and Neosporin-G—trademark of Burroughs Wellcome Corp.
[e] Carmol 20—trademark of Syntex Laboratories.

[f] Domeboro—trademark of Dome Laboratories.
[g] Halotex R—trademark of Mead Johnson & Co.
[h] Lotrimin R—trademark of Schering Corp.

the fluorinated group may permeate the tissues better.

Creams are water miscible, penetrating, nongreasy and nonstaining. Ointments are hydrophobic, greasy, occlusive, and staining. The newest dosage forms are gels. They attempt to combine the best of creams and ointments. Beyond this, creams are better suited to moist lesions and ointments to dry lesions. Also, use of steroid preparations under occlusion increases their penetrability and duration of action. Carmol-HC[i] combines urea with the effectiveness of hydrocortisone.

Hyperhidrosis and bromidrosis are two common conditions seen that respond well to 10% of formalin in rubbing alcohol. The addition of 10% rose water improves the pharmaceutical elegance of the product.

Topical enzymes have marked efficiency in ulcer therapy regardless of etiology, although removal of the causal factors must also be accomplished.

Santyl[j] used in the ulcerative base will clean up the debris and yield a granular base that is more likely to heal. Iodine and heavy metal compounds inactivate the Santyl and must be avoided during therapy. Santyl can be combined with Neosporin. Other agents such as Elase[k] and Biozyme[l] also have usefulness in foot ulcerations. Recent work with Debrisan[m] has yielded some additional results in the removal of debris. Though more expensive than other agents, it may be compensated for by third party plans, as it has been classified as a device (not a drug). Porcine skin covering is used on ulcer sites and acts as a biologic dressing. This covering improves the environment in the ulcer site and as such promotes healing and decreases the risk of infection.

Injectable Products (Prescription)

The most widely used injectable in therapeutic practice is the steroid class. As with the topical agents, the major effectiveness differences are the vehicles in which the steroids are dispersed. The solutions have a rapid onset but short duration of action. They are used in cases where their anti-inflamma-

tory effects are only needed up to a day or so. Decadron[n] or Hexadrol[o] solutions are in this category and are useful for tendonitis and tenosynovitis, as well as in postoperative sites where immediate healing is not imperative. Colloidal or suspension forms of the drug are longer acting and should be used in areas where a longer activity is desired. Decadron-LA,[n] Celestone Soluspan[p] and Aristocort[q] injections are examples. These are not, however, designed to be used in joints. Celestone[p] solution and Aristospan[q] preparations are for intra-articular use.

Local anesthetics are used and may be compatible with several steroid preparations. Examples are Xylocaine[r] as 1 and 2% that also comes with or without epinephrine. Epinephrine is a vasoconstrictor and narrows blood vessels, thus increases the duration of action. In digits, especially those of the elderly, use of epinephrine probably should be avoided.

Marcaine[s] is a newer agent that has a longer duration of action, though it may taken 10–15 minutes for its effect to be appreciated.

Systemic Over-the-counter Preparations

Over-the-counter drugs for analgesia have a wide range of usefulness. One of the most effective is aspirin (325 mg.). Unfortunately, recent work has revealed many interactions between aspirin and other medications. These will be discussed with the individual drug discussions. Acetaminophen in similar doses to aspirin (325 mg.) also has value as a analgesic. However, acetaminophen may also have some risks and has been demonstrated to occasionally cause some blood dyscrasia.

Systemic Prescription Preparations

Frequently prescribed analgesics are sometimes written too often or in too large a quantity for the geriatric patient's good. Pro-

---

[i] Carmol-HC—trademark of Syntex Laboratories.

[j] Santyl—trademark of Knoll Laboratories.

[k] Elase—trademark of Parke, Davis & Co.

[l] Biozyme—trademark of Armour & Co.

[m] Debrisan—trademark of Pharmacia Laboratories.

---

[n] Decadron and Decadron-LA—trademark for Merck Sharp and Dohme.

[o] Hexadrol—trademark of Organon, Inc.

[p] Celestone and Celestone Soluspan—trademark of Schering Corp.

[q] Aristospan and Aristocort—trademark of the Lederle Laboratories.

[r] Xylocaine—trademark of Astra Pharmaceutical Products.

[s] Marcaine—trademark of Winthrop Laboratories.

poxyphene has been widely used but may not be superior to aspirin. Antibiotic agents should be used on the basis of a culture and not just because of clinical impressions. In the geriatric, it is important to realize that the blood levels in the lower extremity may be much lower than in the other parts of the body. Active infections in the foot may require higher dosages to get the wanted results. Some foodstuffs can inactivate oral antibiotics. The tetracycline group is particularly sensitive to milk products and antacids. Approximately 10% of the populace is hypersensitive to the penicillin group. An alternative with appropriate culture is the cephalosporin group. Only 10% of those sensitive to penicillin exhibit cross-sensitivity to the cephalosporins. Keflex[t] (250 mg.) is an example of this class. Should a patient be started on antibiotics empirically while awaiting a culture and with the clinical symptoms improving, it would be advisable to continue and not switch, even though the culture indicates the current medication is not specifically effective. Another standard is due to potential sensitization. Never use any antibiotics topically that may at some point be used systemically. The reasoning behind this has caused penicillin, erythromycin and tetracycline ointments to fall into disuse. Oral griseofulvin incorporates into newly forming epidermis and thereby eliminates fungal infection. A daily dose of the ultrafine form (500 mg.) is effective against skin infections within 30 days, but unless nail avulsions (chemical or surgical) are performed, this systemic agent is not very effective and at best improvement takes many months when used on toenails.

A newer group of drugs are the nonsteroid anti-inflammatory agents. Phenylbutazone (100 mg.) is used for short term inflammatory conditions such as heel bursitis or acute gouty arthritis. Indomethacin (25 mg.) is useful in the class and is currently the drug of choice. Indocin[u] may, like phenylbutazone, cause some stomach upset, so use of antacids or milk may be warranted.

Motrin[v] (400 mg.) is a newer agent that is somewhat safer than the previous two medications. Patients must avoid all use of aspirin with this drug.

Gout has been treated for many years and until the advent of uricosurics little was accomplished. Uricosurics such as probenecid (500 mg.) facilitate urinary excretion of uric acid. Prevention of uric acid production is accomplished with allopurinol, though in the presence of an attack this agent should not be used. The nonsteroidal anti-inflammatory agents also are useful here. Muscle relaxants are very useful for short term spasms seen and their use warranted. Diazepam (5 mg.) is a mild muscle relaxant and tranquilizer that is very popular.

The peripheral vasodilator group has been a much talked about group. Vasodilan[w] (20 mg.) appears to be somewhat effective in the lower extremity when there is enough functional musculature left in the blood vessels. Many geriatrics complain of symptoms consistent with peripheral vascular disease. When confirmed by examination these agents can improve the symptoms. Arlidin[x] (6 mg.), another agent, may act more as a muscular shunting agent for intermittent claudication and night cramps.

Diuretics generally do not pose any problems for the practitioner unless used for over 30 days. Beyond this length of time potassium deficiency may be found, necessitating supplementation, particularly with the thiazide group.

Drug Interactions

Drug interactions are very important to recognize for the practitioner. A good history is essential to determine what other medications the patient may be taking. The following are examples of interactions:

- The hypoglycemic activity of chlorpropamide may be *enhanced* by the concurrent administration of phenylbutazone.

- The hypoglycemic activity of chlorpropamide may be *enhanced* by the concurrent use of aspirin.

- The blood levels of griseofulvin may be *lowered* by phenobarbital.

- The effects of indomethacin will be *decreased* by aspirin.

---

[t] Keflex—trademark of Eli Lilly & Co.
[u] Indocin—trademark of Merck Sharp and Dohme Co.
[v] Motrin—trademark of Upjohn Co.

[w] Vasodilan—trademark of Mead Johnson Co.
[x] Arlidin—trademark of USV Pharmaceutical Corp.

- The blood levels of nitrofurantoin are *increased* by concomitant use of probenecid.

- Penicillin levels are *increased* by concurrent use of probenecid.

- Warfarin activity is *antagonized* by griseofulvin.

- Warfarin activity is *increased* by phenylbutazone.

- Allopurinol activity is *antagonized* by thiazide diuretics.

- Peripheral vasodilators may *lower* blood pressure, necessitating antihypertensive medications.

- Warfarin activity may be *increased* by acetaminophen.

It is easy to extrapolate the following trend in longevity. Two thousand years ago the life span was a mere 25 years. In 1900 people survived to an average age of 49 years. In 1957—67 years, and now over 70 years. If this progression continues, chapters like this one and others contained in this text will become increasingly important to those in medical practice. No longer can the geriatric be lost in the category of adult medical care. He must be considered separately as pediatric cases are. Truly, gerontology has come of age.

chapter 16

Senior Citizen Centers and the Significant Role They Can Play in the Life of the Elderly

Ernestine N. Estes, M.S.W., A.C.S.W.

There are more older people today than ever before. People are living longer.

Advancements in nutrition, sanitation and public health measures have greatly improved living conditions so that we can expect today's life span, which is well over 70 years, to continue to increase. The reduction in infant mortality, continued new medical discoveries and improved delivery of health care will all serve to demand increased concern and knowledge about the elderly and their problems.

The elderly, those persons over 60 years of age, represent a widely different group of individuals with divergent experience and interests.

There is a tendency to categorize the elderly as fragile, frail, senile, immobile without assistance and unable to care for basic needs; a financial and emotional burden on the family and ultimately in need of institutionalization.

While it is true in a broad sense that there are general reactions to old age, the experience of aging is as unique as the individual. People adjust to old age in a manner similar to their adjustment to the experience of living.

As the individual goes through childhood and into adulthood he matures physically and mentally. It is at this time that his basic self is developed and takes the form which will carry him throughout life. This personality represents the way the individual reacts routinely to problems and situations. It influences how he acts, interacts, establishes and maintains relationships. It represents how he perceives himself and others and his way of dealing with his basic instincts and drives.

This personality is determined by heredity and experience. His temperament is manifested by his prevalent mood, the relative liveliness or sluggishness of his motor and intellectual behavior, the relative sensitiveness or dullness of his reaction to stimulations. These are inborn and determined by heredity; equally important are the experiences a person has beginning in infancy and including the significant impact of parental influence.

Attitudes of security or insecurity, ascendancy or submission, optimism or pessimism, confidence in others or distrust of them and many less tangible traits may distinguish the various persons we know. The normal individual who reaches old age will have lived his mature life on the basis of a personality structure which is fixed in a pattern that has worked more or less successfully for the total life situation in which he has found himself. Ultimately, the psychological pattern of the aging person will be determined by his basic personality.

Today, the Older Adult Service (OAS) of the West Philadelphia Community Mental

Health Consortium is actively involved in providing preventive mental health services. In addition to the range of services the Consortium provides for all the residents of southwest Philadelphia, specifically for the elderly there are three multipurpose senior centers and a geriatric day hospital.

The multipurpose senior centers are available for persons 60 years and older who live in southwest Philadelphia. Currently, there are about 2000 individuals actively involved in the program. Another 500 persons are served in information and referral. Staff is made up of 65 persons, professionals; about 50% of staff is over 60 years. Funding for these services is made available through local Area Agency on Aging, i.e., the Philadelphia Corporation for Aging and the Philadelphia County Office of Mental Health/Mental Retardation with a 75%-25% match.

Each of the three multipurpose centers is located within the facilities of a church within the community. They are readily accessible to the elderly and are recognized as a place to meet friends, get help with problems and generally have a good time.

The center is led by a small core of professionals, including a *Center Supervisor* whose primary responsibilities are the direct planning, development and organization of the center, and a *Program Director* who is responsible for planning and implementing meaningful education and recreational activities. The *Social Service Supervisor* has primary responsibility for corrdinating and accessing social service needs of the participants and the *nurse* coordinates medical services.

The actual program activities and direct services are supervised by the professional staff but carried out by a team of senior citizen volunteers. There are nearly 150 senior citizens 60 years and older who serve as volunteers in the older adult programs at the Consortium.

SENIOR CITIZEN AS VOLUNTEER

The volunteers are individuals who are eligible to receive the services of the program and, in fact, are chosen from the participants of the OAS to assist staff in providing the older adult services. When a senior citizen enters the OAS, the volunteer program is explained to him and he is given the opportunity to volunteer his services. Many individuals come to the program with an expectation of functioning as volunteers.

Individuals usually volunteer for a specific task. For one day or a portion of a day he may be functioning as a volunteer and at another point his role is one of participant.

They bring with them the experience of living as well as the specific knowledge of their life's vocation. Volunteers are involved in a wide variety of activities and their participation indeed broadens the scope of the program. They are involved in helping to set up for the noontime meal and the cleanup after. Volunteers run special groups such as sewing, crafts and art. Others assume responsiblity for organizing and running bazaars and other fund raising activities. The homebound participants can expect a friendly visit from a volunteer who has similar interests and concerns. Many act as chaperons for medical appointments while others are involved in assisting with minor home repairs.

The older adult center is an extremely busy and active place and when one enters the facility he is often struck by the sense of purposeful activity, involvement and concern for one another.

The senior volunteers contribute greatly to the environment as they bring exuberance, commitment, energy and a desire to do whatever is necessary to keep things moving.

Their generation is a work oriented one and this is reflected in their strong commitment to keep busy and to be the doer. For many of them employment was the focal point of their lives and the experiences of retirement, if this were to mean inactivity, would be devastating. They are no longer welcome in the world of employment. They are welcome and valued at the Senior Citizen Center. This activity helps them to continue viewing themselves as valuable and valued, useful, individuals.

There are both pluses and minuses to using the senior citizen participant as volunteers.

The senior citizen has more time to give and gives it freely and willingly, making few demands for rewards. He brings a wide range of knowledge and experience with him which adds color and dimension to the program. He can be depended upon to be present to carry out his predetermined task and is willing to assume additional ones should the need arise.

On the other hand, his need for activity, his overexuberance to be involved and active, puts a unique kind of responsibility or pressure on staff to be well organized and in control of the coordination of the program while taking in the needs of all the participants, volunteers as well as nonvolunteers.

Volunteers are identifiable at the center by the volunteer badge which they wear. In addition, names of active volunteers for the day are posted on the bulletin board. They meet monthly to discuss issues common to volunteers and periodically staff plans volunteer recognition activity. There is also an annual affair in recognition of volunteers with plaques or certificates given.

Staff willingly delegates authority to the volunteers to perform certain tasks. There are many volunteers who were experts in their field and have been accustomed to functioning in authority positions. This can be a real asset in that a volunteer can independently plan for and teach a group of his peers to make a vase or a figurine from clay. His delegated authority ends once his designated activity is completed. However, it is difficult sometimes for the volunteer to make the transition from leader to follower and he may alienate the other participants or the volunteer leader of the next activity as he attempts to control this activity also.

It takes skill on the part of the staff to help the teacher of the pottery class to stay within his boundaries without making him feel unwanted.

Some volunteers, because of their close working relationship with staff, will begin to feel superior to be nonvolunteer participant and begin to assume staff functions.

Mrs. Jones volunteers to serve lunch. She eats lunch at the table with Jim Smith whose eating habits leave much to be desired. Instead of discussing the problem with a staff person, as is the expectation of her as a volunteer, she verbally attacks Jim, who is embarrassed and humiliated and stays away from the program until a staff member goes to his home and encourages him to come back.

Some volunteers have been in the program since its inception and have continued performing the same task. However, because of deteriorated physical conditions they are no longer able to perform the task well. An example of this is Tom Coleman, who always poured coffee at lunchtime. Mr. Coleman now has a tremor in his hand. The participants have begun complaining that he spills coffee on them, but he does not willingly give up his task. Although taking this task away from him could be traumatic, staff must intercede for the well-being of the other participants. A task which Mr. Coleman can perform is identified and he is encouraged to give up his endeared responsibility. While each of the above examples seems simple enough to handle, when they are multiplied by the number of individuals who volunteer, they can pose a real problem in running the program.

When one weighs the positive and negative factors involved in using senior citizens as volunteers in an older adult service, it is difficult to get a definitive answer to the question "Is the program better because of the use of the senior citizen volunteers?" However, when one reviews the purpose of the older adult services, which place heavy emphasis on the provision of preventive services to the senior citizen and the process of volunteering is recognized as a preventive services within itself, it is clear that there is real value in using senior citizens as volunteers in an older adult service.

PARTICIPANTS' ADVISORY COUNCIL

Each of the multipurpose centers has a Participants Advisory Council. This council serves in an advisory capacity to the Director of the Older Adult Program. The council is made up of fifteen elected members, all of whom are active participants of the center program. Its purpose is "to advise the staff of the center on all matters having to do with nutrition, recreation, socialization, education, transportation, and other social services provided by the center." The council shall have specific responsibility for advising the Project Director on:

1. Setting suggested contributions for meals
2. Approval of general types of menus that meet required nutrition standards
3. Days and hours of center operations
4. Decor and furnishings at the center
5. Types of programs and social services

The advisory program council is very serious about its work and meets monthly to discuss issues of concern. They take an active role in the functioning of the center and play a significant role in establishing policies within the center. At one point it was necessary to limit the number of days any given participant could get the hot noontime meal at the center because of the large number of participants attending the program. The advisory council played a significant role in establishing guidelines for determining who would receive meals and also for suggesting that other participants bring in a bag lunch on other days.

A member of the Participants' Advisory Council represents the center at the city-wide Philadelphia Senior Centers Council.

The councils are generally clear that the center must function within the guidelines of the Consortium and federal, state and local mandates. However, there are occasions on which they feel very strongly about an issue and staff chooses not to follow their advice. On these infrequent occasions, issues are usually resolved through meetings and negotiations. The Consortium's policy making Board of Directors is available for the resolution of such issues when they are not resolved to the council's satisfaction by administration.

The participants are intelligent, well informed and generally knowledgeable; many of them have been employed in leadership positions for many years. They are a valuable resource to the centers. Reciprocal benefits are derived as the older adult brings wisdom and knowledge to the program; the program provides a setting in which they can continue to experience fulfillment and purposefulness.

SERVICES AT THE CENTER

The centers operate daily from 8:45 A.M. to 4:45 P.M. Monday through Friday, except when there are special events, which frequently take place in late afternoons, evenings and on weekends.

The goal of the multipurpose centers is to assist the older adults in ways that will enable them to retain independent life in their own homes and communities; a life that can become progressively more active, meaningful and characterized by dignity. In order to achieve this goal it was necessary to overcome the following barriers: *

● Isolation, fear, loss of social contact and

lack of information and community resources
● Lack of sound nutrition
● Lack of sound health related services

The Consortium multipurpose center work towards meeting these goals through their program activities.

Isolation, Fear and Loss of Social Contact

An outreach service is provided wherein older adults in the community are identified through contracts with gatekeepers such as clergy, mailmen, physicians, other agencies, and by local publicity and interpretation. These outreach activities include friendly visiting and, where appropriate, follow-up by volunteers and case aides who themselves are older adults. The isolated are informed of community resources, including the multipurpose center services, and are assisted in obtaining necessary services and in participating in various programs, including essential transportation. The multipurpose centers provide daily and special periodic educational and recreational programs in addition to a comfortable facility which provides a comfortable lounge area where individuals can be together outside of their own homes.

The older adult is provided with transportation to enable him or her to become involved in activities and come to the program. These activities are geared toward helping individuals meet and interact with others and establish new relationships which help mitigate fears and isolation. Individual counseling and casework, referrals and follow-up assist those individuals who need help with finances, housing and other personal problems.

The individuals who are involved with the program are stimulated and offered opportunities for socialization, recreation, education, employment, volunteer services, social advocacy, sharing, travel and new experiences. A climate of concern, caring, new opportunities and vitality is fostered throughout the community.

Local neighborhood services include contacts with individuals to inform them of available resources; forums conducted on a regular basis with representative participation from both private and governmental agencies; and use of neighborhood newspapers, printed materials and other appropriate communication methods. Word of mouth is an invaluable tool for spreading the word in the older adult community.

Lack of Sound Nutrition

It is often difficult for the older adult who lives alone to prepare and maintain an adequate diet for himself. In an effort to improve nutrition, the Consortium's senior centers provide 300 meals on a daily basis. About 225 are congregate meals, and 75 are home delivered. Meals for home deliveries are packaged at each center and sent out with a driver and assistant. The R.N. and Social Service Staff determine who should receive home delivered meals.

The hot noontime meals represent the main meal and often the only balanced meal of the day. The meal frequently serves as the impetus for the older adult to come to the center. Once he is there the opportunity to assist him with the many other problems he may present itself.

Home delivered meals are sent to those individuals temporarily unable to leave home for reasons such as a recent hospitalization and to those who are totally unable to prepare their own meals and are unable to leave home. More recently there has been increased recognition of the needs of the homebound elderly. In the past year an active campaign has been established to identify and provide services to those individuals who are unable to come to the center. We have expanded the social service staff of the center and now have service managers whose time is spent exclusively in the home assessing the needs of the frail, elderly, making a service plan and seeing that it is carried out. Providing casework services, supportive counseling, shopping and escort services for the frail, elderly in the home has allowed some of them to improve their functioning so that they are now able to come to the center for services.

All meals are prepared by a caterer and delivered to the center daily. The menu is planned by a joint committee of the caterer, the assistant director, a representative from the participants' advisory council and a nutritionist. The significance of the hot meal was recently highlighted when the partici-

pants attending the center at noontime exceeded the number of meals available. Meals are given out on a first-come-first-served basis. There was a core of participants who attended the program daily and felt that they should be served the meal daily because they arrived early.

If the number of meals was unlimited this would have been acceptable; however, there were other frail individuals who were being denied a meal because of the core group of well elderly.

Some of these individuals had to be transported and had no control of their arrival time. In addition, they were dependent upon the meal for their primary nutrition. An administrative decision was made that the participants would receive three meals per week unless otherwise specified and, while all were welcome to come to the program on a daily basis, it would be necessary to bring in a bagged lunch on 2 days.

They were furious, stating that the meals were their right and organized to fight this inequity. They began by meeting with the center director and after him went through several administrative levels, even approaching the funding agency, the Philadelphia Corporation for the Aging. When it became clear that this was not a capricious decision, they agreed to use their energies toward lobbying for more money for older adult programs through the political sphere.

The situation around the sharing of meals has been resolved; however, it had everyone in an uproar for a period of time.

Lack of Sound Health Related Services

The elderly are prone to have health problems, identified and unidentified. A large part of the service provided through the multipurpose centers is related to the medical needs of the population. The program has a nurse on staff who has responsibility for coordinating the medical needs of the participants. It is clear that the centers cannot assume responsibility for providing the medical needs of the participants. However, the centers play a significant role in identifying that there is the need for medical treatment, directing the individual as to sources of medical treatment and payment for them and assisting the elderly in carrying out the medical directives as prescribed. Although the participants who attend the Older Adult Program come from the same basic geographical area of the city, they are not limited in where they can go to get medical treatment. Consequently, we have a situation where the participants travel throughout the city to meet their medical needs.

With this in mind, transportation becomes an all important factor in the provision of medical care. The program has two full-time and four part-time drivers and currently operates six mini-buses. These vehicles and drivers are essential to meeting the medical needs of the participants as well as many other needs. Transportation to doctors' appointments, clinic appointments and for picking up prescriptions, etc., does much to assure that the elder participant follows through on their medical needs.

In addition to providing transportation to medical resources for the participants, the centers maintain active programs in the education of health issues, in prevention and treatment and just basic education on the body and how to look for and understand the changes it goes through.

There are other occasions on which specific health campaigns are arranged. Recently there was a blood donor campaign where all the older adults worked to get donations of blood. There are other occasions where screening for high blood pressure or foot problems, pap tests or other such tests are provided at the centers.

The Older Adult Program has established ongoing relationships with medical schools, hospitals, clinics and other medical facilities in an effort to maximize the availability of medical resources for its participants.

The fact that the Older Adult Program is an integral part of a comprehensive community mental health center puts its participants at a decided advantage over the average senior citizen center.

The staff of the centers have training in identifying symptoms of mental health problems and there is a full range of mental health services available to the older adult within the same system. Before the older adult centers became a part of the community mental health center only 2% of the individuals served were older adults. Today 80% of the mental health services provided by the Consortium are given to senior citizens.

Conclusion

The Older Adult Services of the West Philadelphia Community Mental Health Consortium clearly identifies that all elderly persons are not fragile, frail, senile, immobile without assistance and unable to care for basic needs; a financial and emotional burden on the family and ultimately in need of institutionalization. In fact, the process of growing old is not necessarily an abrupt, painful period of adjustment to a new phase of the life cycle, but can be a pleasurable transition to increased freedom for recreation and pursuit of avocational interests.

Essentially the way that an individual deals with old age is the way he has dealt with change throughout his life.

While there are many problems associated with the process of aging given the right environment and adequate support systems, these problems can be addressed in an orderly fashion.

The West Philadelphia Community Mental Health Consortium received its initial staffing grant in 1966 and opened its doors for services to the residents of Southwest Philadelphia in July 1967. The Consortium was made up of five area general hospitals, a child guidance clinic, a planning agency, an institute for the mentally retarded and a university department of psychiatry. From the beginning, the Consortium recognized the importance of being a free standing independent agency making use of liaison relationships and of being decentralized, providing services within the community highly accessible to the 203,000 residents to whom it had responsibility for providing mental health and mental retardation services under the mandate of federal, state and local government. It is now a comprehensive community mental health center providing services through 18 facilities to a highly urban population.

The Consortium services include an outpatient system of counseling centers, an impatient unit, partial hospitalization programs, transitional housing, aftercare and rehabilitation, children's services, drug and alcohol programs, specialized services for women, consultation and education, training and, of course, older adult services.

Although older adult services were not

mandated for community mental health centers, as early as 1970 the Consortium was involved in providing some level of preventive services for the elderly residents in the community. The Consortium, along with Community Celebration, a group of local ministers organized to enhance the impact of joint church efforts toward a range of urban and community problems who wanted to develop a program of new, outreaching services for their older parishioners, began a program of services to the aged. The basic concept was that a coalition of community based outreach services could alleviate misfortunes of the aged, that life could be enhanced, and that by mounting an integrated program of casework with individuals, group programs, community action and cooperative comprehensive planning it is possible to serve the total needs of individuals.

Foot health must be a part of the total health effort. It is many times not considered in planning and operations, many times neglected, and many times becomes the catalyst for the elderly to remain active and in their community environment. With proper foot care, patients can usually remain ambulatory and retain their dignity. In one respect we can say that happy feet tend to make happy people.

chapter 17

Education—The Magic Key

Morris Barrett, M.P.H.

HEALTH EDUCATION NEEDS OF THE ELDERLY

Almost any study pertaining to the status of the elderly in America begins with a terse recitation of statistics. Perhaps this dry, digital approach is inescapable. Perhaps to personalize the condition of the aged among us would be to indict the national conscience beyond tolerance. Perhaps the abstraction of figures serves as a shield against the searing reality of human need. Even so, the numbers tell a tale.

According to the United States Census, there were in 1980 over 25 million persons aged 65 years or older in America. Of these, 80% were chronically ill. Over a million lived in nursing homes or homes for the aged. Close to 4 million lived "independently" in substandard housing. About 10% were seldom or never seen by their children. Over half of a million were under treatment in mental institutions. Another 10% had emotional problems apparently severe enough to require psychiatric care. Statistically, at least, there seems to be little "light" in the twilight years.

But to present these statistics apart from the factors of swift social and technological evolution that underlie them would be an unfair condemnation of our civilization.

To begin with, longevity is a modern phenomenon. Mathematicians estimate that, of all the people who since the dawn of mankind have reached 65 years of age, more than one-quarter are living today. We are just beginning to learn to live with older people in our midst.

With a progressively older population, people 65 and over are the fastest growing group in American society. The population of elderly persons is expected to be 12% of the total population in the year 2000 and 16% in 2020.

As recently as 1900, the life expectancy of the average American was 49 years. In those days tuberculosis and pneumonia were the "captains of death." It was not uncommon for many Americans to die young. A fractricidal war that ended just 35 years earlier may have removed from the population most of those hardier persons who might otherwise have survived to old age. The wave of immigrants from Eastern Europe around the turn of the century was composed almost entirely of younger stock.

America was then a youthful nation, populated by youthful people; a sparsely settled, predominantly rural, agricultural society in which "economic productivity" was measured by the output of human hands. And many hands were needed.

The "typical" turn-of-the-century American family was a multigenerational, self-contained, farm-based unit in which each member, through manual labor, contributed to the economic health of the family and the economic growth of the nation. Rarely in the early 20th century did an American live beyond the age of economic productivity. Retirement from the work force was economically undesirable, if not morally impossible. In the eight decades since 1900, the life span of the average American has increased to age 74. The "killer" diseases of former years can hardly be found on today's lists of causes of death. The nation's total population, which at the turn of the century was 76 million, is now over 225 million, of which more than 25 million are aged 65 and over. It is this sizable group of people who have the very questionable privilege of being America's first true generation of "senior citizens." And they, probably more than any other segment of our population, have been affected by the incredible changes that have taken place within their life spans.

The health status of the elderly has changed considerably. Over the past half-century, the major thrust of medical progress has been at the communicable diseases and acute conditions. These swift and deadly foes have for the most part been conquered. At the present time the major health enemies are diseases of the heart and circulatory system, conditions that frequently bring chronic illness and disability before ultimately resulting in death.

The illnesses can affect persons of any age, but they are seen overwhelmingly in the age groups of 55 and over. Though Americans do live longer, they tend with increasing years to have increasing rates of physical impairment, morbidity and medical care utilization.

Even so, most of the American elderly are not severely impaired. Public Health Service statistics show that only a relatively small portion of Americans in the 65–74 age group are disabled severely enough to prohibit them from carrying out major activities.

Then, too, no longer is America the comfortably open and placidly pleasant collection of small towns and clustered farms that it was a generation ago. The direction of our national growth has converted us to a conglomerate of massive metropolitan centers where, for better or worse, the overwhelming majority of our people—young and old—are concentrated. The fact that our cities are in a state of grave crisis needs no elaboration here. Overcrowded, decaying, dirty, polluted and tense, the cities offer their inhabitants a frightening lack of housing, health care, social services, recreational facilities and other vital resources. No one needs those resources more nor can afford them less than the elderly.

In our present-day society technological advances have substituted mechanical devices for human labor. Though we have need for far fewer "hands" today, there are now far more "hands" available. But economic resources still are distributed on the basis of contribution to production, mostly through wages and other related means. Partly as a reward for loyal service and partly as a pragmatic means of reducing a too abundant manual labor force, American industry has devised a system of compulsory retirement at the arbitrary age of 70. Sometimes long before biophysiological conditions require it, older persons are removed from that group of our population rewarded for contribution to a growing economy. Instead, some older people become dependent upon obviously inadequate substitute income programs, such as social security, private pension funds and, in a growing number of cases, public assistance. One authority in the field of gerontology estimates that the majority of our aged citizens live in some degree of dependency.

We have created out of the later years of life a kind of anticlimatic superfluousness, an "outliving of usefulness" that is reflected in our distribution of economic resources. Though income projections do see improvement in the economic status of the elderly in future years, inflation could counteract most of the projected gains, particularly since much of the income of the aged is in fixed dollars. If the same average price level rise which occurred in the years 1970–1980 continues, there will be little if any improvement in the real income of retired persons in the 1980's.

In our fickle work- and achievement-oriented society, lack of employment can often be a psychological catastrophe. Work holds an important place in mankind's emotional balance ... it is its bond with reality, its contact with the community and its form of participation in purposeful existence. Through their work men and women maintain contact with society. Its loss isolates them. Removal from the companionship, the status, the purposefulness of work leaves feelings of stagnation and unworthiness and sometimes results in the clinical syndrome known to physicians as "retirement shock." As commonly seen, the symptoms include anxiety neuroses, depression, despair and, at times, self-destruction, as well as a variety of physical complaints.

Another mutation in the basic American culture brought about by technology and bringing mixed blessings to the elderly is our astonishingly improved level of mobility. Americans have the means to travel relatively quickly, easily and inexpensively from one edge of the continent to the other. Many do. Though our economy as a whole is remarkably stable, employment opportunities can fluctuate from area to area. Young Americans go where the jobs are. Older Americans tend to "stay put."

Thus, spatial separation fragments family life, depriving both young and old of the security of continuing family ties and, perhaps even more significantly, depriving the young of the opportunity to witness the natural and inevitable process of aging within their own families. Too many Americans never know what it is to grow old until they themselves are the aging ones.

This endemic ignorance of aging, possibly more than any other factor, has contributed to the national delusion of the desirability of eternal "youth" and the concomitant alienation of the aged from total American society.

The aged population has a variety of special health needs. While it is probably too late to change deep rooted habits and practices, it is apparent that this group is receptive to new information regarding health practices and could benefit from much advice relating to their stage in life and their condition.

Health education for the aged is not a new endeavor. Public agencies have had health course offerings for many years. Many concerned agencies have distributed leaflets, used television and radio spot announcements, public billboards and other media to dispense health education. Many physicians, dentists, nurses, pharmacists, and other health professionals have engaged in health education activities. Yet, it is generally recognized that this nation's citizens' knowledge of the fundamentals of health, so necessary for their own contribution to their health, is abysmally inadequate. There is also a consensus that these efforts are either ineffective, insufficient, or both.

Any recommendations dealing with health education have to take into consideration existing health education delivery systems. Some delivery mechanisms are highly motivating, others can reach larger numbers of people, all have advantages and disadvantages.

As Victor Fuchs has stated:

The greatest potential for improving the health of the American people is not to be found in increasing the number of physicians or in forcing them into groups, or even in increasing hospital productivity, but is to be found in what people do and don't do to, and for, themselves. With so much attention given to medical care and so little to health education and individual responsibility for personal health, we run the danger of pandering to the urge to buy a quick solution to a difficult problem.

Given the present "crisis" in health care, the need for a major effort directed at consumer health education, and the capability and capacity of health planners, it is appropriate that health planning personnel now engage their efforts in a common quest. Together, these groups can reach out to include the consumer, not as the object of but as the active subject and participant in, health care.

The day of the podiatrist being only a "repair mechanic" where ailing people have their acute foot problems patched up with no thought given to prevention, education, or follow-up is rapidly departing. The move toward "consumerism" in health care, as in other aspects of American life, now places the podiatrist-patient in a priority role as a partner in the health care system.

To that end, this chapter develops several program models in community foot health education which can serve as a guide for the podiatrist in considering the following:

1. Greater concern for personal health.
2. Positive steps to prevent foot illness; to prevent progression of illnesses; and to prevent dependency on long term treatment.
3. A better understanding of the changing health education delivery system and how to obtain access to it most effectively and efficiently.

Background

Changing personal attitudes requires educating people, both individually and collectively, not only in terms of personal habits but, just as importantly, in terms of community-wide health "consumership." Developing consumer health education programs where virtually none exist now (in schools, offices, factories and homes), forming active neighborhood groups and involving people in the health care process are vital actions of good health consumership.

Efforts to change health behavior must be seen in the same light as efforts to change any other form of human behavior: resistance to change exists; apathy is remarkably strong. This is evidenced by weaknesses in past programs designed to improve behavior with respect to smoking, exercise, weight reduction, chemical abuse, and use of occupational and vehicular safety devices as well as foot problems. Some success has been achieved, but there is a great deal of room for improvement. Where any of those programs have been at least partially effective, the ingredients of success and/or failure have not been sufficiently researched. Where they have been, the means for making the results widely known have not seemed to exist.

While a community podiatric health education is not a panacea that will solve all foot problems, it is undeniably a fundamental part of any logical attack on them.

However, while the demand for health care services has been rising, consumer health education has been neglected. The whole field of health education has been fragmented and largely unevaluated. There is no agency inside or outside of government that is either responsible for, or assists in, setting goals or maintaining criteria for performance. One result has been a health care system overburdened with patients who know too little about themselves and the things they could do to prevent illness.

It is the individual's daily living habits which often bring about illness (e.g., eating too much, drinking too much, resting too little, exercising too little, driving too fast and ignoring early symptoms that warn him to seek medical attention). Once he seeks care, it is the individual's lack of knowledge during or after treatment which may blunt the impact of even the greatest of medical skills.

In essence, making a total health care system work means joint acceptance of responsibility by both the providers of health care and the people they hope to serve. If either group fails to live up to its share of the obligation, total benefits to society will be reduced to that degree. A community podiatric health education can play a tremendous role in making that total system work, for it can at the same time stimulate and be stimulated by both parties: health care providers and health care consumers.

For many years it was too often assumed that if people were told what was good for them they would take correct action. The response to the voluntary mass immunization against infantile paralysis was very favorable, but the response to other programs was not. Many people who had access to health information maintained an indifferent attitude, in spite of the potential threat to their well-being. Consequently, the consumer, the person to be educated, can no longer be considered merely a recipient of information. He must become motivated and actively involved.

Although the problems are great and diverse, the opportunities for a community foot health education have never been greater. One encouraging factor is the continuing increase of all age groups in running and jogging. Generally speaking, however, the more affluent, the better educated, the more sophisticated and the better informed enjoy better health and seek better health care. If a person knows what is good and what is bad for him; if he knows how to protect himself and his family; and if he is in a position to take advantage of the best health care available, his chances of serious illness or premature death are significantly less than those of the ignorant, the apathetic, the confused, the poor, the uprooted or the alienated.

This is not to imply that health education should be confined to the latter groups. The benefits of affluence, education and sophistication favorably affect a person's health only if he knows what is helpful, and does what is helpful.

Thomas W. Elwood, in an excellent article entitled "Older Persons' Concerns About Foot Care," written in the Journal of the American Podiatry Association, reported on a program of health education for the elderly called Vigor In Maturity (VIM).

The program involved 25,000 older persons who were given information on foot care along with other health subjects. The project was sponsored by the National Retired Teachers Association-American Association of Retired Persons, an organization of 8 million persons.

The study revealed the nine most common questions on foot problems affecting older individuals. The subject areas included: corns

Table 17.1.

A Study of Common Foot Problems Involving Elderly Persons

Corns and bunions
   What are corns and bunions?
   What causes them?
   Is it advisable to remove them?
Arthritis
   Can it occur in the feet?
   Will it cause the joints to enlarge?
   Is there a cure?
Toes
   What is the best way to trim an elderly person's toenails?
   Is it safe to file a thick nail down rather than cut it?
   Should the nail be cut straight across or in a V?
Fallen arches
   Is there any pain that accompanies fallen arches?
   Does old age itself cause an arch to fall?
   Will this lead to a lengthening of the foot?
Heels
   What causes a spur on the heel?
   Can anything be done for it other than surgery?
   If removed, will the spur return at a later time?
Footwear
   Is any one kind of shoe recommended?
   What shoes should be avoided?
   Should an elderly person wear tennis shoes frequently?
Exercise
   Is exercising the feet a good thing to be doing?
   Is walking a beneficial exercise for the feet?
   What causes the feet to be so stiff that they resist exercise?
Foot care
   Should the feet be soaked in hot water when they hurt?
   Is it good to rub peroxide on them?
   Is vaseline good for use on the feet?
Miscellaneous
   How can people of low income obtain care for their foot problems?
   Can damage to the foot cause a deterioration of the bones?
   What treatment is available for a plantar wart?

and bunions, arthritis, toes, fallen arches, heels, footwear, exercise, foot care and a miscellaneous category. This information is shown more descriptively in Table 17.1.

DEVELOPING A COMMUNITY FOOT HEALTH EDUCATION MODEL

Basic to further discussion of health education at this time is a definition. People tend to confuse health "information" with health "education." Health education is a process that bridges the gap between health information and health practices. Health education motivates the person to take the information and do something with it—to keep himself healthier by avoiding actions that are harmful and by forming habits that are beneficial.

It is a frustrating paradox, given their relative effectiveness in bringing about change, that while health information has grown year by year in volume and in excellence, health education has developed much more slowly. The public must be made clearly aware of the profound difference between health information (disseminating facts) and health education (persuading people to change their lifestyles). They must also be encouraged to accept the fact that health education is a longer, costlier, broader, deeper and more complicated process. The health care delivery system can do a great deal to help solve health problems. But it cannot do everything. People must meet it at least halfway.

The complete range of comprehensive prevention services to meet the needs of the aged and their families and the provisions for correlating them and assuring continuity of service, do not now exist in any community. Every community has a core of medical and social services, however, and it is primarily within these existing services that the comprehensive structure may be built.

"Whole Person" Approach

With individuals and families in need of service all aspects of each situation must be examined. With comprehensive service goals in mind, physical health needs are assessed and resources are found to achieve better total physical health. Simultaneously, social and emotional components are parts of a whole person, and the plan must take into consideration all of these components.

Although this concept underlies the "whole person" approach, the interservice linkage necessary for total care in almost any situation has not yet been worked out as a community-wide pattern. Workers in the field of podiatry may not be able to create such a community-wide approach, but they can begin to demonstrate it by bringing together existing services, by making adaptations, and by emphasizing the need for coordination on behalf of the aged and his family.

Services which are essential components of a comprehensive community network include emergency (or acute care), diagnostic and referral inpatient and outpatient intermediate care facilities, rehabilitation services, counseling and protective services, financial assistance, employment and training services, housing and legal, social and recreational, and consultation and education services. These may be needed in varying combinations and in different sequence by the aged and their families. A comprehensive network is geared to the effort to assure that they are available when needed, and to assist the aged and his family to use them.

This same range of services is also needed by persons with many other problems. Many of the services may be incidental to the aged, yet essential to a total approach to care for the aged. The development of a parallel system of services is not advocated because such a system must inevitably be less effective in dealing with total need. It is important, however, that special attention be given to the problem of foot care in each community through the use of one or more individuals who serve as advocates for the aged and as catalysts for the development of needed services. Most communities need the aid of such catalysts to "make things happen," to assure that essential services are developed and provided.

Health problems of the feet constitute a compound problem and this fact in itself creates considerable difficulty for those who would deal with it.

- It is a problem for the patient.
- It is a problem for his family and for those who are intimately related to him.
- It is a problem for his community, for the neighborhood in which he lives.
- It is a problem for the state and for the nation which must pay the human costs, the costs of personal and community disruption, and the costs of planning for prevention and control measures.

- It is a problem for the professionals and those allied to them in the provision of treatment services for the victims of foot problems.

Although it is complex, the prevention, treatment and control of foot problems is not an impossible goal. At the individual level we know that patients can be helped. They are as rewarding, as challenging to those in the helping professions as any other patient or client. They present the same individual variety, the same range in their capacity to use treatment, the same range in their potential for growth. Professionals who are increasing their knowledge and skills in the treatment of patients and their families know this. Communities, when they are concerned with the problem and are actively involved in the development of services, see the positive effects of a community approach in dealing with this as with any other problem.

Problem of Chronic Foot Disease

The human foot has been called the mirror of health. In the broadest sense of the word chronic foot disease is a series of multiphasic illnesses, progressive in nature, but having prevention strategies.

Screening, Diagnostic and Referral Services

Definitive diagnosis with respect to the social, medical and psychological aspects of the problem of the aged is necessary if appropriate services and care are to be provided. This requires for each community the availability of competent screening, diagnostic and referral resources. These may be provided in a community health center, a hospital, outpatient clinics or in other community agencies. When necessary, collaborative arrangements may be developed among the private physician, the public health nurse, a consulting social worker and other professionals so that their joint skills may be brought to bear in determining the diagnosis and the aspects of need around which a treatment plan and appropriate referrals may be made.

Services are usually initiated on the basis of the presenting problem. In emergencies these may begin as a part of the diagnostic process. Immediate response to the patient's presenting need is essential in order to engage him in the treatment process. If he is put off and his immediate need is ignored pending complete diagnosis, his motivation to seek treatment may be extinguished and the opportunity to a prevention program lost.

Consultation and Community Education

Every health education service or treatment program has an important responsibility to community agencies and organizations in the development of increased knowledge and skill related to foot disease and its treatment. Podiatrists can help generalists to identify foot problems and provide appropriate help.

Podiatrists should encourage and help others to provide services appropriate to their organizations and professional roles. Such education, when it is directed to enlarging the understanding of professions and the general public and diminishing their frustration and consequent rejection of the aged, is an important approach to the development of needed foot health services. As members of the community and its services see that help is possible—that the aged want help and are worth helping—they become more willing and able to work with those persons suffering from foot problems.

Training

Foot health programs can and do provide a variety of training opportunities for other agency staffs as part of their continuing education programs. Generally, these are in the form of seminars, field observation, and similar opportunities. They can and do provide field placements as a part of their professional training for social work students, nurses, medical students, psychiatric and psychological interns, and vocational counselors. It is important that additional opportunities be provided in hospitals, community health centers, and specialized podiatry programs where those who have some expertise in working with the foot illness may share their knowledge and experience.

It is obvious from the review of these elements of a community podiatric health education program that they are not essentially different from those needed to meet other chronic health and social disabilities and handicaps. It is equally obvious that provision of such services requires a multidisciplinary approach.

Although all of the above services essential to a comprehensive prevention service network are listed individually, this should not imply fragmentary or unconnected delivery of service. The "whole person" approach means that all needs of the aged and his family are identified and given their proper consideration; that the problem of foot disorders takes its place among other problems and that this may not be first or second place; that continuity of services is assured; that referral relationships among agencies provide coordinated planning for the family as well as the patient and for appropriate movement from one service to another or between levels of service.

Communities now have the kinds of agencies and facilities which are able, with a little special education in respect to foot health, to give needed services to the patients and their families, just as they do to others in need. The services themselves are not new or different from those now offered in most communities to persons with like needs.

The podiatrist is the one professional who holds the key. All other professions are needed, in varying combinations at various points, in the processes of treatment and care. A total community podiatric health education program that is dynamic will modify methods and activities as the patient needs change. A major requirement of the podiatrist is the ability to work with other professionals and with nonprofessionals in a climate of mutual regard and trust. As E. A. Hooton has stated,

The medical profession has a very myopic viewpoint when it starts at the autopsy table and works backward. It would be most desirable to start with a healthy infant and healthy parents and promote a program of positive health. In this way, many of the nuisance disorders would be eliminated and a generally more healthy population would result.

THE PODIATRIST AS A COUNSELOR IN PATIENT EDUCATION

A gap exists between knowledge and practice. Has health education failed because members of our community fail to follow our teachings? Priorities are necessary in program planning. On what should health education priorities be based—the number and type of deaths; the number and type of communicable disease; monies spent foolishly by the public; chronic conditions limiting activities; what people think and talk about? There is need for the podiatrist to serve as a health counselor in selecting health education priorities and make community-wide efforts more effective.

The podiatrist, although increasingly required to serve as health counselor, receives very little preparation in this practice. This is a serious omission. The majority of the leading causes of foot disease today are intimately related to personal habits and behavior. Counseling is essential for attempting alterations in these forms of behavior. Primary disease prevention and successful maintenance of patients on long term regimens of treatment likewise are dependent upon the podiatrist's role as counselor even more than upon his traditional roles as a "healer."

The podiatrist may receive little preparation for the practice of being a counselor, but he does find himself involved in this practice by demands placed upon him by his patients and their families. If not by academic preparation, then through trial and error he is involved as a counselor, and his success is reflected by the scope of his counseling. A review of the results of his treatment program often indicates the failure on his part when he sees his patients return with the same old problems.

The health appraisal concept has three facets, namely,

1. *Health history*, "Past"—What a Patient Was!
2. *Health examination*, "Present"—What a Patient Is!
3. *Counseling*, "Future"—What a Patient Can Be!

Often the appraisal process ends after the examination. Ideally, the following kinds of interaction take place.

1. The patient-doctor relationship is a two-way process. Patients should get information from the doctor as the doctor obtains information from them.
2. Patients want to get their health information from podiatrists or to be referred by their podiatrist to other members of the health team. The podiatrist can "open up the doors" to knowledge.
3. The podiatrist has several roles outside his office:
   a. To get involved in the community process.
   b. To serve on health boards, be a resource person.
   c. To refer patients to community resources, after he learns about them himself.
   d. To present group talks and lectures and participate in health education.
   e. To set an example with respect to health for the community.
   f. To ask community health workers for help.
   g. To serve as an information and referral agency.
   h. To set up group education situations.
   i. To participate in the school health program.
   j. To not be an "aginer," but provide leadership as a "forer."
4. Health education considerations:
   a. People tend to react more rapidly to recommendations from a physician.
   b. The physician must learn that when this information doesn't get across, his methods may be at fault.
   c. In regard to foot health, patients must be instructed to better understand what their doctor has said.
   d. What kinds of allied health personnel would help the health education process and in what manner would they function? Reference was made to the use of the professional health educator in group practice situations.
   e. The physician and the pharmacist might play a role in education regarding drug therapy, at least for selected patients.
   f. Repetitive types of educational materials are needed.
   g. Medicine cannot be practiced without relating to or practicing health education.

The need for counseling is great. People—the patients—need and desire and seek information from the physician. The physician has the information to give, but needs to develop skills in its delivery. The physician has the image, the respect, and must take his place in the health education process.

PATIENT EDUCATION PROGRAMS IN HOSPITAL SETTINGS

Programs of patient education in hospitals are the exception rather than the rule. A review of the literature over 15 years reveals much on roles, responsibilities and unique opportunities, but little on actual practices. Here are both a need and an opportunity for the trained health educator. Undeveloped professional staff perception of and interest in the education component of quality health care are reasons for slow expansion of educational services in the hospital setting. Systematic goal setting, means of financing programs, greater interest of the hospital administrator and more program descriptions in the literature are among current needs.

To develop the concept of health education in a hospital program one must consider the roles of the physician, the hospital, the consumer of health services, the nurse, the hospital administrator, the medical school and the government on the national, state and local level.

The availability of medical care to the public will differ in accordance with the area being considered—rural, suburban or urban.

1. Hospital administration—health education relationship.
2. Community hospital as a health education center.
3. Aids to teaching the patient and consumer.
4. Auxiliary health aids.
5. Positive community health education programs.
6. Role of the physician, hospital administration and county medical society.
7. Cooperative arrangements with hospital regional programs and the federal government.
8. Changing image and role of hospital.

The role of the hospital is changing to that of an intensive care unit to serve those patients who need acute care, surgical services and diagnositc services.

There is direct evidence that planned health education programs, such as the following, for the patients and community at large will eventually reduce the high cost of hospital and medical care.

1. New health education materials with which special groups will identify and which they will use in developing new attitudes leading to possible changes in behavior.
2. The addition of trained health educators in general hospitals whose responsibility will be to plan, organize and assist in the implementation of programs.
3. Structuring the administration of comprehensive health planning to include the hospital as an integral agency in furthering health education.
4. The ability of the practicing health educator to assume a new role as an innovator with the daring and willingness to try new approaches and techniques which may lead to a changed system, a change in the role of the professional, and a change in ourselves.

Interest areas needing development or further consideration:

1. Clinic and hospital program.
2. Hospital administrator support.
3. Hospital-patient education programs using learning and teaching machines.
4. Hospital-community health programs involving the board of directors, the administrator, and inservice staff training.
5. Programs that can be developed from a hospital setting.
6. Patient-hospital costs. Effectiveness of health education program in regard to costs.
7. Hospital costs reduction through health education.
8. Hospital as a resource in social development, patient care and after care—follow-up.
9. Availability of health services—location of service in relation to the consumer.
10. Hospital in a cooperative relationship to regional medical program.

In the hospital the podiatrist must be sensitive to the beliefs, opinions and knowledge regarding health and illness held by the patients. He also must understand the "system" of institutional health service. Not only is he concerned with the health education of the patient by various individual and group techniques, but by periodic surveys he identifies needs and evaluates programs, participates in teaching educational methods to the health professionals, stimulates programs of patient teaching, and develops reference materials for the benefit of all involved in patient teaching.

There is a health education component in patient care. The podiatrist has a responsibility to help those who provide patient services to become aware of the educational component in their work and to assist them to fulfill their educational role.

It is recognized that the importance of staff, patient and community attitudes, beliefs and expectations; of leadership in, and the climate of, the patient-care setting; of communication, nonverbal as well as verbal; of feedback; of changing others—and ourselves; of *caring* about the patient; and of remembering that mankind, be it patient, institution staff member, or health educator, is a polyphasic learner, and is extremely adept at learning more than one thing at a time.

The patient care institution provides a learning experience, whether planned or unplanned, for the patient, his family, and his friends. But what accounts for the variance between what the "teacher" teaches and the learner learns? Whom does the patient "hear"? What medical expertise and authority is vested by the patient in the professional staff, in lower echelon staff, in other patients?

A teachable moment occurs each time a patient enters a patient-care facility whether as an inpatient or outpatient. But teaching is a dialogue, yet who "listens" to the patient? Who checks to see if the patient knows what has been said, if the patient understands?

There is a need to reexamine the patient-care facility's goals in the light of community and patient goals. But if the goals of the patient-care facility are in conflict with the community's or patients' goals, who gives in, who resists? Who wins, who loses?

Patient education is not the exclusive purview of the patient-care facility's professional staff. Everyone who handles and/or relates to the patient plays a role in patient education. But do the program planners, the administrators, know what this role is? Do the dispensers of patient-care services, themselves, know their educational role? Every staff member has an educational function that flows naturally from his contact with the patient. But how can each staff member be helped to see and understand this function,

and the uniqueness of his individual contribution to patient education?

With expanding demands for patient-care services, time is increasingly important. But whose time, that of the staff or that of the patient? Does the saving of staff time, at the expense of patient time, in fact, increase rather than decrease the requirement for staff time?

The patient needs to know certain things in respect to his illness to enable him to better cooperate with his treatment. But what are the things he needs to know? Do they vary with each illness, with each patient, or are they attitudes toward health, toward illness, that can be "taught" to all patients?

Priorities of patient care should be established. But on what basis and by whom will the priorities be set? Is the determinant the number of like patients, the interest and/or ability of staff, the captiveness of the patient population, the seriousness of the condition, the patient's needs as seen by the patient, or as seen by the staff?

Podiatrists in training have to understand the new role of the physician. But what is this "new role" and who will teach it to the patient? Traditional or new, is it the podiatrist's responsibility to educate the patient himself or to see that the information needed by the patient is given to him by others? Is the physician's educational role one of sharing or directing? All of us need to be reeducated. But do we know how to change ourselves— or others?

We need a program that would seek to educate the patient-care facility's total staff. We need staff orientation to the importance of patient education and we need inservice attitudinal education. But how can a program of staff education be started? Who will convince the administration that it's needed? Who will convince the staff? Who will plan and conduct the program? The staff is the key to effective patient education. But the staff is also the key to other responsibilities in the patient-care facility. Who will help them to recognize the importance of the patient's educational needs? And the importance of their involvement in patient education?

The climate in which patient care takes place affects the way of the patient accepts the care. But if the climate is not a favorable one, what can be done to change it? How can the channels of communication within the patient-care facility be opened? How can rapport between staff members be fostered? How can resistance to change be reduced?

An educational diagnosis is needed for each patient if we are to provide total patient-care services. But who shall make this diagnosis? And when shall it be made? Effective patient care includes the mapping out of an educational program, as well as a treatment program, to meet the patient's needs. But how and by whom is the patient's educational prescription prepared? Who supervises its application? Who measures its effectiveness? Organized patient education programs should be an integral part of comprehensive care. But where and by whom will such programs be carried on? Is the hospital the "best" setting? do we need a full-time person assigned to the hospital for patient education, or could the community educator conduct such a program?

There are exciting beginnings in patient education which need to be measured objectively; beginnings which include the expansion of the treatment team, the reliance on the insight to be gained from appraisal of the patient-care setting, staff needs, and patient needs by the psychological disciplines; the delivery of services where the patient is, the sharing of the development of the treatment plan with the patient himself, and the acceptance of our failures in patient education as a source of new knowledge.

There are also some apparent successes in patient education which need to be studied further. Chief among these are rehabilitation centers with their extensive retraining programs and self-help groups of patients with similar problems who, by joining together, support and reinforce each others' learning.

From studies that have been carried on, there are clues to areas that need to be studied further.

chapter 18

Foot Health Education—Podiatric Considerations

Arthur E. Helfand, D.P.M.

During the past decade, many changes have taken place in the concepts of total health services. The marked growth of population and the rising economic and educational levels of our population have created new demands for additional health programs and facilities. The most dramatic change in disease patterns, during this time, has been the tremendous reduction of the infectious diseases and the resultant emergence of chronic disease as our number one health problem. There is no question that the association of chronic disease and aging has placed an increased burden on many programs and has necessitated the inclusion of all facets in patient care.

We know that a healthy population is our most important natural resource and that a person's health is dependent upon a wide variety of the physical and social influences of his environment. One of the most interesting findings is that senior citizens are not particularly interested in chronic disease, per se. They have achieved their goal in life by the mere fact that they have lived to be golden agers. Their chief concerns are retaining their ability to see, hear and walk about.

Maintaining an ambulatory population is one of the responsibilities of the podiatry profession. If a community loses its ambulatory citizens, the resultant socioeconomic changes can create wards of society.

The initial step in the spectrum of health care is prevention. We know that chronic disease and aging cannot be prevented at this time. However, if through public health education and continuous evaluation, early diagnosis can be made prior to the onset of symptoms, and overt abnormalities can be prevented. This concept of secondary prevention when applied to foot health would increase the life span by maintaining an ambulatory and useful population.

There are many facets to programs for the aged. These generally involve the following areas: research, diagnosis, treatment, followup, rehabilitation, education and custodial care. In a sense, the initial phase is education; educating the community as to the program and need for the particular health service. Programs must include a complex of multiagencies, as no one agency or one profession can solve the many related health problems. It is obvious that the development of foot health educational programs and material over the next decade will be evolutionary. The foot is seldom the cause for mortality. However, we know that the foot is many times the site of morbidity and often the cause of morbidity, disability and limitation of activity.

Thus, in taking the initial step toward the prevention of pedal pathology, "Protect What Can Not Be Replaced" becomes exceedingly meaningful, especially with the emphasis now being placed on outpatient and home care programs. In a sense, podiatry and foot health can put "life into living" and permit a population to maintain a useful and productive life by "keeping them walking."

We can define foot health education as "the sum of experiences of podiatry and related health fields which favorably influence the habits, attitudes and knowledge relating to the individual and his community." This definition applied to geriatrics and chronic disease opens the door to a broader concept of total health service and total personal health.

The basic objective of any health education program is to do things with people and to get people to do things about their own personal health. To reach this goal, communities must be evaluated. The existing health facilities, personnel, the rates of illness which present pedal manifestations or complications, and the population characteristics are all important aids in analyzing public health needs with relation to foot health education.

We must consider the education of the patient. The ability of patients to cope with their health problems is directly related to their education. We also know that groups within the community also vary in educational background. As older citizens will generally have far less formal education than younger people, special consideration must be given to their special needs.

We must also consider the customs, culture and social influences which frequently form barriers to the acceptance of a particular health service and health education program.

The most important single individual in the promotion of any foot health educational program is the family podiatrist. His daily person-to-person contacts with patients are responsible for the daily transmission of foot health information. By adding large scale health department educational programs to this community health service, the population will be increasingly motivated. In these projects attention must be focused on remaining ambulatory, as the foot is an indicator of body health. Program planning and consultation must be sought to develop the materials to be utilized in any expanded program. Personnel, other than podiatrists, must be indoctrinated as to the need for foot health and the relationship of the foot to aging and the chronically ill patient.

There is no one method of providing patients with foot health education. These programs are multiphased and each segment is related to and overlaps other aspects of the program. The initial phase is informational and might be termed sensitization. It is not the purpose of this segment to increase the health knowledge of the individual or to change the health habits of the people exposed to the program. Rather, before people accept or reject a program they must be made aware of the need for the service and the existence of facilities, and understand the particular health service. Audiovisual methods such as spot radio announcements, posters and slogans provide an excellent medium to create a community need. This phase merely provides the individuals with enough information so that they will be more receptive to further detailed information.

The second phase is really an expansion of the informational segment. Publicity for particular programs, services and other aspects must emphasize to the community the importance of foot health. We know, for example, that once a patient is moving about he will accept other forms of therapy more readily. Care must be exercised in the preparation, presentation, explanation and demonstration of materials and information.

People must understand why foot trouble is more common in older people and, to some degree, the relationship of the foot to chronic disease. The need to be able to move about, visit friends, pursue a hobby, lead a useful life and, in fact, put life into living, must be stressed. Patients must understand the role of their family podiatrist as part of the health team. By emphasizing podiatry as an integral link in the health chain, the senior citizen will begin to see the need for foot health.

Foot health is a basic and needed service. To develop a community foot health educational program, the elderly and the patient with chronic disease must be impressed with this personal health need. Examples of personal health benefits are:

1. Increased personal comfort.
2. Lessened possibility of additional medical or surgical complications.
3. Reduced institutional and confined care.
4. Reduction or elimination of hospitalization due to a foot condition.
5. Increased life span with added mental health benefits by reducing a stress or strain.
6. Providing an increased diagnostic pro-

gram to follow the concept of secondary prevention of chronic disease.

7. Keeping the individual and the community foot healthy and ambulatory.

This phase of the educational program must be extended to all health professions within the community as well as to the individual citizens.

To reach this goal of improved community and personal service, cooperation between the podiatrist, other professionals and the citizens must be maintained. Full use should be made of audiovisual facilities to make the individual conscious of his foot health. Interest must be maintained and emotional barriers removed. The individual must be made to feel that he wants to do something about his personal foot health and the foot health of the entire community. He must want to practice foot health. In a sense, he must be motivated to seek health education material. By utilizing existing information and past experience, and by demonstrating common conditions, a community will learn to appreciate the need for good foot health care.

The third phase is the actual preparation and presentation of the educational information. By sensitizing and publicizing foot health, the individual is ready to accept and make changes in his personal health habits. Realizing that learning takes place through the learner, and that through personal contact with people, unwillingness is overcome, specific information can be presented to the community. These programs should be extended to family group therapy and utilize terms familiar to the listener and related to their personality and circumstances.

The mere fact that an individual believes in foot health and has been exposed to a program does not mean that he will act. The fourth phase of foot health education is motivation. People have basic emotional drives: jealousy, determination, pride, malice or combinations of the above and other feelings. Some assist in motivation, others prevent it. Personal contact, group therapy and audiovisual presentations persuade individuals to take action.

In motivating a group to change health habits, the individuals must make a conscious efffort to learn. There must be a continuous effort to maintain interest, demonstrate need and remove the emotional barriers which might be associated with a foot health education program. The individual must feel that he must practice foot health to reach his own personal goal of maximum physical fitness. Inactivity can foster mental and emotional fatigue. The mere fact that an individual has nothing to do, or is simply bored, might be the forerunner of physical disability and a marked limitation of activity. Older people and those with chronic disease must be made to realize that a person is never too old to participate in some form of recreational activity that includes exercise, and that the ability to participate depends a great deal on foot health and the ability to move about. Even the less active sports, such as golf and fishing, require ambulation. If the entire foot health education program only achieves one goal— making the individual look at his feet and observe changes—serious complications can be eliminated through follow-up professional care.

Through the maximum cooperation of the community, its health department and the health profession, foot health education programs will provide many benefits. These are:

1. For the individual—better health, greater self-sufficiency, higher morale and lower medical costs.
2. For his family—less dependence, reduced medical costs and minimal psychological problems.
3. For his community—a healthier, more productive citizenry with marked socioeconomic advantages.

If we recognize that health education significantly is a first line of prevention, then we can view health promotion as a form of prevention and a form of health education. Many older people are unaware of what is even expected to be good health or good foot health habits. They may seek services from areas other than those technically qualified and may turn to over-the-counter medical goods or home remedies as a means of treating their own self-diagnosed problem.

The types of questions that many elderly patients require assistance with deal with the management of many common foot problems. One of the most common questions that elderly patients require assistance with is in defining the term "bunion." Elderly patients generally are interested in knowing what causes a bunion. They need to receive information on the hereditary tendency toward this type of foot. They need to clearly understand the relationship of walking to the changes that occur in the first metatarsal phalangeal joint. They need to have a clear understanding of the degenerative changes that can take place at the first metatarsal phalangeal joint. They need to understand the somewhat irreversible pattern of a hallux valgus deformity and need to recognize that a surgical approach is elective and should be based upon difficulty in ambulation and pain rather than a concern for the cosmetic appearance of the foot. Elderly patients tend to recognize that the term bunion means many things. They are not sure whether it represents deformity, hyperkeratosis, soft tissue swelling or arthritic changes. They need to be clearly informed as to the long range ambulatory goals when surgical repair is contemplated.

Elderly patients do need to know the difference between a bunion and a corn. They need to recognize that a hyperkeratotic area with a central core, is effectively known as a heloma or corn. Elderly patients do have concerns about footwear and the selection of footwear needs to based upon the functional needs of the individual as well as his environmental activities. For example, individuals living in nursing homes or long-term care institutions require a different conceptual model of footwear and ambulation than those living in the community who still are maintaining their own destinies. Elderly patients should be given advice on walking and the relationship of ambulation to the development of hyperkeratotic tissue. They should be clearly informed as to the hazards of walking barefoot and the hazards of loose footwear. Elderly patients should be given instruction on the appropriate mechanism of the management of hyperkeratotic tissue. They should be told not to provide any degree of self-treatment, be it through over-the-counter chemical remedies or self-surgical reduction.

Elderly patients are also concerned about the permanent removal of cornified tissue. A clear and practical demonstration that identifies the presence of osseous abnormalities and pressure points, along with biomechanical problems, should be included in the health educational approach to the elderly patient.

Elderly patients need to recognize that the residuals of rheumatoid arthritis and the changes that occur in degenerative joint disease affect the joints of the foot. They need to recognize that the management of arthritis is in fact management and does not represent a cure or a regeneration to a normal position without some surgical activity. They need to understand simple drugs for the management of pain, as most elderly patients have different responses to medication than the young individuals and require generally less medication to achieve a therapeutic level. Elderly patients with severe arthritic changes should be made aware of the need for the use of orthotics and special changes in footwear. However, it might be wise to consider an educational approach to permit the elderly patients to utilize an appropriate orthosis for most of their activities but retain some degree of style for special activities.

Many times in the elderly patient, toenails become a focal point for questions. Older patients can be instructed in the proper management of normal nails. In many cases elderly patients are unable to see properly or bend properly. The use of an emery board periodically is one method of getting elderly patients involved in their own foot care. Where nails are thickened, patients must be informed that they should seek initial professional care to properly diagnose and treat the condition and then begin a program of home care and education. Patients should be instructed not to cut abnormal shapes into nails and not to remove a nail as a result of their own diagnosis. Where fungus toenails are a problem, the elderly patient needs to be aware of the ramifications of neglect and needs to be made aware of the various aspects of treatment. Where deformity is such that surgical removal is appropriate, the elective aspects of the procedure and the informed consent should not only deal with the provisions of the surgical procedure itself, but significant discussion of the postoperative management. Many patients are unaware that when nails are removed, they may or may not grow back. Elderly patients may be unaware of the fact that the nail grows from a matrix or root and they must clearly receive a proper explanation of these facts. Patients should be told that ingrown toenails are not quite as common as they appear to be; that there are many other conditions that can produce a similar pressure-like pain, such as incurvated nails or onychophosis; and that appropriate care depends upon the proper diagnosis. Elderly patients are many times concerned about deformities of their toes such as hammer toes. They recognize that a surgical approach is one method of correcting or modifying the deformity. However, they also need to be given an alternative mechanism of treatment to permit them to determine the relationship of the elective procedure to pain and difficulty in ambulation. Proper information concerning the use of silicone molds, other orthodigital devices and footwear changes should be included in the total discussion with the patient. Patients with hyperkeratotic lesions or calluses on hammer toes should be instructed in the appropriate self-care of these lesions. They should be advised not to provide any degree of self-treatment but to limit their activity to the protective activities of lamb's wool and the use of an emollient to maintain appropriate lubrication of the skin itself. Where the deformities are related to pain and difficulty in ambulation, surgical considerations would be appropriate, as age itself should not be a contraindication for surgical revision. Many elderly patients can remain quite active if their feet are pain free and every effort should be made to permit elderly patients to achieve a pain free status for the balance of their years in order to maintain their dignity.

There is much myth pertaining to the height of an arch in the foot. Many patients believe that arches fall. They need to have clear and concise information on the broad biomechanical concepts of foot motion to understand the compensating factors involved in foot deformity and the rotational activities that take place to create an illusion of deformity. Arthritic changes which occur tend to change joint structure and in fact may not only produce pain and changes in gait but may produce compensatory changes in footwear. A full explanation of proper treatment dealing with orthotics and footwear would be appropriate for the geriatric patient prior to the institution of any therapeutic regimen.

Many elderly patients are concerned about heel spurs. They believe that the bony projection is in a plantar mode and only when it is x-rayed and demonstrated are they able to accept the anterior projection of the spur itself. There needs to be a clear understanding on the part of the geriatric patient as to the years of abuse that create the fascial strain which produces the bony abnormality. Elderly patients should be aware that treatment, for the most part, can be managed in a non-surgical manner and that there may be a need for various types of heel cups, orthotics and special footwear changes.

The changing economy and inflationary spiral have produced significant changes in the concerns of the elderly towards footwear. An approach to educating patients for proper footwear depends on whether or not the individual is institutionalized or living in the community. For those institutionalized, foot covering should be considered that will permit the patient to ambulate based upon his needs, and secondarily may, in fact, be modified to avoid all pressure from the dorsum of the foot.

Many times a sneaker may in fact be the best type of footwear for many of these patients. For patients living in the community, one consideration of footwear selections should be based upon the ability of the patient to bend. Where arthritic changes are such that the patients are unable to properly use a lace shoe, then a slip-on with a long shoe horn would be appropriate. Where range of motion is normal, then a conservative shoe generally fits the needs of most patients. It should be noted, however, that all patients require some degree of style consciousness and the compromise of having an individual wear adequate walking shoes for 95% of the time is much more acceptable than a patient who refuses to make any changes based upon a concern for dress. Patients should be instructed in the proper method of selecting a fit and given to understand that special shoes may not be needed for most elderly patients. Patients should be instructed that shoes are basically articles of clothing and should meet the needs of the activity that is contemplated. They should be instructed as to the various segments of shoes and that modification should not be made without appropriate evaluation and/or prescription. Elderly patients also need to understand the relationship of hosiery to footwear and to ambulation. They should be instructed that the indiscriminate use of support hose without an appropriate diagnosis may be detrimental to their foot health and to their ambulatory status.

Elderly patients should be informed that walking is perhaps the best form of exercise that they can deal with. Special exercises may also be prescribed to eliminate some of the stiffness that is present in the geriatric foot. The patients need to understand what causes stiffness and what causes leg cramps both at night and during walking. They need to be given clear information on the etiologic activities of swelling under the ankles that occurs both at rest and in walking.

The elderly need to be given some specific instructions that would constitute a basic foot health leaflet. The attached information has been utilized and provides such an approach. If we view the concept of education, health promotion and prevention as a singular approach to patient management, we can recognize that an informed patient will be a therapeutically better patient.

RULES FOR FOOT HEALTH

How To Prevent Foot Problems In Aging Feet

Foot care for patients who are aging is an essential part of the total care of patients. Much of the ability to remain active and productive rests with good foot health.

First, you must avoid doing those things which add to the danger of decreasing the circulation in your feet. Pressure, cold and smoking generally have the same localized effect. They are harmful because they tend to decrease blood flow. The everyday activities that can produce pressure on blood vessels include sitting with your legs crossed, wearing socks with elastic tops, and wearing round elastic garters. In addition, wading, swimming or bathing in cold water should be avoided. Exposure to cold and refraining from smoking is essential in managing the pedal complications of aging.

A second major area of prevention includes breaks in the skin and infection. Any disruption in the skin surface can produce an infective process unless care is instituted. You can avoid such breaks from burns, irritations, cuts and/or other injuries by a variety of methods. For example, do not put your feet in hot water or add hot water to your bath without testing the temperature of the water. Generally, your bath temperature should be between 85 and 90°. If you do not have a proper thermometer, test it with your elbow. Use extreme care if you use a hot water bottle or heating pad. It is generally best to avoid their use entirely.

Do not use corn plasters or commercial corn cures. These preparations are acid in nature and destroy tissue. In all cases, these preparations produce tissue destruction far beyond their original intent. Once there is tissue loss, breaks in the skin occur and some form of infection usually results. Caution labels, when present, usually indicate that such preparations should not be used by people who are elderly, have diabetes mellitus or poor circulation.

Other warnings include excessive sunburn, wearing run-down shoes, wearing worn-out stockings, treating your own foot problems with sharp instruments and digging into the corners of your toenails, and walking barefoot, even at home.

Washing your feet daily and wearing clean stockings are musts. You should inspect your feet at least twice a week and look for things such as redness, blisters, cuts or scratches or cracks between your toes. Any discolorations or other changes should also be noted. Because you are aging, you may have some loss of sensation in your feet, making inspection essential. Help your family doctor and podiatrist help you by reporting any change to them. If you do notice any change or abnormality, early reporting and care can usually prevent serious trouble. You should remember that all health professionals work together to help keep you healthy and walking.

You should wear shoes that not only fit your feet but fit the occasion. Selecting a shoe is important. The widest part of the shoe should match the widest part of your foot. The shoe should follow the natural outline of your foot and fit snugly but not be tight.

If you have some existing deformity, special lasts or shoes may be needed.

In general, shoes for general use should have a firm counter that will keep your foot in position in the shoe. The heel should have a wide support (about 1½ inches for women). There should be about ¾ inch of space beyond your big toe (longest toe) when you stand. The toe box should be round and high to allow space for your toes. The shoe upper should be soft and flexible. The lining should be smooth and free of ridges and wrinkles. Wear new shoes for short periods of time until you are used to the change.

Our purpose is to help you understand why your feet need special care and how to help prevent problems. The next job is up to you. Only you can try to remember and follow these simple rules—and thus prevent the serious trouble you could have. We sincerely hope you do.

chapter 19

Podiatry's Role in the Nursing Home

Edward L. Tarara, D.P.M.

In 1960 Tarara conducted a survey of a sample group of podiatrists in the United States. He found at that time, of 182 returns from an inquiry of 500 podiatrists, that 27.67% of patients seen were over age 65.

Less striking, however, was the result of another survey that showed podiatric care in the nursing home. Twenty-eight states replied to a questionnaire. Five states reported that no podiatrists were making nursing home calls. The other states reported that anywhere from 1 to 48 podiatrists were spending time caring for such persons. Fourteen states reported that fewer than 10 podiatrists were doing this work, two states reported 46 to 48 podiatrists, respectively, working in nursing homes. The time spent in these institutions ranged from 1 to 16 hours per week and from 3 to 35 patients were being cared for in this amount of time.

Liss reported the first instance of a podiatry clinic in a nursing home expanding into an externship program and being integrated into a part of a course in hospital podiatry at the California College of Podiatric Medicine.

Merrill et al. reported on a survey of 1011 nursing home patients in 1967. The objectives of the survey were (1) to determine the prevalence of foot problems among nursing home patients in Minnesota; (2) to determine the need for providing podiatric care in nursing homes; 3) to classify the foot conditions in nursing home patients on the basis of indicated care and treatment; and (4) at a later date, to offer a curriculum for the teaching of basic information to nursing home personnel

in the prevention and rehabilitation of common foot problems of patients.

The survey identified the prevalence of nursing home patients with foot problems that was consistent with the percentage of an aged population that was not in a nursing home or extended care facility, as Helfand's "Keep Them Walking" program in Philadelphia.

The survey found that those needing routine hygienic care in most instances were receiving such care by their physician, podiatrist, or by the staff of the institution. The survey pointed out, however, that only 44% (163 of 364 patients) who needed professional care by their podiatrist or physician were receiving the needed care.

Lastly, the development of a curriculum for the teaching of basic information to nursing home personnel in the prevention and rehabilitation of common foot problems was started and tested by a team of podiatrists in Minnesota. They gave a series of 1-day seminars in five different areas of the state that were evaluated by the Northlands Regional Medical Program, Inc. Later this same team of podiatrists gave a series of 2-day seminars to nurses in nursing homes that became the basic outline of an inservice program developed by the American Podiatry Association. This will be discussed later in this chapter.

In 1973 Helfand, in his report *At the Foot of South Mountain* reinforced the findings of the Minnesota group and demonstrated the need for podiatric programs and consultations in all similar programs, if truly comprehensive health care were to be accomplished.

The foot problems of the geriatric patient stem from a lifetime of use and abuse. Unless a toe or foot is swollen or painful, little attention is paid to it. Poor vision, arthritis, obesity and an inability to bend downward because of dizziness or breathlessness prevent elderly patients from taking proper care of their feet. In old age there is an increase in the incidence of foot infections, ulcerations, gangrene and limb amputations as chronic disease inevitably progresses toward its terminal phase. Arthur E. Helfand has written:

Foot trouble is generally common in this group because of lowered vitality, impaired circulation, retarded healing, and a variety of associated changes in the anatomic structure of the foot.

The skin is among the first structures to demonstrate changes. The earliest sign is usually the loss of hair along the outer side of the leg and on the dorsum of the foot. Brownish pigmentations follow with an associated increase in the presence of hyperkeratotic areas, due to keratin dysfunction. There is also a loss of muscle mass and soft tissue in the foot so that even minor lesions can limit activity. The nails have a tendency to become brittle and thickened, and onychomycosis seems to be more prevalent in the aged.

There are numerous changes in the musculoskeletal structures of the foot. Due to wear and tear, repeated trauma, years of abuse, and a decreasing arterial supply, patients are easily fatigued and there is a marked decrease in work tolerance. With the associated loss of muscle and soft tissue mass, there are frequent complaints of leg cramps and foot cramps, which may or may not be associated with arteriosclerosis. Osteoarthritis, hyperostosis, senile osteoporosis, fixed deformities and marked limitation of motion are also noted and contribute further to the problems of ambulation.

The vascular system demonstrates trophic changes, intermittent claudication, rest pain, coldness, pulse changes, and color variations. These pathologies can turn simple abrasions into gangrenous lesions.

Aging and chronic disease produce many degenerative changes in the foot, such as a loss of sensation, complex gaits, reduced agility and atrophy. If we add the complications of systemic disease, such as diabetes, arteriosclerosis and arthritis, the need for early diagnosis of foot pathology, maintenance and rehabilitation becomes obvious.

A podiatry service in an extended care facility is essential to provide adequate health care to the patient. If the podiatric portion of total health care is not provided, the facility is not fulfulling its duty to the aged community.

In setting up a podiatric care program the ideal would contain the following:

1. As soon as possible after admission each patient should receive a complete podiatric screening. This evaluation should include past history of foot care, status of circulation, neurologic manifestations, foot orthopedic complications, and dermatologic and personal hygiene information. In this way the podiatrist can determine whether the patient needs routine hygienic care by the nursing staff, including care of nonpathogenic nails; professional podiatric service on a periodic basis; or extensive rehabilitation, including shoes, orthotics, and/or surgery.

In this way a comprehensive program can be set up for each patient in the facility. The podiatrist can then outline a care program for each patient and set up a tentative schedule of visits. Most podiatrists attending nursing homes have a definite schedule of timed visits, whether it be once a week, twice a month or once a month. They then can set up their schedule for the patient, if she needs extensive care or professional palliative care once a month or once every six weeks, or if the nursing staff can handle the routine care with the podiatrist examining and caring for the patient every 3 or 4 months.

2. Ambulatory patients (wheelchair, crutch patients, and those with walkers) could be transported to a private office or area where portable equipment could be available. An aide can accompany the patients to help remove shoes and stockings in preparation for foot care. The presence of a ward secretary to make notes for the attending podiatrist is of great help and also would help facilitate rescheduling of the patient at a proper interval. For the bedfast patient, it is usually suggested that an aide or nurse accompany the podiatrist to the patient's room and help prepare the patient by removing bedclothes and/or stockings if the patient is wearing them.

3. At the end of a clinical session all patients' charts should be available for pertinent notes or requests for follow-up care that the podiatrist may want the nursing staff to accomplish.

The nurse in the extended care facility is a very important part of the team effort. She is the liaison between the patient and the doctor. It is she who hears daily the complaints of the patient and can screen such complaints as to whether or not to relay them on to the doctor or if she can handle the minor problems herself. Therefore, I feel it is very important in any comprehensive podiatry program in an extended care facility that a good inservice program be set up.

To this end the American Podiatry Association has produced two brochures as foot health training guides for long term care personnel. These brochures are the culmination of work and experience of the Minnesota group, Helfand and others and are the most complete, step-by-step guides available for inservice training to extended care personnel.

Since the nurse is an important member of the health care team, it is important that she understand all the complications and ravages that systemic diseases can wreak upon the lower extremity of the geriatric patient. These inservice programs are designed to give the nursing personnel a basic overview of the foot and the problems that can occur in the geriatric foot. They outline the common foot problems in the aged, the anomalies that often occur and the complications of the many systemic diseases that are manifested in the feet and the lower extremity.

The most important objectives of all inservice programs should be fourfold: (1) to teach the nurse to recognize serious pedal problems such as infections, pregangrenous lesions and gangrene, so that the podiatrist can be made aware of any complication. As the liaison between the patient and the doctor, the nurse must be able to decide when to call the doctor for an emergency problem and when to wait for visits for foot care. She must be able to evaluate when the diabetic or vascularly embarrassed patient needs immediate emergency attention or if the problem can wait until the podiatrist's regular visiting session.

2. The nurse should be taught the prophylactic care of nonpathogenic nails. She should be aware of which nails she or her staff can trim and which nails need the professional care of the podiatrist.

3. She should be taught simple first aid to corns and calluses. Instructions should point toward use of protective paddings with moleskin, lamb's wool or sponge rubber protectors.

4. Finally, a most important aspect of the inservice training program should be the nurse's advice to her patients. She should be able to explain the advantages of daily foot care, using creams, antiseptics, foot powders and soaps. She should be able to tell her patients about the harmful effects of the extremes of temperature, why hot water bottles, hot foot soaks, electric pads, hot compresses and the like can be dangerous to the lower extremity. She should be able to explain why extra foot covering in the cold weather is necessary to prevent frostbite or freezing of the feet. She can caution her patients about walking barefoot, and about the danger that exists of cutting a foot or breaking a toe by striking a bed or dresser. She can explain the dangers of corn cures and ingrown nail medicine and the dangers of being one's own podiatrist by trying to use razor blades or cuticle scissors. She can also explain why the use of rubberbands or circular garters should be discarded as a means of holding the stockings up. Also leg crossing for long periods of time can cut off the blood supply and limit sensations to the legs. She can instruct the patient in the use of bed socks to provide warmth and comfort for poor circulation or arthritis.

In summary then, I feel the *role of the podiatrist* in the nursing home should be threefold:

1. *Prevention.* Through the routine screening of all admissions to a nursing home, a podiatrist can set up a treatment program for each patient.

2. *Early detection of foot pathology.* Thorough careful history, examination and testing can alert the podiatrist to a patient with a foot problem. Many systemic diseases are manifested in the feet.

3. *A planned program of treatment* for those patients who need preventive maintenance and those who need more specific care such as foot prosthetics, special medications, and/or surgical intervention.

The three key functions of the nurse in foot health care are:

1. *Detection and inspection.* Early detection of foot problems can often be accomplished during the bathing period without adding to

the work schedule. She can observe the nails, skin texture, temperature, color, hue and swelling; and check between the toes for signs of soft corns or cracking or athlete's foot; and observe the nails for discoloration, irritation or infection.

2. *Administering basic foot health care.* After the patient's bath, make sure that the feet are properly dried, especially between the toes to prevent maceration. The nurse can massage the feet with foot lotion to help maintain a soft supple skin tone. She can use powder between the toes to help keep the skin dry and prevent skin cracks and infection. Lastly, she can trim the simple, uncomplicated toenails, by cutting them straight across and avoiding probing of the corners.

3. *Advise the patients on foot health.* The nurse can advise the patient about helpful drugs, the advantages of daily foot care, using creams, antiseptics, foot powders and soaps. She can explain the harmful effects of the extremes of temperature, why hot water bottles, hot foot soaks, electric pads and the like can be dangerous to the lower extremity. She can explain the dangers of corn cures and ingrown nail medicines.

The team effort of the podiatrist and the nurse plays an important part in the well-being and foot comfort of the nursing home patient. The inclusion of podiatric services in extended care facilities will often produce dramatic benefits and effects. Individuals can be returned from long-standing, and at times absolute, immobility due to relative freedom that new-found ease brings.

chapter 20

Guidelines for Podiatric Programs in Long-Term Care Facilities

Arthur E. Helfand, D.P.M.

CONTRIBUTIONS OF A PODIATRY STAFF AND SERVICE TO AN EXTENDED CARE FACILITY

In long-term care facilities, the trend is toward offering a complete health service, with the total health care of the individual patient as the ultimate objective. Podiatrists, as members of the health team, work cooperatively with all types of institutions and facilities in attaining this objective and in turn expect reasonable cooperation from other members of the health team, including the facility staff. Greater utilization of podiatric service is the best demonstration of the contribution the podiatry staff can make to the total health care of the patient.

COMPREHENSIVE HEALTH CARE OF THE PATIENT

A podiatric service and staff in a long-term care facility are essential to provide adequate health care to the patient. If the podiatric portion of total health care is not provided, the facility is not fulfilling its duty as a service organization to the community. When reference is made to a podiatric program or service, all phases of podiatry for the chronically ill and the aged, i.e., diagnostic, preventive, rehabilitative and corrective are included. Podiatric services should be available consistent with the needs of the community and the needs of the institution or facility.

It is well recognized that patients are more easily motivated to accept appropriate therapy when they are able to walk and remain active members of the community even if that community is a hospital or long-term care facility. The various pedal complications associated with chronic disease, aging, the handicapped and the mentally ill further stress the need for comprehensive services to include podiatry and so further the quality of care provided the patient.

As soon as possible after admission, each patient should receive a complete podiatric screening. This evaluation should include statistical data, history, and circulatory, neurologic, foot orthopedic, dermatologic, and personal hygiene data. This evaluation is in addition to the general physical and dental examinations and should provide recommendations for a treatment program and maximum rehabilitation.

Ambulatory patients may be transported to a private office or clinical facility. This again should be determined by the size and needs of the institution. Portable equipment should be available to render necessary treatment in the long term care facility for non-ambulatory patients.

Methods of providing payment should be established, compatible with and supportive of existing financing of health programs. Methods must also be established to provide payment for those residents who require and desire care, but who are not financially able to assume its cost. These methods should be determined at the community level.

In addition, a program of foot hygiene should be instituted in all institutions and facilities. This regimen of daily care is the starting point for the entire podiatric or foot health program.

In extended care facilities, many patients do not have the strength or emotional stability to maintain good foot hygiene. The nursing staff, through proper staff education, should aid and instruct the patient in foot baths and other allied procedures, under the supervision of the staff podiatrist. The nursing staff should be trained to assist the patient in caring for biomechanical orthotic molds which may have been prescribed. The nursing staff should be trained to identify pedal lesions, swellings and other irregularities and to call the podiatrist when such findings are noted. Proper foot health will depend upon full cooperation between the professional and allied staffs, as well as from the patient.

In order to encourage full cooperation, the patient should be instructed in the following areas of personal hygiene:

1. The methods of washing and drying the feet.
2. The role of emollients and foot powders.
3. The proper methods of cleaning prosthetic devices.
4. The proper type of footwear and hose.
5. The proper exercise to stimulate circulation.
6. How to maintain muscle tone and encourage ambulation.
7. The importance of daily hygiene to maintain his well-being.

HOW TO PREVENT FOOT PROBLEMS IN AGING FEET AND PROVIDE A WORKING MODEL AS A BASE

The American Red Cross, in its *Fitness for the Future Program*, recommends the following foot health exercises:

1. Extend the legs horizontally, pull feet forward and downward. Hold and release.
2. Walk on tiptoe in your stocking feet around the room.
3. Standing in one spot, raise and lower the body, never coming down entirely on the heels.
4. Stand with your feet apart, straddling a seam or rug line. Force your feet to roll, throwing your weight to the outer borders of your feet.
5. Straddling a rug line, walk across the room on the outer borders of your feet.
6. Place marbles of various sizes on a rug. Sit on a chair and pick up the marbles with your toes.
7. Roll up a towel with your toes while sitting on a chair.
8. Raise yourself on tiptoes and rock from heel to toe, while holding onto a chair for support.

The proper exercise should be prescribed based on the individual patient's needs and ability to perform.

Diagnostic and Consultative Service

Podiatrists can carry out a useful role in the diagnostic service. Since many systemic diseases and conditions present pedal manifestations which are often the first signs of disease, it is difficult to visualize a complete physical survey of the patient without an adequate podiatric evaluation. It is therefore recommended that all patients of long-term care facilities receive a podiatric examination as part of their admission to the facility. This segment can best be completed by a member of the podiatric staff.

The podiatrist, as an integral part of the health team, can render a great service to the patient when the pedal condition or complication is the primary complaint. Proper treatment and management of the pedal complications, of diabetes and arteriosclerosis, for example, require full cooperation between the admitting practitioner, consulting podiatrist, patient and facility staff. This combined cooperation can radically reduce the period of bed confinement and permit the patient to again become a part of his particular community.

Consultative services should be widely used. Members of the professional staff should welcome the specialized training presented by the podiatrist and, likewise, podiatrists should welcome the training offered by other members of the professional and allied staffs. By sharing knowledge in a facility atmosphere, each profession can contribute to the overall understanding, diagnosis and treatment of the patient.

Research

Research activities are becoming more and more established as a vital part of staff functions in all health care facilities. With a greater number of qualified members of the health professions being trained to do research, this important phase should be included and expanded.

There are projects in many areas which may be considered. A few suggestions are:

1. Diabetes screening and its pedal complications.
2. Arthritis screening and complications.
3. Arteriosclerosis and its pedal complications.
4. Neurologic and sensory disease screening.
5. Training programs in applied gerontology.
6. Service patterns associated with long term care.
7. Onychomycosis and its relationship to general health.
8. Patient and professional education programs.
9. The functional management of foot pathology to increase ambulation.

Contributions to Administration

Administrators are becoming more aware of the importance of foot health as it pertains to the general well-being of the patient, and therefore of the need for podiatry programs as vital health services in health care facilities of all types. The members of the podiatry staff can aid the administrator in the broad areas of long-term care facility administration.

The podiatry staff should take an active part in staff conferences and seminars. Individual members should take an active part in the discussion of clinical problems, procedures, and in case presentations. Such cases should be carefully selected for their interest to the entire institution or facility staff. Senior members of the podiatry staff could serve on various committees of the institution, such as the records committee and training committee.

The podiatry staff should establish its administrative policy, and maintain its own audit of service consistent with the administrative policies of the facility.

Continuing Educational Programs

With long-term care facilities and hospitals now closely affiliated, these institutions will also serve as educational centers in the care of geriatric and chronically ill patient for all professions. Many such educational programs are now being established in the field of podiatry. In addition, a well organized podiatry staff may be used to train podiatry students and students of related professions in foot health. With the prospect of chronic disease and aging becoming an increasingly larger segment of professional education, exposure in extended care facilities will provide a more comprehensive interprofessional education. These facilities provide the appropriate atmosphere for training, and this results in improved service to patients.

The professions allied to podiatry have, in general, received little in the way of foot health education. The podiatry staff can provide this training for the nursing and other personnel. Such training will be beneficial to patients and to professional personnel and will help make the practical measures of pedal hygiene a daily routine.

PLANNING A PODIATRY PROGRAM FOR A LONG-TERM CARE FACILITY

In planning podiatry programs or services for a long-term facility, three major factors must be considered. These are:

1. The type and size of the facility.
2. The needs of the community for podiatric programs in nursing homes and related facilities.
3. The type of podiatry program to be carried out.

Knowledge of what other facilities of similar size and type have done can be of great assistance and a useful guide in the consideration of these factors.

The facilities for the podiatry program should receive the same consideration accorded other professional health services. It is ideal when each particular specialty has its own particular equipment, but when space is at a premium, the room and equipment can be shared with other health services. As demands on the podiatry service are increased, specialized facilities and programs may become necessary.

The floor plans of a podiatry operatory and the equipment needed will depend on the size of the facility and the extent of the podiatry service rendered. It is recommended that consideration be given to a waiting area, treatment area and mechanical laboratory. Other requirements such as physical therapy and radiology can usually be met by sharing facilities with other health services.

Modern concepts of diagnosis and therapy require modern equipment. It is recommended that all of the needed diagnostic facilities and equipment be available for the podiatry program. Podiatry is a basic health service. It requires and deserves careful planning and consideration to achieve optimum facility utilization.

Guidelines for Staff Structure and Service

The following is intended as a guide in the establishment of a podiatry staff, service or department.

I. *Definition of Podiatry*
Podiatry can broadly be defined as that profession of health sciences which deals with the examination, diagnosis, treatment and prevention of diseases and malfunctions affecting the human foot and its related or governing structures, by the employment of medical, surgical or other means. The applicable state statute, in addition, forms the basis for scope of practice and services.

II. *Intent and Purpose of the Guidelines*
In any facility, podiatry programs should have adequate facilities and high levels of professional conduct and proficiency to insure an optimum level of care to the patient. Establishing criteria or requirements for a podiatric program provides a measure of basic fundamental principles and essentials for the best possible care of patients.

III. *Prerequisites for a Podiatry Program*
A. The facility should have a physical plant free from hazards and properly equipped for the adequate care and comfort of the patient.
B. Bylaws, rules and regulations pertaining to podiatric services should conform to local statutory requirements.

C. All regulations for podiatric services should describe organization, duties, responsibilities and professional relationships.

IV. *Podiatry Staff*
A. Definition
The podiatry staff is defined as all those podiatrists privileged to work in the particular facility. Privileges are granted, at the discretion of the governing body. A written application, on a prescribed form, should designate the applicant's qualifications as a podiatrist. If acceptable to the governing body, the podiatrist may be granted privileges in podiatry, with tenure similar to other professional staffs.

B. Functions
1. Organizational
a. Establish bylaws, rules and regulations to govern the podiatry staff in a manner compatible with and supportive to other departments.
b. Provide podiatric services comparable to other professional health services.
2. Administrative
a. Conduct the activities of the podiatric program in a manner amicable and consistent with the administrative policies of the facility.
b. Aid in the selection of podiatric personnel.
3. Clinical
a. Render professional care to patients in accordance with the precepts of modern scientific podiatry.
b. Audit the clinical work of the podiatry staff and maintain the qualitative efficiency of podiatric care to patients.
c. Attend regular professional staff conferences.
4. Education and research
a. Provide education to allied professional staffs and other personnel of the facility and such patient education as is necessary to maintain an optimum level of foot health.

b. Provide or participate in podiatric research programs where possible.

C. The podiatry privilege
Privileges granted podiatrists shall be in accordance with local statutes and accrediting guidelines, equal to other professional disciplines.

D. Advisory committee
Each facility should have an advisory podiatrist or podiatry advisory committee to advise the administrator concerning podiatric services and policies. This committee shall make every effort to see that appropriate foot health programs are provided for the facility.

E. Qualifications for Membership
Membership on the podiatry staff shall be restricted to podiatrists who are:
1. Graduates of accredited colleges of podiatric medicine.
2. Legally licensed to practice in their respective states.
3. Members, or eligible for membership, in the American Podiatry Association and subscribers to the Code of Ethics as set forth by the American Podiatry Association.
4. Worthy in character and manners.
5. Competent in the practice of podiatry. All podiatrists engaging in the practice of a recognized special area of podiatry practice should meet, insofar as possible, requirements established for that special area of practice.

F. Methods of appointment
Podiatry staff appointments are made officially by the governing body of the institution or facility. Applications should designate the applicant's credentials as a podiatrist. This form should include:
1. Identification data.
2. Podiatry college and year of graduation.
3. Postdoctoral training.
4. Additional training and experience.
5. Names of professional societies and associations in which the applicant is a member in good standing.

6. A list of scientific papers the applicant has published.
7. Scientific meetings the applicant has attended in recent years.

Podiatry Program

All podiatric examinations and treatment should be entered on a standard record and made a permanent part of the patient's record. Records should include: complaints, history, examination, diagnostic findings, consultations, treatment, final results and recommendations.

Periodic foot examinations should be made as often as indicated by the foot health needs of the patient. Such examinations and follow-up treatments are essential to the care of the patient and can prevent complications from local foot conditions or from pedal manifestations of chronic diseases. Such programs will also provide a maximum degree of ambulation for the patient. Written instructions and prescriptions of the consulting podiatrists should be followed by the facility staff.

Podiatry Service in Mental Health Facilities

The various chronic and transitory foot problems which occur in any segment of the population often create a need for special consideration. In the mental health patient, the presence of physical pain, and particularly the discomfort of a chronic foot problem, can incapacitate the patient. Foot problems can further diminish his ability to think for himself or to concentrate and can lessen the effectiveness of other therapeutic regimens.

Members of the podiatry staff should be aware that the patient population referred to them for treatment presents a variety of psychiatric problems and symptoms, which complicate diagnosis and treatment. Some such symptoms are poor contact, limitation in the ability to communicate verbally, withdrawal, negativism, excessive fear and apprehension, paranoid ideation, and somatic delusions. Limitations in emotional controls exist typically in these patients. Sensitivity and skill in dealing with psychologic techniques should be acquired to initiate and maintain podiatric diagnosis and treatment. The podiatrist, in obtaining histories, should be aware that there is often a distorted reference from factors arising from the patient's mental state. The reliability of the patient's verbalized subjective complaints is questionable.

The podiatry service should provide for the prevention, examination, diagnosis and treatment of local foot conditions and the complications or pedal manifestations of the various systemic, cutaneous and functional diseases and conditions of the human body. The utilization of adequate foot health programs will decrease, and may even eliminate physical discomfort and help keep patients ambulatory. The programs contribute to easier motivation of the patient to accept other therapeutic regimens, increasing their effectiveness. Comprehensive foot health care can provide additional diagnostic, consultative and therapeutic service; aid in administration; and aid in clinical research and educational programs.

Foot examinations of new patients should be a part of the initial medical history and examination. Periodic evaluations should be performed and therapy instituted as indicated. The diagnosis and treatment of acute foot conditions and indicated consultations should be a part of the regular foot health program.

Other considerations for psychiatric and mental retardation facilities are:

1. Programs on foot health education for the staff, hospital and allied clinic personnel.
2. Foot health education for patients in groups where feasible.
3. Footwear for patients.
4. Additional and special podiatric care for patients with severe deformities or those with neuromuscular disorders.
5. Additional and special podiatric care for patients with diabetes, arthritis, peripheral vascular disease, strokes, etc.

Cooperation between the medical, nursing, podiatric and other clinical personnel is the key to an adequate foot health program. The objective of the podiatry program is to keep patients ambulatory.

A Curriculum Outline for Foot Health Care

Training of Personnel in an Extended Care Facility

The following outline is intended to assist in the establishment of inservice training.

I. Introduction
  A. The profession of podiatry.
    1. Definition: Podiatry is that profession of health science which deals with the examination, diagnosis, treatment and prevention of diseases and malfunctions affecting the human foot and its related or governing structures, by the employment of medical, surgical or other means.
  B. Education of podiatrists and their role in a total health effort.
  C. The need for podiatric services in geriatric programs.
  D. The contributions of podiatry to a total geriatric health program.
II. Basic Essential Points
  A. Many major foot problems are inherent in or the result of a complication of a systemic, cutaneous or functional disease.
  B. Many foot problems may be acquired through improper personal hygiene and care.
  C. Discussion of "secondary prevention of chronic disease" through screening and early detection prior to onset of symptoms or the presence of overt abnormalities.
    Examples: diabetes, arteriosclerosis and arthritis, all of which, many times, present foot symptoms as the initial sign of the disease.
III. Evolutionary factors which influence foot health
    Examples: Metatarsus varus, hallux valgus, short first metatarsal, Morton's syndrome, plantigrade calcaneus, pes cavus, etc.
IV. Anatomy
    Review the anatomy of the foot with the extent of review determined by the level of the class. Material: osteology, arthrology, syndesmology, myology, neurology and angiology.
V. Physiology
    Functions of the human foot: support, propulsion of locomotion, shock absorption. Gait: discussion of ambulatory process, the type of gait and the conditions which can affect it.
VI. Basic sciences
    Review of the basic sciences as they

relate to foot health, i.e., anatomy, histology, embryology, physiology, biochemistry, pathology, microbiology, mycology and pharmacology. Laboratory evaluations utilized in the diagnosis and treatment of foot conditions.

VII. Clinical sciences

A review of internal medicine, surgery, roentgenology and related clinical areas. Dermatology: special consideration in a geriatric program to the anatomy, physiology and care of skin conditions of the human foot. Particular stress on the first line of defense.

VIII. Common foot problems in the aged

A. Sweat glands: bromidrosis, hyperhidrosis, anidrosis.

Skin: dry skin, fissured heels, tinea pedis, contact dermatitis, psoriasis, pyodermas, ulcerations; diabetic, arteriosclerotic, etc.

B. Nails: onychauxis; onychomyosis, onychophosis, onychogryphosis, onycholysis, onychocryptosis— granuloma, inversion, hypertrophy, improper hygiene, subungual heloma, subungual exostosis, effects of trauma, manifestations of systemic or cutaneous diseases.

C. Hyperkeratotic lesions

D. Mechanical problems: pes planus, pes valgo planus, imbalance, acute strain, fascitis, myositis, tendinitis, heloma, tyloma, hallux valgus, digiti flexus, digiti quiniti varus, metatarsal length patterns, Morton's syndrome, Morton's toe, anterior metatarsal bursitis, absence of plantar soft tissue, bursitis, calcaneal spurs, hallus limitus and rigidus.

E. Anomalies: injuries and effects of trauma: contusions, lacerations, dislocations, fractures.

F. Systemic diseases manifest in the foot: most common diabetes, arthritis, (degenerative, traumatic, rheumatoid, gouty), arteriosclerosis, Bueger's disease, Raynaud's disease, gout, nutritional disorders, osteoporosis, cardiovascular disease and strokes.

In each of the above listed common problems, discussion will include the following: definition, etiology, location, diagnosis, including laboratory and x-ray findings, treatment, complications and functional management.

Essentials of proper footwear: heel to ball length, last compatibility, heel height, shank construction and stockings.

Total foot health programs for the patients in extended care facilities will include: podiatric services, consultations, physical medicine, rehabilitation, nursing services, social services, clerical assistance, follow-up technique, appointment systems, clinical space, clinical facilities, research; health education for patients, their families and allied health personnel; prosthetics, records, statistics, surgery, roentgenology, special clinics, interpreters, conferences, teaching, and pharmaceutical services.

SUMMARY

The podiatrist should provide periodic examinations and relief from pain by rendering the necessary professional service. The podiatrist and the other members of the professional staff must work together to insure the best possible patient care. Through this joint effort, many benefits can be provided, including:

1. Greater self-sufficiency
2. Higher morale
3. Lower medical costs
4. Less dependence
5. Minimized psychologic problems
6. More productive citizen with associated socioeconomic advantages

The inclusion of podiatric services in extended programs will often produce dramatic benefits and effects. Individuals can be returned from long-standing and, at times, absolute immobility due to the relative freedom that new found foot care brings. The adoption of foot health programs will insure a facility and community with many more ambulatory citizens.

chapter 21

A Conceptual Model for Medical Assistance Programs for the Elderly

Arthur E. Helfand, D.P.M.

Disability, illness and the inability to remain active are often related to dependency. Foot conditions are among the most common health problems of man. It is the rare individual who does not have a "foot condition" sometime during his life. No one is immune and hereditary factors combined with the environmental changes of a modern society contribute to their development. It has been estimated that the majority of children are born free of foot problems; however, by the time retirement years are reached, as high as 95% of the population will have developed some chronic foot condition which will require continued management if the individual is to remain an active and productive member of his community. Foot conditions are not self-limiting. They may be local in nature or they may be the complication of some other systemic disease. Thus, podiatric treatment needs are cumulative and become more complex in the aged, unless management is planned on a regular basis.

It has been demonstrated in the Philadelphia program "Keep Them Walking" that persons of the lower socioeconomic status fall short of receiving the podiatric care they need. This would seem to be confirmed by the absence of appropriate and total care in almost all welfare programs. Podiatric needs of public assistance recipients should, therefore, receive special recognition from state medical care programs. Adequate care of the pedal extremities is as important to general health as many of the other medical services provided for the rest of the body. Programs which fail to include podiatric care are seriously deficient, as foot health care must be a part of the total health care of the individual.

SCOPE OF PODIATRIC SERVICE

The scope of services which should be included in a podiatry program should be wide and, to a large extent, is dependent upon the availability of funds. A basic program for the elderly requires that provision be made for (1) relief of pain; (2) treatment of acute foot conditions; (3) foot health education; (4) institutional service programs; and (5) special programs related to chronic disease control and adult health.

A basic program should also provide for such radiographic and laboratory services as may be needed. Funding of basic programs must also include recommended orthomechanical devices and prescription services.

When funds are made available for additional podiatric services, it is desirable to assign priorities. These can include home care programs, and special programs for state hospitals and clinics, as well as total cooperation in all phases of geriatrics and adult health. Even though total podiatric care for all age groups may be impossible because of limited funds, some practical and systematic approach to care, based upon the immediate projected needs of particular communities, should be developed to insure total care as a supplement to Medicare coverage.

Complete programs should include education, both public and professional, screening, diagnostic (including laboratory and radiographic) services, and other identified needs, such as podiatric rehabilitation. Foot defects frequently are contributing factors in immobility. Podiatric rehabilitation can help these people maintain their ability to remain non-institutionalized and retain their dignity.

The lack of pre-Medicare coverage for medical assistance recipients increases the cost of Medicare.

QUALITY OF SERVICE

Obviously, any service provided should be of high quality. It is recommended that each state agency have a podiatrist serve as a podiatric consultant on a full or part time basis to (a) assist in developing and maintaining constructive relationships and understanding with the podiatry profession; (b) assure a program of podiatric services of high quality by developing policy and establishing standards; (c) participate in inservice training programs; and (d) provide case consultation when required. The following are some suggested guidelines regarding standards of quality of service.

1. The podiatrist should be a graduate of a podiatry college which is accredited by the Council on Education of the American Podiatry Association at the time of his graduation; licensed to practice podiatry in the state; and a respected member of the podiatry profession. He should possess superior knowledge in areas of podiatry practice, podiatric research, public health and podiatric education.

2. A podiatric advisory group should be appointed to help the state agency in its work of providing effective podiatric services. The committee members should be drawn from the podiatry profession in cooperation with the state podiatry association. Specifically, the group should advise the podiatric consultant and the state agency director regarding (a) the scope of services to be provided; (b) fees to be paid; (c) the methods of providing services; (d) evaluation of the effectiveness of the podiatry program; (e) desirable changes in the program; and (f) relationships with the state podiatry association.

3. To assure that only qualified practitioners participate in the program, licensure to practice within the state should be a basic requisite for services to welfare recipients. Experience has shown that individuals in the low income group of the population are especially prone to become prey to unethical or illegal practitioners. To prevent this and promote high quality of care, it is necessary to enlist the support and participation of qualified, ethical podiatric practitioners, in public assistance programs. When a state elects to use only certain podiatrists rather than to open the program to all licensed podiatrists, it should consider whether this decision will adversely affect the quality of podiatric care rendered. If a program is offered which permits the patient to go to a podiatrist of his own choice, it will be necessary to ascertain the willingness of podiatrists in all parts of the state to participate. In some areas, transportation will need to be provided for the patient.

4. Departments of health, local podiatry societies, voluntary agencies and vocational rehabilitation divisions are among the agencies which should provide podiatric care for the elderly to augment the Medicare program. At present, some agencies provide maximum podiatric programs, some minimal, and some, none at all. The prime concern should be to have all maintain a high standard for foot health.

5. Arrangements should be made for the local caseworkers to participate in inservice training programs in the essentials of foot health. A program should be provided to familiarize the workers with current facts on the relationships between pedal hygiene, local foot conditions, and the pedal complications of the various cutaneous, systemic and functional diseases. The case workers should also be aware of the merit of providing for preventive foot care, health maintenance and the treatment program. The local caseworker could then assist the client and receive appropriate podiatric care. In this effort, cooperation with the public health nurse, public health podiatrists and the podiatry profession is of great importance.

ADMINISTRATION

Payment for podiatric care can be arranged by the same methods which are used to provide other medical supplies and services. The "fee for service" method is one of the most commonly employed by states, By this method, the podiatrist is paid directly by the state agency on the basis of units of service rendered. Providers of care include private practicing podiatrists, podiatry clinics and hospitals.

As with other types of health care, the state agency may also contract with other organizations to provide services. Contracts may be made with podiatry societies, clinics or the state's own health department. When this method is used, the state welfare agency should certify eligible recipients to the contracting agency. The contractor arranges and provides for services and is reimbursed by the state welfare agency.

Regardless of the administrative method used, it is important that payment be at a level sufficient to promote high quality services and that the fees be established in consultation with appropriate podiatric representatives of the state podiatry association and the appropriate state agency, equal to levels for other providers.

It is desirable that administrative controls on costs of services be maintained by establishing the priorities of service described in the section "Scope of the Podiatric Service." The range of podiatric services, the groups to be served and podiatric procedures for which payment is provided should be specified. If cost controls are established by priorities of types of service to various groups, the program can be expanded as more funds become available. This method avoids the problems that arise when broad coverage has been offered initially, but funds prove insufficient to finance the services covered.

When a schedule of fees is used, it should be based upon the recommendation of the state and local podiatric advisory committees, podiatry societies, and associations, or other professionally qualified podiatric representatives who have responsibility for determining realistic podiatry fees as they relate to the costs of providing services. When a state agency attempts to adopt fees that are inconsistent with the costs of services, many members of the organized podiatry profession may choose not to participate in the program. It is essential that realistic podiatry fees be paid in order to insure broad participation and high quality podiatry care.

The state agency should maintain an administrative record of services rendered. Some state agencies have instituted computer tabulations of medical services. Forms for podiatric records are readily available for all types of mechanical systems and can be used to advantage in a podiatric care program. Podiatrists may indicate on podiatry record sheets the services provided and the charges for them. Each bill should indicate precisely what services were provided and the usual and customary charges for services.

These data may be used to determine the total costs of the program, utilization rates, types of services provided or other program statistics needed by the state agency. Periodic checks of these records provide a means for administrative evaluation of the quality and types of podiatric care provided and will suggest methods by which the program may be improved or extended.

UTILIZATION

Information suggests that utilization is higher in older age groups and in patients with chronic disease. The Committee on Public Health and Preventive Podiatric Medicine of the American Podiatry Association has estimated that rarely do more than 10% of the eligible persons in a program receive podiatric care.

The low rate of utlization is probably due in part to a lack of interest in receiving podiatric care and partly to a lack of awareness by eligible recipients that a podiatry program is available. In addition, unprofessional decisions that podiatric care is or is not needed for a given individual undoubtedly reduce utilization among the elderly. Judgments on the need for care should be made only be qualified podiatrists.

When a state agency offers a comprehensive range of services, it should be careful to inform recipients of the permissible levels of podiatric services in order to distribute podiatric care equitably and in accordance with established priorities.

SUMMARY

Podiatric services should be available to public assistance recipients as a part of a state's medical assistance program. Priorities for service have been suggested with objectives aimed at care and prevention.

To secure the highest possible quality of podiatric care, recommendations of the state podiatry consultant should be followed. Together with the advisory group and state association, programs can be developed to meet the public needs in keeping with available funds and facilities.

The importance of providing payments for podiatric care at rates which will promote high quality care is essential. Suggestions have been offered as to how such rate setting may be established in consultation with the podiatry profession.

Recent studies have identified many gaps in relation to foot health. The provision of podiatric programs will help maintain ambulation with psychosocioeconomic and medical benefits to the individual and his community.

chapter 22

Utilization Factors for Foot Care for the Elderly

Arthur E. Helfand, D.P.M.

As of January 1981, the current Medicare Guidelines provide for the payment for conditions and diseases of the foot with certain exclusions. It should be noted that the exclusions in general for conditions of the foot do not apply to the same diagnostic categories made for any other portion of the body. Perhaps the limitations were made because there was an inappropriate estimate that many elderly people did not have foot problems. But it also should be noted that because of the high percentage of foot conditions in the elderly patient, essential care in many cases was limited or eliminated.

One of the conditions which is listed as an exclusion is the treatment of flatfoot. The term flatfoot has been defined by some carriers as a condition in which one or more of the arches of the foot have flattened out. Medicare has indicated that services directed towards the care or correction of such a condition are not covered, unless surgery is employed.

The second major categorical exclusion includes the treatment of subluxations of the foot. Some carriers define these conditions as partial dislocations or displacements of joint surfaces, tendons, ligaments or muscles of the foot. They have further indicated that surgical or nonsurgical treatment undertaken for the sole purpose of correcting such a subluxated structure in the foot as an isolated entity may not be covered. Some carriers have further identified as covered services reasonable diagnostic and treatment programs except by

the use of orthopedic or other supportive devices for the effects of osteoarthritis, bursitis (including bunion), tendonitis, etc., that result from or are associated with such subluxed structures. Some carriers have also indicated that surgical correction of such structures which are an integral part of the treatment of a foot injury or are undertaken to improve the function of the foot or to alleviate an induced or associated symptomatic condition becomes a covered service. It should be noted however, that the exclusions listed do not apply to the ankle joint.

The third categorical exclusion is a poor term included in regulations as "Routine Foot Care." Routine foot care has been defined as the cutting or removal of corns or calluses, the trimming of nails and other hygienic and preventive maintenance that might be defined as self-care. Skin care for both ambulatory and bedfast patients in the absence of localized illness, injury or symptoms involving the foot is also a noncovered service. Care provided as soaking and topical medication on a physician's orders between visits to a practitioner is also not covered.

It should be noted at this point that when Medicare was originally adopted in 1965, these exclusions were not present. When the payment for podiatric services was added in 1967, these exclusions were adopted.

We have been unable to uncover any data which would demonstrate that the exclusions were based upon any reliable charges or utilization patterns, based upon the initial two years of the Medicare program. It is also interesting to note that many of the broad categorical exclusions represent areas which serve as predisposing lesions to more serious foot problems that generally require hospitalization and expensive long term care and are, many times, the very conditions which limit the ambulatory status of an elderly individual, reducing their ability to remain active and in the community, and predisposing the elderly patient to becoming a ward of society or becoming institutionalized.

Medicare subsequently identified that certain foot care procedures generally considered by definition to be routine usually pose a hazard when performed by a nonprofessional person or when there is a specific systemic disease that creates an area of either circulatory embarrassment or desensitization of the legs or feet. Although not intended to be comprehensive, by any means, Medicare did identify that a series of metabolic, neurological and peripheral vascular diseases (with synonyms listed) most commonly represented the underlying conditions that were to be included as exceptions to the exclusion rule. Medicare also identified that, in order to be a covered service, the patient also was required to be under active general medical care prior to and during any management of the pedal complication or condition.

The exceptions to the exclusion included conditions such as foot problems associated with diabetes mellitus, arteriosclerosis obliterans (ASO, arteriosclerosis of the extremities, occlusive peripheral arteriosclerosis), Berger's disease (thromboangiitis obliterans), chronic thrombophlebitis, peripheral neuropathies, including the feet, associated with malnutrition and vitamin deficiency malnutrition (general pellagra), alcoholism, malabsorption and pernicious anemia, carcinoma, diabetes mellitus, drugs and toxins, multiple sclerosis, uremia (chronic renal disease), traumatic injury, leprosy or neurosyphilis, and hereditary disorders such as radicular neuropathy and amyloid neuropathy.

Another exception to the exclusion is that services defined as routine would be covered if they were performed as a necessary and integral part of an otherwise covered service such as the diagnosis and treatment of diabetic ulcers, wounds, and infections. Medicare has identified that fungal (mycotic) and other infections of the feet and toenails require professional services and therefore are defined as covered services. It should be noted that such diagnostic and treatment services of foot infections are covered in an identical manner for the treatment of infections occurring elsewhere on the body and that the same general types of coverage rules apply. This is particularly important when one deals with the reasonable and necessary limitations for care.

Guidelines have identified that supportive devices for the feet, such as orthopedic shoes and other supportive devices, are not covered items. However, the exclusion for orthopedic shoes has an exemption if the shoe is an integral part of a leg brace.

Additional comments relating to the exceptions to the exclusions indicate that when a portion of a service which is noncovered is performed incidental to those services which are covered, and the charges reflect only the covered service, only the covered section of the treatment would be reimbursable. However, if, for example, a secondary service includes both noncovered and covered services in the same charge, the primary charge generally is acceptable.

When a primary procedure on the foot is covered, the administration necessary for the performance of such a procedure also becomes a covered service.

Payment may also be made for initial diagnostic services that are performed in conjunction with a specific symptom or complaint, even if it seems likely that the treatment for future services would be classed as an exclusion by virtue of the final determination for a noncovered service.

We have identified that there are certain exemptions to the exclusions for the basic management of debridement of hyperkeratotic tissue and nails. When a patient has one of the listed systemic diseases and is under the treatment of an appropriate medical practitioner, such conditions become an exemption. Such activities have been included in a listing of clinical findings which are used to support the exemption. They include a nontraumatic amputation of the foot or integral skeletal portion thereof. They include two of the following changes: absence of posterior tibial pulse, advanced trophic changes such as a decrease or absence of hair growth, thickening of toenails, pigmentary changes and discolorations, skin atrophy which appears thin and shiny, and skin color which appears as rubor or redness; and the absence of a dorsalis pedis pulse. The third major classification of clinical findings include: claudication, temperature changes such as cold feet, edema, parathesias, or abnormal spontaneous sensations in the feet, and burning. These clinical findings tend to substantiate the severity of the condition of patients requiring care that would add to the presence of the appropriate systemic disease. In general it is presumed that having appropriate medical treatment and/or evaluation for a complicating systemic disease should have taken place during the 6-month period prior to the treatment of a noncovered foot care service for the management of hyperkeratotic lesions and nail disorders to provide the exemption to the exception.

The utilization of services to deliver foot care should be both reasonable and necessary for the diagnosis and treatment of an illness or injury of the foot or to improve the functioning of a malformed body member. The levels of care should conform to the same general audit principles that are applied to the management of conditions and diseases of other portions of the body. For example, infections of the feet and toenails may require a wide variety of services such as examination, laboratory tests and cultures, the prescribing of a plan of treatment, periodic review and examination throughout the course of treatment to evaluate the status of the problem and minimize complications of a condition and the active treatment by many modalities such as surgical intervention, mechanical debridement, topical treatment or systemic treatment.

There are several other specific entities which carry some additional guidelines in relation to the delivery of care. The following segments of this chapter will deal with several of the specifics and their general utilization principles.

When prescribed by an appropriate practitioner, the lymphedema pump or intermittent compression unit would be appropriate as an inhouse or home unit when used for the management of lymphedema of the leg that may accompany carcinoma of the bladder with metastasis and edema of the foot as seen in reflex sympathetic dystrophy and Sudeck's atrophy. Intermittent compression therapy can also be provided as part of a physical therapy modality, during a spell of illness which is generally a 30-day period, as therapy three times a week. This would include such conditions as hematomas, where there has been trauma and ruptured tissue, lymphedema of the leg, and venous insufficiency.

In general, where treatment is utilized for the management of tinea pedis and tinea unguium, it is generally accepted that three cultures over a 12-month period would be acceptable utilization to add to the clinical impression of the disease and to permit an ongoing review of the patient's progress. It should be noted, however, that clinical judgment should support any laboratory diagnostic entities and, in fact, where the clinical diagnosis is clear, adequate laboratory studies may increase costs, particularly where the clinical management has stabilized or limited the condition.

Plethysmography is the measurement and recording of the changes that relate to the size of a part, as modified by the circulation of blood to that part. When surgery is projected involving the lower extremity in the elderly patient, various forms of plethysmography may be useful in the preoperative and postoperative evaluation of the patient with peripheral vascular disease and in the preoperative management of the diabetic patient, or one with intermittent claudication. The hemorheograph is a diagnostic instrument used to determine skin perfusion and may also be used prior to surgical intervention in the lower extremities. It measures surface blood flow but does not generally measure the total blood flow in a digit or limb. It is useful in the preoperative and postoperative diagnostic evaluation of patients with suspected peripheral artery disease.

In an earlier section of this chapter, we identified the various exceptions to the exclusions for foot care under Medicare. The misnomer of routine foot care has been defined to include the treatment of corns, calluses, clavus, tyloma, plantar keratosis, hyperkeratosis, and keratotic lesions, bunions (except by surgery), nails, (except for surgery for ingrown or mycotic nails). The term "routine foot care" is a misnomer because of the fact that procedures termed routine are, in fact, peculiar to many professions and many specialities in the health care fields. It would be difficult to imagine a geriatric patient who is not under active care for diseases such as arteriosclerosis obliterans, diabetes mellitus, ischemia, edema of the feet secondary to diseases such as congestive heart failure, hypothyroidism, kidney disease, Milroy's disease, patients receiving anticoagulant therapy, or peripheral neuropathies involving the feet. There are also some diseases which have been identified as those not being on the excluded list. These conditions include blindness, Parkinson's disease, arthritis, (rheumatoid or osteoarthritis), mental retardation, psychiatric disorders, and Huntington's disease. Practitioners in the field of mental retardation and mental health are quick to recognize that foot problems are common and the resultant immobility created by painful feet precludes activity on the part of patients for a more normal regimen or life style.

The conditions identified by Medicare as being classed "routine foot care" are generally reimbursable when the exceptions to the exclusions are met and when there is a determination of medical necessity. It is generally believed that one treatment per month categorically provides the basis for medical necessity. It should be noted that these categorical listings are not employed on any other segment of the human body and would not be precluded as necessary treatment programs for other areas.

It has been generally accepted by many that the debridement of mycotic nails should be based upon one visit per twenty-eight to sixty days dependent on the degree of involved tissue. It should also be noted that effective treatment should be instituted upon the appropriate clinical diagnosis and may include the use of topical antifungal agents in addition to debridement. In addition, the debridement of mycotic nails, as is the case in the debridement of ulcers or repeated chemo-, cryo-, or electrosurgical techniques, generally cannot be performed at one time and may require subsequent procedures in the management of these conditions. Such conditions and procedures should not be considered as serial but should reflect visits based on the severity of the individual condition.

The management of fungal or mycotic infections of the feet, exclusive of the toenails, requires special care in the geriatric patient. If the infection becomes well organized, secondary bacterial involvement may be precipitated and require vigorous antibiotic therapy in addition to fungal management, and requires periodic examinations throughout the course of the treatment to evaluate the status of the infection, to review the case for complicating factors, and to consider hospital admission early if the bacterial infection becomes significant.

The management of ulcers of the foot depends upon the etiologic characteristics of the specific ulcerative site. It has generally been accepted that an initial debridement is acceptable once during a three-week period per ulcer site. Subsequent debridements generally are listed as subsequent visits. In addition, appropriate medical management should be included to coordinate the effective utilization of services between all practitioners involved in managing the patient. This may include periodic debridement of any lesion where necrotic, devitalized, and/or contaminated tissue may be present.

It is generally accepted that the injection and needling of bursae, the injection of heel spurs, the injection of ganglionic cysts of the foot, and other related conditions may be utilized as singular treatment or in conjunction with other types of visits. The injection of a neuroma may be classified as an intralesional injection and should conform to the existing diagnostic treatment programs for these conditions.

The effective utilization of physical modalities in the management of foot conditions may require a treatment program to provide adequate care for the patient. Generally speaking, most diagnostic categories include a spell of illness which should be reevaluated at the end of each thirty-day period. It is generally accepted that, on an outpatient basis, a maximum of fifteen treatments during that thirty-day period or one treatment three times per week, may be considered as appropriate. The diagnostic categories of the foot, which should be included in these types of considerations, include the following: adhesive capsulitis, arthritis (acute or severe), arthritis with nerve root pressure, ataxic gait, burns, bursitis, capsulitis, contusions, residuals of stroke or CVA, degenerative joint disease (acute or severe), dislocations, fascitis, fibrositis, flexion contractures, foot drop, (peroneal palsy), fractures, hemiplegia, inflammation, (acute), muscle spasm (acute or severe), muscular dysfunction or paralysis from nerve disease or injury, nerve palsy, neuralgia, osteoarthritis, (acute or severe), osteomyelitis, periostitis, peripheral neuritis (acute or severe), peripheral neuropathy, postjoint surgery, sesamoiditis, sprains, strains, Sudeck's atrophy, synovitis, tendonitis, tenosynovitis; and, with supporting documentation, osteoporosis, pain, severe generalized weakness, post-trauma and ulceration.

We have attempted to outline some of the utilization concerns dealing with the management of foot problems and foot conditions as they are delineated under health insurance programs for the aged and chronically ill.

In order to appropriately review the effect of utilization of most conditions dealing with the foot, it is important to consider those items or areas which would demonstrate appropriate documentation or appropriate care by a retrospective audit of foot care. Some of the areas that would be included would be as follows.

Part of the review should include the record involving the patient. It should be able to demonstrate an appropriate history, physical examination, proper progress notes, a record that is properly organized, and justification of the recorded tentative diagnosis based upon proper documentation of the record. A second segment of review should include the diagnostic management of the case. Items such as the time involved in obtaining indicated procedures, the appropriately indicated laboratory studies, radiographic examinations, if indicated, to include comparison studies, if indicated, appropriate consultations, and a summary of the overall diagnostic handling of the patient. The third primary area for consideration should be the treatment and follow-up, including the therapy prescribed, follow-up laboratory and radiographic studies, adequacy of the follow-up visits, and the overall management of the patient.

It should be noted that the triads of prevention, i.e., primary, secondary and tertiary, mean little per se when we deal with foot problems in the geriatric patient; only through effective management and care of existing conditions can we prevent minor foot problems from becoming major expensive medical and social dilemmas that create wards of society.

In conclusion, most geriatric foot problems are chronic in nature and require continued management. The total cost of such management over a geriatric lifetime is less than the cost of one hospital admission and rehabilitation period for a singular amputation of the foot or leg.

Bibliography

Abramson, D.I., Circulatory Diseases of the Limbs. Grune & Stratton, New York, 1978.

Abramson, D.I., Vascular Disorders of the Extremities, 2nd ed. Harper & Row, Hagerstown, Md., 1974.

Albanese, J.A., Bond, T., Drug Interactions. McGraw-Hill, New York, 1978.

Alvarez, W., The value of foot care to the aged, Editorial. Geriatrics, 16:104, 1961.

American College of Foot Surgeons, Complications in Foot Surgery; Prevention and Management. Williams & Wilkins, Baltimore, 1976.

American Podiatry Association, Foot Health Training: Guide for Long-Term Care Personnel. Washington, D.C., 1977.

American Podiatry Association, Interpretations and Guidelines for Podiatrists Services under Medicare. Washington, D.C., 1978.

American Podiatry Association, Podiatry in Institutional Services, reprint No. 7:65:02. Washington, D.C., 1965.

American Public Health Association, Functions and educational qualifications of podiatrists in public health, Podiatric Health Section. Am. J. Public Health 65(9), 1975.

Amundsen, L.R., Assessing exercise tolerance. Phys. Ther., 59:534–537, 1979.

Andelman, S., Public health and the aged. J. Am. Podiatry Assoc., 50:967, 1960.

Anderson, M.H., A Manual of Lower Extremity Orthotics. Charles C. Thomas, Springfield, Ill., 1972.

Azarnoff, D.L., Yearbook of Drug Therapy. Year Book Medical Publishers, Chicago, 1978.

Barnes, R.W., Noninvasive evaluation of peripheral arterial disease. Angiology, 29:631, 1978.

Barrett, M., Health Education Guide, A Design for Teaching K-12, 2nd ed. Lea and Febiger, Philadelphia, 1974.

Basmajian, J.V., Muscles Alive, 2nd ed. Williams & Wilkins, Baltimore, 1967.

Berlin, S.J., Soft Somatic Tumors of the Foot; Diagnosis and Surgical Management. Futura Publishing Co., Mt. Kisco, N.Y., 1976.

Bistrain, B.R., Blackburn G.L., Hallowell E., et al.: Protein status of general surgical patients. J.A.M.A., 230:858, 1974.

Bonney, G., McNab, L.: Hallux valgus and hallux rigidus-a critical survey of operative results. J. Bone Joint Surg., 34B:366, 1952.

Brachman, P.R., Mechanical Foot Therapy. Podiatry Books Co., Chicago, 1966.

Brachman, P.R., Foot Orthopedics. Podiatry Books Co., Chicago, 1966.

Brand, P., Insensitive Feet, A Practical Handbook on Foot Problems in Leprosy. The Leprosy Mission, London, 1977.

Bruno, J., Gross muscle evaluation by the podiatrist. J. Am. Podiatry Assoc., 57:309, 1967.

Bruno, J., Helfand, A.E., A positive approach to rehabilitation, J. Am. Podiatry Assoc., 60(6), June 1970.

Bruno, J., Helfand, A.E., Some physical therapy concepts in managing the podiatric complications of diabetes, in Modern Therapeutic Approaches to Foot Problems. Futura Publishing Co., Mount Kisco, N.Y., 1973.

Butler, R.N. Mission of the National Institute on Aging. J. Am. Geriatr. Soc. 25(3), March, 1977.

Butler, R.N., Lewis, M.I. Aging & Mental Health: Positive Psycho-social Approaches. C.V. Mosby Co., St. Louis, 1973.

Caillet, R., Foot and Ankle Pain. F.A. Davis Co., Philadelphia, 1968.

Campbell, G.M., Hill, R.N., Deschler, M., Kiley, K., An Appraisal of a Series of One-Day Seminars Directed at Improvement of Pedal Care in Minnesota Nursing Homes. Northlands Regional Medical Program, St. Paul, 1973.

Carron, H., Relieving pain with nerve blocks. Geriatrics, 33:49–57, 1978.

Cash, J.A., Yeoman, P.A. The painful foot. J. Rep. Rheum. Dis., 26:1–2, 1966.

Charlesworth, F., Chiropody, Theory and Practice, 5th ed. Actinic Press, London, 1961.

Clayton, M.L., Surgery of the forefoot in rheumatoid arthritis. Clin. Orthop., 16:136–140, 1960.

Clayton, M.L., Surgery of the lower extremity in rheumatoid arthritis. J. Bone Joint Surg., 45-A:1517–1536, 1963.

Clemmsen, S.A. The influence of shoes on deportment and gait. J. Postgrad. Med., 21:43, 1956.

Close, J.R., Motor Function in the Lower Extremity: Analysis by Electronic Instrumentation. Charles C. Thomas, Springfield, Ill., 1964.

Cluff, L.E., Petrie, J.C. (eds), Clinical Effects of Interaction Between Drugs. Excerpta Medica, Amsterdam, 1975.

Coffman, I.D., Mannick, J.A., Failure of vasodilator drugs in arteriosclerosis obliterans. Ann. Intern. Med., 76:35, 1972.

Coffman, J.D., Vasodilator drugs in peripheral vascular disease. N. Engl. J. Med., 300:713, 1979.

Coilliet, R., Foot & Ankle Pain. F.A. Davis Co., Philadelphia, 1975.

Collins, V.J., Principles of Anesthesiology, 2nd ed. Lea & Febiger, Philadelphia, 1976.

Comroe, B.I., Arthritis, 3rd ed. Lea & Febiger, Philadelphia, 1944.

Conforti, J.A., Foot care for mental patients. Ment. Hosp., 10:42, 1961.

Cowdry, E.V., Steinberg, F.U. (eds), The Care of the Geriatric Patient. C.V. Mosby, St. Louis, 1971.

Cozen, L. Office Orthopedics, 4th ed. Charles C. Thomas, Springfield, Ill., 1974.

Cranley, J. J., Arterial embolism, in Advances in Surgery, edited by Rob, C., Vol. 11. Year Book Medical Publishers, Chicago, 1977.

Cranley, J.J., Extending the vascular examination by noninvasive means. Am. J. Surg., 134:179, 1977.

Dagher, F.J., Alongi, R.N., Smith, A., Bacterial studies of leg ulcers. Angiology, 29:641, 1978.

Dale, W.A. (ed), Management of Arterial Occlusive Disease. Year Book Medical Publishers, Chicago, 1971.

Daniels, L., Williams, M., Worthington, C., Muscle Testing, 2nd ed. W.B. Saunders, Philadelphia, 1958.

Dasco, M.M., Restorative Medicine in Geriatrics. Charles C. Thomas, Springfield, Ill., 1963.

DeBakey, M.E., Patterns of atherosclerosis and rates of progression, in Atherosclerosis Reviews, edited by Paoletti, R., Gotto, A.M., Vol. 3. Raven Press, New York, 1978.

Deaven, G.G., Brown, M.E., The Challenge of Crutches. Institute for Crippled and Disabled, New York, Reprinted from Archives of Physical Medicine, July 1945.

De Lorme, T.L., Watkins, A.L., Progressive Resistance Exercise. Appleton-Century-Crofts, New York, 1951.

Dix, R., Freeman, J., Systemically related foot disorders: The podiatrist's role. N.Y. State J. Med., 74(9):1645–1647, 1974.

Donick, I.I., Podiatry for the Assistant. Futura Publishing Co., Mount Kisco, N.Y., 1977.

Downer, A.H., Physical Therapy Procedures, 2nd ed. Charles C. Thomas, Springfield, Ill., 1971.

Downey, J.A., Darling, R.C., Physiological basis of rehabilitation medicine. W.B. Saunders, Philadelphia, 1971.

Durbin, F.C., Afflictions of the toes. Practitioner, 201(205):749–754, 1968.

DuVries, H.L., Hypertrophy of ungualabia. Chiropody Rec., 16:13–15, 1933.

DuVries, H.L., Surgery of the Foot, 2nd ed. C.V. Mosby Co., St. Louis, 1965.

Ellenberg, M., Rifkin, H. (eds), Diabetes Mellitus; Theory & Practice. McGraw-Hill, New York, 1970.

Elwood, T.W., Older persons' concerns about foot care. J. Am. Podiatry Assoc. 65:490–494, 1975.

Facts About Older Americans. Administration on Aging, Department of H.E.W., Washington, D.C., 1970.

Facts on Aging. Administration on Aging, Publication no. 146, Department of H.E.W., May, 1970.

Fairbairn, J.F., Bernatz, P.E., Acute arterial occlusion, in Peripheral Vascular Diseases, edited by Fairbairn, J.F., Juergens, J.J., Spittell, J.A., 4th ed. W.B. Saunders, Philadelphia, 1972.

Fairbairn, J.F., Juergens, J.J., Spittell, J.A., Peripheral Vascular Diseases, 4th ed. W.B. Saunders, Philadelphia, 1972.

Falconer, M.W., Allamura, M.V., Behnke, H.D. Aging Patients: A Guide to their Care. New York, Springer Publishing Co., 1976.

Farber, E.M., Soth, D.A., Urea ointment in the nonsurgical avulsion of nail dystrophies. Cutis, 22:689, 1978.

Feigenbaum, E.M., Ambulatory Treatment of the Elderly in Mental Illness in Later Life, in Mental Illness in Later Life, edited by E. Busse, E. Pfeiffer. American Psychiatric Association, Washington, D.C., 1973.

Fielding, M.D. (ed), The Surgical Treatment of the Hallux-Abducto-Valgus and Allied Deformities. Futura Publishing Co., Mt. Kisco, N.Y., 1973.

Fielding, M.D., Skin Tumors of the Foot, Diagnosis and Treatment. Futura Publishing Co., Mt. Kisco, N.Y., 1974.

Fielding, M.D., The Surgical Treatment of the Contractable Plantar Keratoma. Futura Publishing Co., Mt. Kisco, N.Y., 1974.

Forster, F.M., Synopsis of Neurology. C.V. Mosby Co., St. Louis, 1962.

Frost, L., Nursing home foot problems and the geriatric patient. J. Am. Podiatry Assoc., 49:26, 1959.

Fuery, J.G., Plantar fasciitis: The painful heel syndrome. J. Bone Joint Surg., 57:672–673, 1975.

Gamble, F.O., Yale, I., Clinical Foot Roentgenology. R.E. Krieger Pub. Co., Huntington, N.Y., 1975.

Gartland, J.J., Fundamentals of Orthopedics. W.B. Saunders, Philadelphia, 1979.

Gersh, M.R., Postoperative pain and transcutaneous electrical nerve stimulation: A model to critique literature and develop documentation schemes. Phys. Ther., 58(12):1463, 1978.

Giannestras, N.J., Foot Disorders, Medical and Surgical Management, 2nd ed. Lea and Febiger Co., Philadelphia, 1973.

Gibbard, L.C., Charlesworth's Chiropodial Orthopedics. Balliere, Tindall and Cassell, London, 1968.

Gibbs, Richard C., Skin Diseases of the Feet. W.H. Green, St. Louis, 1974.

Gibbs, R.C., Costello, M.J., The Palms and Soles In Medicine. C.C. Thomas, Springfield, Ill., 1969.

Gitelson, M., The emotional problems of elderly people. Geriatric, 3, 1948.

Goldfort, A.I., A Psychosocial & Sociophysiological Approach to Aging, in Normal Psychology of the Aging Process, edited by Zimberg, N.E., Kaufman, I. International University Press, 1963.

Goodhart, R.S., Wohz, M.G., Manual of Clinical Nutrition. Lea and Febiger, Philadelphia, 1964.

Gordon, D. (ed), Ultrasound-As a Diagnostic and Surgical Tool. Williams & Wilkins, Baltimore, 1964.

Gorecki, G.A., Bryzyski, T.P., Podiatric medicine: A new threshold in health manpower. Am. J. Public Health, 65(11), 1975.

Gotz, B.E., Gotz, V.P., Drugs and elderly. Am. J. Nurs., 78:1347–1351, 1978.

Griffin, J.E., Kavselis, T.C., Physical Agents for Physical Therapists. Charles C. Thomas, Springfield, Ill., 1978.

Grollman, J.H., Webber, M.M., Gomes, A.S., Phlebography and radionuclide clot localization in the lower extremities. Radiol Clin North Am, 14:371, 1976.

Gruber, H.W., Geriatrics-Physician Attitudes and Medical School Training. American Geriatric Society Conferences on Geriatric Education, Vol. 25, 1977.

Gruntzig, A., Kumpe, D.A., Technique of percutaneous transluminai angioplasty with the Gruntzig balloon catheter. Am. J. Roentgenol., 132:547, 1979.

Guttmann, D., Patterns of legal drug use by older americans. Addict. Dis., 3:337–355, 1978.

Hamer, D.H., Howson, D.C., Bibliography on Electroanalgesic. Phys. Ther., 58(12):1485, 1978.

Hanby, J.H., Walker, H.E., The Principles and Practice of Chiropody, 2nd ed. Balliere, Tindall and Cox, London, 1960.

Hatcher, R., Goller, W., Weil, S., Intractable plantar keratosis—a review of surgical corrections. J. Am. Podiatry Assoc., 68:377, 1978.

Hauser, E.D.W., Disease of the Foot, 2nd ed. W.B. Saunders, Philadelphia, 1950.

Helfand, A.E., A study in podogeriatrics. J. Am. Podiatry Assoc., 51:655, 1961.

Helfand, A.E., The relationship of chronic disease to mechanical problems in health studies. J. Am. Podiatry Assoc., 52:587, 1962.

Helfand, A.E., Podiatry—a basic long-term need for the chronically ill and the aged. Nurs. Homes, 12:9, 1963.

Helfand, A.E., Foot health education—a community health need for the aged and chronically ill. J. Am. Podiatry Assoc., 54:178, 1964.

Helfand, A.E., Guide to a methodological approach for a community foot health study for the chronically ill and the aged. J. Am. Podiatry Assoc., 54:465, 1964.

Helfand, A.E., Hunting diabetics by foot. Med. World News, 5:107, 1964.

Helfand, A.E., Diabetic screening in a hospital podiatry clinic. J. Am. Podiatry Assoc., 55:38, 1965.

Helfand, A.E., Guidelines for podiatry service in nursing homes and related facilities. Nurs. Homes, 14:25, 1965.

Helfand, A.E., A survey of podiatric service in some Pennsylvania nursing homes. J. Am. Podiatry Assoc., 55:440, 1965.

Helfand, A.E., Podiatrist looks at public health in diabetes and arthritis control, state of New Jersey. Public Health News, 46:131, 1965.

Helfand, A.E., Assessing podiatric clinic care and referral patterns for the chronically ill and the aged. J. Am. Podiatry Assoc., 56:56, 1966.

Helfand, A.E., Practice Guide for Podiatric Programs in Extended Care Facilities. J. Am. Podiatry Assoc., 56:221, 1966.

Helfand, A.E., The Responsibility of Podiatry in Aging Problems. J. Am. Podiatry Assoc., 56(9):401–407, 1966.

Helfand, A.E., Foot Impairment—an etiologic factor in falls in the aged. J. Am. Podiatry Assoc., 56:326, 1966.

Helfand, A.E., Guidelines for podiatric programs in extended care facilities. Hosp. Top., 44:26, 1966.

Helfand, A.E., The responsibility of podiatry in aging programs. J. Am. Podiatry Assoc., 56:401, 1966.

Helfand, A.E., Arthritis in older people as seen in podiatry practice. J. Am. Podiatry Assoc., 57:82, 1967.

Helfand, A.E., Podiatry in a total geriatric health program—common foot problems of the aged. J. Am. Geriatr. Soc., 15:593, 1967.

Helfand, A.E., Podiatry in a total geriatric health program: Common foot problems of the aged. J. Am. Geriatr. Soc., 15(6):593–599, 1967.

Helfand, A.E., Podiatry in public health. J. Am. Podiatry Assoc., 57:338, 1967.

Helfand, A.E., Keep them walking. J. Am. Podiatry Assoc., 58:117, 1968.

Helfand, A.E., Rules for foot health. J. Pract. Nurs., 18:25, 1968.

Helfand, A.E., Guidelines for podiatric services in medical assistance programs. J. Am. Podiatry Assoc., 58:262, 1968.

Helfand, A.E., Reflections on "Keep Them Walking." Geriatr. Institut., 16(1), 1969.

Helfand, A.E., The principles and techniques of podogeriatric management. J. Am. Podiatry Assoc., 59:295–299, 1969.

Helfand, A.E., The Foot of South Mountain: A foot health survey of the residents of a state geriatric institution. J. Am. Podiatry Assoc., 59:131–139, 1969.

Helfand, A.E., Podiatric case studies. J. Am. Podiatry Assoc., 59(6), 1969.

Helfand, A.E., U.S. Department of Health, Education, and Welfare, Public Health Service, Health Services and Mental Health Administration, Community Health Service, Long-Term Care Facility Administration, Case Study Manual, Podiatry, March 1970.

Helfand, A.E., Podiatry—essential nursing home care—your patient's care. Nurs. Homes, 19(5):35–37, 1970.

Helfand, A.E., A positive approach to rehabilitation, with Bruno, J. J. Am. Podiatry Assoc., 60(6), 1970.

Helfand, A.E., Evaluating the foot health status of the residents of a state restoration center—intermediate report. J. Am. Podiatry Assoc., 61(7), 1971.

Helfand, A.E., Podiatric considerations for the aged patient. Nurs. Homes, 20:30–31, 1971.

Helfand, A.E., Working with Older People, Vol. IV—Podiatry and the Elderly Patient, Dept. HEW, PHS, PHSP No. 1459, Vol. IV, Washington, D.C., 1971.

Helfand, A.E., Modern Therapeutic Approaches to Foot Problems: Some Physical Therapy Concepts in Managing the Podiatric Complications of Diabetes, with Bruno, J. Futura Publishing Co., Mount Kisco, N.Y., 1973.

Helfand, A.E., How to prevent foot problems in people who have diabetes. Newsletter, Delaware Valley Diabetes Association, February-March, 1973.

Helfand, A.E., Podiatric services for the aged. J. Am. Podiatry Assoc., 63:368, 1973.

Helfand, A.E., At the foot of south mountain: A 5 year longitudinal study of foot problems and screening in an elderly population. J. Am. Podiatry Assoc., *63:*512–521, 1973.

Helfand, A.E., Treating foot problems, geriatric issue. Med. World News, October, 1973.

Helfand, A.E., The diabetic foot, guidelines for care. Chron. Dis., March, 1974.

Helfand, A.E., Podogeriatrics: Historical review. J. Am. Podiatry Assoc., *64*(5):357–363, 1974.

Helfand, A.E., Alive and Well, Diabetics, Take Care of Your Feet, *1*(6): February 1975.

Helfand, A.E., Consumer's guide to podiatric services. J. Health Ed., Jan.-Feb., 1976.

Helfand, A.E., On your feet. Diabetes Forecast, *32:*23, 1979.

Helfand, A.E., Primary podiatric care for the elderly. J. Am. Podiatry Assoc., *69*(8):471–474, 1979.

Hirschberg, G.G., Lewis, L., Thomas, D., Rehabilitation. J.B. Lippincott Co., Philadelphia, 1964.

Hollander, J.L., Arthritis and Allied Conditions. Lea & Febiger, Philadelphia, 1966.

Hollander, J.L. (ed.), The Arthritis Handbook. Merck, Sharp & Dohme, West Point, Pa., 1974.

Holling, H.E., Peripheral Vascular Diseases: Diagnosis and Management. J.B. Lippincott Co., Philadelphia, 1972.

Horner, M.T., Minor foot lesions with diabetes mellitus and peripheral vascular disease. Geriatrics, *12:*164, 1967.

Howard, R., Herbold, N., Nutrition in Clinical Care. McGraw Hill, New York, 1978.

Howson, D.C., Peripheral Neural Excitability—Implications for Transcutaneous Electrical Nerve Stimulation. Phys. Ther., *58*(12):1467, 1978.

Hsu, J.D., Foot problems in the elderly patient. J. Am. Geriatr. Soc., *19*(10):880–886, 1971.

Hymes, L., Forefoot Minimum: Incision Surgery in Podiatric Medicine. Futura Publishing Co., Mt. Kisco, N.Y., 1977.

Imperato, A.J., Lumbar sympathectomy: Role in the treatment of occlusive arterial disease in the lower extremities. Surg Clin North Am, *59:*719, 1979.

Inman, V.T., DuVries Surgery of the Foot, 3rd ed. C.V. Mosby Co., St. Louis, 1973.

Jackson, D.S., Flickinger, D.B., Dunphy, J.E., Biochemical studies of connective tissue repair. Am. N.Y. Acad. Sci., *86:*943–947, 1960.

Joint Motion: Method of Measuring and Recording. American Academy of Orthopedic Surgeons, Chicago, 1965.

Joseph, J., Man's Posture: Electromyographic Studies. Charles C. Thomas, Springfield, Ill., 1960.

Juergens, J.L., Spittell, J.A. Jr., Fairbairn, J.F. (eds), Allen-Barker-Hines Peripheral Vascular Diseases, 5th ed. W.B. Saunders, Philadelphia, in press, 1981.

Kart, C.S., Metress, E.S., Aging & Health: Biological and Social Perspectives. Addision-Wesley Publishing Co., Reading, Mass., 1978.

Kelikian, H., Hallux Valgus: Allied Deformities of the Forefoot and Metatarsalgia. W.B. Saunders, Philadelphia, 1965.

Keller, W.L., Further observations on the surgical treatment of hallux valgus or bunions, J. Med. N.Y., *95:* 696–698, 1912.

Kempczinski, R.F., Rutherford, R.B., Current status of the vascular diagnostic laboratory, in Advances in Surgery, edited by Rob, C., Vol. 12. Year Book, Chicago, 1978.

Kendall, H.O., Kendall, F.P., Boynton, D.A., Posture and Pain. Williams & Wilkins, Baltimore, 1952.

Klenerman, L. (ed), The Foot and Its Disorders. Blackwell Scientific Publications, London, 1976.

Krall, L.P. (ed), Joslin Diabetes Manual, 11th ed. Lea & Febiger, Philadelphia, 1978.

Krehl, W., The influence of nutritional environment on aging. Geriatrics, *29:*65, 1974.

Krusen, F.H., Kotthe, F.J., Ellwood, P.M. Jr., Hand Book of Physical Medicine and Rehabilitation, 2nd ed. W.B. Saunders, Philadelphia, 1971.

Kubler-Ross, E., On Death and Dying. MacMillan Co., New York, 1970.

Lampe, G.N., Introduction to the use of transcutaneous electrical nerve stimulation devices. Phys. Ther. *58*(12):1450, 1978.

Lee, P.V., Drug therapy in the elderly: Clinical pharmacology of aging. Clin. Exp. Res. *2:*39–41, 1978.

Levin, M.E., O'Neal, L.W., The Diabetic Foot, 2nd ed. C.V. Mosby Co., St. Louis, 1977.

Levin, M.E., Medical evaluation and treatment, in The Diabetic Foot, edited by Levin, M.E., O'Neal, L.W. C.V. Mosby Co., St. Louis, 1973.

Levy, S., Foot care for the patient with diabetes and/or impaired circulation. J. Am. Podiatry Assoc., *49:*32, 1959.

Lewin, P., The Foot and Ankle, 4th ed. Lea and Febiger, Philadelphia, 1959.

Licht, S. (ed), Electrodiagnosis and Electromyography. Elizabeth Licht, New Haven, Conn., 1961.

Licht, S. (ed), Therapeutic Electricity and Ultraviolet Radiation, 2nd ed. Williams & Wilkins, Baltimore, 1967.

Licht, S. (ed.), Therapeutic Heat & Cold. Elizabeth Licht, New Haven, Conn., 1965.

Lippmow, A.J., Must loss of limb be a consequence of diabetes mellitus? Diabetes Care, *2:*432, 1979.

Liss, L., Twenty-two years of podogeriatrics. J. Am. Podiatry Assoc., *50:*963, 1960.

Locke, R.K., Foot care for diabetics. Am. J. Nurs., *63:* 107, 1963.

Louis, T.J., *et al.,* Aerobic and anaerobic bacteria in diabetic foot ulcers. Ann. Intern. Med., *85:*461, 1976.

Lowenthal, M.F., Thinker, M., Chiriboga, D., et al., Four Stages of Life. Jossey-Bass, San Francisco, 1975.

Mann, R.A., DuVries Surgery of the Foot. C.V. Mosby Co., St. Louis, 1978.

Mannheimer, J.S., Electrode placements for transcutaneous electrical nerve stimulation, Phys. Ther., *58*(12): 1455, 1978.

March, D.C., Handbook, Interactions of Selected Drugs with Nutrition Status in Man. American Dietetic Association, Oct. 1976.

Marmor, L., The rheumatoid foot. Geriatrics, *11:*132, 1966.

Marr, S.J., The Problem Foot. Austr. Fam. Phys., *7:* 1031–1036, 1978.

Martin, E.W., Hazards of Medication. J.B. Lippincott Co., Philadelphia, 1971.

Mayo, C.H., The surgical treatment of bunion. Ann. Surg., *48:*300–302, 1908.

McGill, H.C. Atherosclerosis: Problems in pathogenesis. In Atherosclerosis Reviews, edited by Paoletti, R., Gotto, A.M., Vol. 2. Raven Press, New York, 1977, pp. 27–65.

McGregor, R.R., Geriatric foot care. Nurs. Clin. North Am., *3:*687, 1968.

McKelvy, P.L., Clinical reports on the use of specific TENS units. p. 1474. Phys. Ther., *58*(12)*:*1474, 1978.

Mendoza, C.B., Postlethwait, R.W., Johnson, W.D., II. Incident of wound disruption following operation. Arch. Surg., *101:*396, 1970.

Mennell, J., Mc M., Foot Pain. Little, Brown and Co., Boston, 1969.

Merrill, H.E., Frankson, J. Jr., Tarara, E.L., Podiatry survey of 1011 nursing home patients in Minnesota. J. Am. Podiatry Assoc., *57:*57–64, 1967.

Minaker, K., Little, H., Painful feet in rheumatoid arthritis. J. Can. Med. Assoc., *109:*724–725, 1973.

Moeller, F., Surgical Treatment of Digital Deformities. Futura Publishing Co., Mt. Kisco, N.Y., 1975.

Montgomery, R.N., Foot complaints of the elderly. Cutis *18:*462–463, 1976.

Montgomery, R.N., Relieving painful feet. Geriatrics, *29:*137–138, 1974.

Moorehead, L.E., Miller, A.T., Jr., Physiology of Exercise. C.V. Mosby Co., St. Louis, 1963.

Morris, J.D., Brash, L.F., Hird, M.D., Chiropodial survey of geriatric and psychiatric hospital in-patients—Angus District. Health Bull. (Edinb.), *36:*241–250, 1978.

Mueller, C.B., Foot infections in the elderly. Postgrad. Med., *55:*111–115, 1974.

Murray, J.G., Tender heels due to Padget's disease. J. Bone Joint Surg., *34:*440–441, 1952.

National Academy of Sciences, National Research Council, Division of Medical Sciences, Ad Hoc Committee of the Committee on Trauma, Postoperative wound infections: The influence of ultraviolet irradiation of the operating room and of various other factors. Am Surg., *160*(suppl 2)*:*192, 1964.

Neale, D., Care of the feet in the elderly. Practitioner, *220:*253, 1968.

New Jersey State Department of Health, Foot care for people with diabetes. Trenton, N.J., 1963.

Neugarden, B.L., Personality in Middle and Late Life. Atherton Press, New York, 1964.

Nightingale, A., Physics and Electronics in Physical Medicine. G. Bell and Sons, London, 1959.

Ochsner, A., Circulatory disturbances of the foot, in Foot Disorders, Medical and Surgical Management, edited by Giannestias N.J., 2nd ed. Lea and Febiger, Philadelphia, 1973.

Palmberg, S., Hirsjarvi, E., Mortality in geriatric surgery. Gerontology, *25:*103–112, 1979.

Pardo-Castello, V., Pardo, O.A., Disease of the Nails, 3rd ed. Charles C. Thomas, Springfield, Ill., 1960.

Payton, O.D., Hirt, S., Mewton, R.A., Neurophysiological Approaches to Therapeutic Exercise. F.A. Davis, Philadelphia, 1977.

Penna, R.P., Handbook of Non-Rx Drugs, 5th ed. American Pharmaceutical Association, Washington, D.C., 1977.

Pennsylvania College of Podiatric Medicine, Screening forms, evaluation forms, foot care leaflets, aging, Philadelphia, 1965–1970.

Perkins, G., Rest and movement. J. Bone Joint Surg., *35B:*521–539, 1953.

Petrin, T., Sjostrand, T., Sylven B., Der Einfluss des Trainings auf die Haufigkeit der Capillaren in Herz- und Skeletmuskulatur (The Influence of Exercise on the Frequency of Capillaries in Cardiac and Skeletal Musculature). Arbertsphysiol., *9:*376–386, 1936.

Philadelphia Department of Public Health, Keep them walking project. Philadelphia, 1962–1965.

Prinsley, D., Pitfalls in geriatric medicine. Aust. Family Phys., *7:*1317–1323, 1978.

Pomeroy, L.R., Practical Preventive Medicine, Vol. 3. Symposia Specialists, Miami, 1975.

Pories, W.J. (ed), Clinical Application of Zinc Metabolism. Charles C. Thomas, Springfield, Ill., 1974.

Rakow, R., Podiatric Management of the Diabetic Foot. Futura Publishing Co., Mt. Kisco, N.Y., 1979.

Rakow, R.D., Friedman, S.A., The significance of trophic foot changes in the aged. Geriatrics, *24:*134–145, 1969.

Rush, H.A., Rehabilitation Medicine, 4th ed. C.V. Mosby Co., St. Louis, 1977.

Reichel, W. (ed), Clinical Aspects of Aging. Williams & Wilkins, Baltimore, 1978.

Reichel, W., The Geriatric Patient. HP Publishing Co., New York, 1978.

Riccitelli, M.C., Foot problems of the aged and infirm. J. Am. Geriatr. Soc., *14:*1058–1066, 1969.

Richle, F.A., Rankin, K.P., Shuman, C.R., Salvage of extremities with ischemic necrosis in diabetic patients by intrapopliteal arterial bypass. Diabetes Care, *2:*396, 1979.

Roberts, E.H., On Your Feet. Rodale Press, Emmanus, Pa., 1975.

Robertson, A.L., The spectrum of arterial disease. Atheroscler. Rev., *3,* 1978.

Rogers, D.E., 1979 Year Book of Medicine. Year Book Medical Publishers, Chicago, 1979.

Root, M.L., Orien, W.P., Weed, J.H., Normal and Abnormal Functions of the Foot. Clinical Biomechanics Corporation, Los Angeles, 1977.

Rosow, I. Socialization to Old Age. University of California Press, Berkeley, Calif., 1974.

Rossman, I., Clinical Geriatrics. J.B. Lippincott Co., Philadelphia, 1971.

Rovin, M., Non-Disabling Surgical Rehabilitation of the Forefoot. W.H. Green, St. Louis, 1976.

Rusk, H.A., Rehabilitation Medicine, 2nd ed. C.V. Mosby, St. Louis, 1964.

Samitz, M.H., Dana, A.S., Jr., Cutaneous Lesions of the Lower Extremities. J.B. Lippincott Co., Philadelphia, 1971.

Samman, P.D., The Nails in Disease. William Heinemann Medical Books, London, 1965.

Sarason, S.B., Work Aging and Social Change. Macmillan Publishing Company, New York, 1977.

Sauer, G.C., Manual of Skin Diseases, 3rd ed. J.B. Lippincott Co., Philadelphia, 1973.

Schifferes, J.J., Peterson, L.J., Essentials of Healthier Living, 4th ed. John Wiley & Sons, New York, 1972.

Sgarlato, T., A Compendium of Podiatric Biomechanics. California College of Podiatric Medicine, San Francisco, 1971.

Simard, T.G., Basmajian, J.V., Methods in training the conscious control of motor units. Arch. Phys. Med., 48:12–19, 1967.

Simko, M.V., Foot concerns in the aging process. J. Am. Podiatry Assoc., 61:399–400, 1971.

Simonson, W., Medication in the elderly. Phys. Ther., 58:178–179, 1978.

Smiler, I., Geriatric Foot Care: An Aging Challenge. Penna. Podiatry Assoc. and Penna. College of Podiatric Medicine, Philadelphia, 1979.

Smiler, I., Horwitz, R., The medical aspect of foot and leg problems in geriatrics. J. Am. Podiatry Assoc., 51: 559, 1961.

Smiler, I., Horwitz, R., The role of the podiatrist in nursing homes. Geriatr. Institut., 8:5, 1965–1966.

Smith, L.H., Antimicrobial Drug Therapy, Vol. 8. W.B. Saunders, Philadelphia, 1976, pp. 100–143.

Somers, A.P., Promoting Health Consumer Education and National Policy. Aspen Publication, Boulder, Colo., 1976.

Spencer, O.M., Practical Podiatric Orthopedic Procedures. Ohio College of Podiatric Medicine, Cleveland, 1978.

Stern, F.H., Leg cramps in geriatric diabetics with peripheral vascular ischemia, treatment. J. Am. Geriatr. Soc., 14:609, 1966.

Strandress, D.E., Peripheral arterial disease. Little, Brown and Co., Boston, 1969.

Strandress, D.E., The use and abuse of the vascular laboratory. Surg. Clin. North Am., 49:707, 1979.

Subotnick, S.L., Digital deformities: Etiology and treatment. J. Am. Podiatry Assoc., 65:542–555, 1975.

Swanson, A.B., Implant arthroplasty for the great toe. Clin. Orthop., 85:75–81, 1972.

Tarara, E.L., Podiatry's role in the care of the aged. J. Am. Podiatry Assoc., 50:972, 1960.

Tarara, E.L., Merrill, H.E., Frankson, J., Jr., Podiatry survey of 1011 nursing home patients in Minnesota. J. Am. Podiatry Assoc., 57:57, 1967.

Tarara, E.L., Spittell, J.A., Jr., Clues to systemic diseases from examination of the foot in geriatric patients. J. Am. Podiatry Assoc., 68:424–430, 1978.

Taretz, P., Two conceptual models of the senior centers. J. Gerontol., 31:219–222, 1976.

U.S. Department of Health, Education and Welfare, Feet First. (Stanford, E.D., Lithgow, C.H., and Helfand, A.E., consultants.) Washington, D.C., U.S. GPO-1970-0388-126.

U.S. Department of Health, Education and Welfare, Foot Care for the Diabetic Patient, Public Health Service Publication No. 1153, Superintendent of Documents, Government Printing Office, Washington, D.C., 1964.

U.S. Department of Health, Education and Welfare, Long-Term Care Facility Administration, Case Study Manual, GPO-1970-384-034/922.

Veterans Administration, Department of Medicine and Surgery, Program Guide, Nursing Service, Nursing Care of the Long-Term Patient, G-8, M-2 part V. Veterans Administration, Washington, D.C., 1963.

Vancura, E.J., Unpredictable drug response in the aging. Geriatrics, 34:63–73, 1979.

Vener, A.M., Krupka, L.R., Climo, J. J., Drug usage and health characteristics in non-institutionalized persons. J. Am. Geriatr. Soc., 27:83–90, 1979.

Waisman, M., A clinical look at the aging skin. Postgrad. Med., 66:87, 1979.

Watson-Jones, R., Fractures and Joint Injuries, Vol. I, 4th ed., Williams & Wilkins, Baltimore, 1952, p. 5.

Weiner, B.E., Ross, A.S., Bogdan, R.J., Biomechanical heel pain: A case study. J. Am. Podiatry Assoc., 69: 723–726, 1979.

Weinstein, F. (ed), Principles and Practice of Podiatry. Lea and Febiger, Philadelphia, 1968.

Weinstein, F., Roentgenology of the Foot. Warren H. Green, St. Louis, 1974.

Weiss, E., Spurgeon, E.V., Psychosomatic Medicine, 3rd ed. W.B. Saunders, Philadelphia, 1957.

Wenger, R.J.J., Whalley, R.C., Total replacement of the first metatarsophalangeal joint. J. Bone Joint Surg., 60-B:88–92, 1978.

Wheat, L.J., Infection and diabetes mellitus. Diabetes Care, 3:191, 1980.

Whitehouse, F.W. Saving a foot and salvaging a limb. Diabetes Care, 2:453, 1979.

Williams, M., Lissner, H.R., Biomechanics of Human Motion. W.B. Saunders Co., Philadelphia, 1962.

Wolf, S.L., Perspectives on Central Nervous System Responsiveness to Transcutaneous Electrical Nerve Stimulation, p. 1443.

Wolf, S.L., Gersh, M.R., Kutner, M., Relationship of selected clinical variables to current delivered during transcutaneous electrical nerve stimulation. Phys. Ther., 58(12):1478, 1978.

Woodside, N.B., Shapiro, J., Podiatry services at clinics of a local health department. Public Health Rep., 82: 389, 1967.

Yale, I., Clinical and Roentgenological Interpretations in the Lower Extremities. Chiropody Literature, Ansonia, Conn., 1952.

Yale, I., Podiatric Medicine. Williams & Wilkins, Baltimore, 1974.

Yater, W., Symptoms and Diagnosis, 4th ed. Appleton-Century Crofts, New York, 1954.

A Consumer's Guide to Podiatric Care

Arthur E. Helfand, D.P.M.

Today, foot health has become a major concern to many population groups. The demand for health services in general has placed many stresses on the total delivery system, and the projections for new forms of delivery and financing mandate equal concern for quality care. Foot care services available today suffer from a major manpower shortage, a poor distribution of professionals and facilities, and a marked limitation on prevention and health education. Perhaps what is most striking is that foot care for the elderly and certain disease categories has been emphasized, but no major attempt has been made to provide similar services for the young. If we as a society wait until we are old to consider the need for mobility, we shall never begin to cope with preventing disability and impairment among the elderly. We must begin to think of children's foot health in its proper light.

Today, there is perhaps more commercialism in foot care products than ever before. The controls and evaluative standards on most of these products are nonexistent. Many segments of the American population are not exposed to any foot health programs until they reach their later years and are perhaps institutionalized for the balance of their lives. Thus, during the productive years, the ounce of prevention is missing. Governmental foot health programs are too few in number. When they do exist, they also tend to focus on the elderly, as is true for most governmental health publications on foot care.

Some direction is needed for the consumer of foot care and health services, if for no other reason than as a potential patient. Essentially, good foot health begins with the individual. When he and his family podiatrist work together, foot health can be maintained.

Today's podiatrist is a professionally educated foot care practitioner who delivers clinical services. The podiatric degree, Doctor of Podiatric Medicine (D.P.M.), requires the successful completion of 4 years study at a college of podiatric medicine accredited by the Council on Podiatry Education of the American Podiatry Association. Prepodiatry education consists of a minimum of 3 years collegiate education, although 86% of students entering colleges of podiatric medicine have attained a baccalaureate or higher degree. The Council on Podiatry Education is recognized by both the U.S. Office of Education and the National Commission on Accrediting as the accrediting agency for professional podiatric education, thus providing a base for similarity with other health care disciplines and providers. Today, there are about 8,200 podiatrists in the United States and there are five schools of podiatric medicine. The curriculum is similar to medicine and dentistry, with much emphasis on the basic sciences, medical and surgical elements, podiatric segments, and the social sciences, in an effort to product a community-oriented family practioner who can deliver primary foot care services. Podiatrists are licensed in all states and the District of Columbia and must meet quality and ethical standards.

Podiatrists are not all equal in the quality of their work. As in other fields, some practioners excel and some fall below or are at the minimum level of care. Fortunately, the incompetent and dishonest are comparatively small in number. There are methods through the state licensing body and the state podiatry associations to deal with such situations, and with increasing third party payment for health services, there is an increasing level of peer review. Continuing education in the future will be a means to document continued study. The American Podiatry Association is now developing standards to evaluate such programs, and some states now require a prescribed period of continuing education for relicensure.

What step can the public take to ensure adequate foot care? Perhaps the best approach would be to identify and explore the situation at two levels, the individual consumer or patient and the community as a whole.

THE CONSUMER AND THE PODIATRIST

How do you find a podiatrist and how do you evaluate the individual?

The number of practitioners in some parts of the country is quite small. The state licensing agency has a list of the licensed practitioners in the area, or the local or state podiatry association can provide a list of the membership. Being a member of an association does not imply competence; however, it does indicate that the doctor does maintain an ethical and moral practice, as judged by his/her peers. If located near a college of podiatric medicine, e.g., New York City, Philadelphia, Cleveland, Chicago, or San Francisco, the consumer can obtain a list of the faculty associated or affiliated with the college. The consumer can also contact the American Podiatry Association at 20 Chevy Chase Circle, NW, Washington, DC 20015 to obtain a list of those podiatrists affiliated with groups in the special areas of podiatry practice—foot orthopedics, foot surgery, foot radiology, podiatric dermatology, and podiatric medicine. Such affiliation usually means advanced training and a qualifying examination. Local hospitals list the names of podiatrists who are on staff. The family doctor can be a source of information about podiatric practitioners, which might be the best approach, as it permits a continuum of care by both health disciplines.

Once you find your personal podiatrist, you can ask to see an educational background. Today, most podiatrists completing their professional education go on for an additional period of in-hospital residency training. In addition, ask if they participate in the third-party payment programs, such as Blue Shield or other similar state plans. Participation permits peer review of claim forms and provides some measure of quality care. You can contact the insurance company in your state and obtain a list of the participating podiatrists.

Try to find prevention oriented podiatrists who will discuss long-range needs and solutions and will provide information on preventing foot problems in the future. They will be concerned about health education and will recommend appropriate literature on foot health for the family in general.

It is important to find a podiatrist who provides total foot health care and initiates a conservative but appropriate method of treatment. If surgical treatment is recommended, your podiatrist should explain alternative methods of care. If you have reservations about the procedures suggested, seek consultation and inform your podiatrist of your concerns. Most practitioners welcome consultation, as additional opinion usually improves the patient's understanding of the problem and the ultimate quality of care. When surgery is suggested, it is appropriate to review the x-rays as part of the total discussion of care and these should be available to the consultants if requested.

Any podiatrist should first tell you what has been found and what he plans to do. Before starting diagnostic studies and/or treatment you must grant permission. When you discuss the treatment plan, the alternatives should be fully explored together with their benefits and complications. Do not be afraid to ask questions. You have a right to know. If you have doubts, seek an independent consultation.

Before treating you, the podiatrist should complete a past podiatric and medical history. This will identify your past foot care and results and indicate any medical conditions that may require special care and/or precautions, such as history of diabetes mellitus, heart disease, peripheral vascular disease, or drug allergies, to mention a few. Many times, patients tend to minimize a foot problem and may even be reluctant to provide an adequate medical history. In the interest of total patient care and prevention, these facts are vital. In fact, the podiatrist may refuse to accept you as a patient under these circumstances. This is a plus in his or her favor, as the podiatrist has demonstrated concern for your total health.

The family podiatrist should provide a telephone number for emergency care when needed. You should also be able to contact him or her about treatment programs at mutually convenient times. If your podiatrist is away, generally someone will take the calls. Availability is one of the concerns utilized to select any health professional.

Avoid professionals who refuse to discuss charges. A frank discussion of fees and itemized services provides an easy breakdown in relation to care needs and particular family situations. Before you conclude that you may be overcharged, you might check with the state Medicare carrier, who generally has a list of most reasonable and usual charges. They can also give you some idea of the charges for other podiatrists in the same special area of practice in the same community. If you feel that you have been overcharged, contact your state podiatry association. They have a committee that can review the case with the podiatrist in question. The procedure should be employed after you have discussed the problem with your personal podiatrist. If you still feel that you have a problem, the

state licensing agency can also be contacted.

Most practitioners will use consultation in appropriate specialties as the need arises. Making x-ray and examination reports available to consultants is a clear indication that your podiatrist is attempting to provide the best possible foot care for you.

All of the health professions are aware of the need to avoid unnecessary x-ray examinations and exposure. Your podiatrist has information on special precautions and appropriate protective measures; equipment standards are generally part of state regulatory acts. X-rays are used when needed to rule out or confirm a clinical diagnosis. They may be taken in the office or another facility for special studies. A review of the films and reports with you will help you better understand your problems and the projected solutions.

There are some other points that you can look for from a family podiatrist. They should be concerned about health education as the first avenue of prevention. They should be able to recommend literature to you on foot health. The American Podiatry Association has a large number of publications available, without charge, on request. In addition, the U.S. Public Health Service publishes a booklet entitled *Feet First* which is available through the Government Printing Office. Although designed for people with diabetes, the aged, and people with peripheral vascular disease, the booklet provides an excellent health educational base and one which needs to be publicly expanded to include all populations.

In addition, you and your family podiatrist should be working together to preserve your foot health. An annual checkup should be considered as part of your total physical evaluation. Your podiatrist should demonstrate compassion about your foot health problems and concerns, answer questions about prevention, and provide advice on footwear needs.

STATUS OF FOOT HEALTH IN THE COMMUNITY

Does your state or local health department have a podiatric service? Does your local hospital provide for podiatric services? What level of foot health education is provided by your local school system? Are foot health examinations provided to all school children in your community? Is foot health informa-

tion available at all of the health fairs in your community? Are podiatric services covered by your health insurance policy and what kinds of services are provided?

The needs for the future are quite clear. The American Public Health Association at its 1973 annual meeting passed a significant resolution, calling for foot health as public policy. To achieve that goal, much work needs to be done. The level of foot health education needs to be extended to all population groups, especially the young. Podiatric services should be available to all segments of population and provided as part of primary health care services in future health delivery and financing systems. Governmental and administrative agencies must begin to include foot health as part of their regular program activities, even if only on a consultant basis to begin with. The services should include preventive, diagnostic, and therapeutic personal services; program administration; program development and consultative services; public health education; expanded professional education to increase the manpower available; and research into financing and delivery.

If consumers do not provide adequate levels of foot health today, the patients of tomorrow will have to pay the price, not only for the acute health care needed, but to provide the funds to manage the social complications of disease. The foot is many times not a matter of life and death, but foot comfort has a most important relationship to the quality of life and occupational productivity.

Selected Reading

The Functions and Educational Qualifications for Podiatrists in Public Health, American Public Health Association, Podiatric Health Section, 1975.

Feet First, U.S. Department of Health, Education and Welfare, Public Health Service, Government Printing Office.

On Your Feet, E.H. Roberts, Rodale Press, Emmaus, PA., 1975.

A Shopper's Guide to Surgery, H. S. Dennenberg, Commonwealth of Pennsylvania, Insurance Department, 1972.

A Shopper's Guide to Dentistry, H. S. Dennenberg, Commonwealth of Pennsylvania, Insurance Department, 1973.

Consumer's Guide to Dentistry, Connecticut Citizen Action Group, 1974.

Podiatry, Health Careers Guidebook, U.S. Department of Labor, Third Edition, 1972, pp. 121–22.

The Potential of Podiatric Medicine in Comprehensive Health Care, L. A. Levy, Public Health Reports, Sept.–Oct. 1974, Vol. 89, No. 5, pp. 451–455.

Podiatric Medicine: A New Threshold in Health Manpower, G. A. Gorecki, and T. P. Brzyski, presented 1974 Annual Meeting, American Public Health Association, New Orleans, Louisiana.

What Can A Podiatrist Do For You?, R. S. Lepow, Alive and Well, April 1975, pp. 69–70.

Foot Complaints ... "Doctor, my feet are killing me," R. K. Locke, J. McM. Mennell, and T. E. Sgarlato, Patient Care, March 1975, pp. 20–47.

The Podiatric Aspects of Geriatric Care, A. E. Helfand, to be published, 5th Edition, The Care of the Geriatric Patient, by Cowdry and Steinberg, 1975, Mosby.

Reprinted from HEALTH EDUCATION—January/February 1976

Foot Health Training Guide for Long-Term Care Personnel*

Prepared by
Arthur E. Helfand, D.P.M.
Chairman, Long-Term Care Project Advisory Committee
Chairman, Department of Community Health
Pennsylvania College of Podiatric Medicine

*with the assistance of Long-Term Care
Project Advisory Committee Members*
Raymond Benack, M.D., Medical Director
Bel Pre Health Center

Robert W. Brumeister, Ph.D., Director of
  Education, Research and Development
American College of Nursing Home
  Administrators

Roberta Conti, R.N., M.S., F.A.A.N.,
  Director of Nursing
Anne Arundel General Hospital

Rev. William P. Harris, Administrator
Baptist Home of D.C.

Robert Heil, Executive Director
American Association of Colleges of
  Podiatric Medicine

Adelaide Lloyd, R.D., Division of Licensing
  and Certification
Maryland State Department of Health and
  Mental Hygiene

Shirley McKnight, Administrator
Wildwood Health Center

Jerome Shapiro, D.P.M., Supervisory
  Podiatrist
Washington, D.C. Department of Public
  Health

Marcile Backs, R.N., M.P.H., Project
  Officer
HRA Division of Long-Term Care, DHEW

Merle Adrian, Project Staff
American Podiatry Association

---

* Reprinted by permission of the American Podiatry Association, Contract No. HRA-230-76-0177 DHEW-HRA Division of Long Term Care.

FOREWORD

The Department of Health, Education, and Welfare has for many years had a commitment to upgrading the quality of care offered by nursing homes and related long-term care facilities. Certain specific aspects of program efforts directed toward this goal have been assigned to the Division of Long Term Care, Health Resources Administration. These program areas are research and development and provider training. In the area of research and development the program thrust is to learn more about systems of care, quality of care and alternatives in long-term care. In the area of short term training the Division carries out a broad range of activities aimed at improvement of provider knowledge and skills. Short term courses have been offered to physicians, nurses, dietitians, social workers, and others who are regularly involved in furnishing services to nursing home patients. Appropriate professional organizations have been involved, and course materials have included the latest research findings.

It has long been recognized that pedal health is necessary to independent activity, individ-ual dignity, and the general well-being of long term care patients. Problems contributing to disability and pain commonly lead to inactivity, listlessness, and deterioration of mental as well as physical health. The Division of Long Term Care, through Contract No. HRA 230-76-0177 with the American Podiatry Association, is attempting to increase the involvement of podiatrists in long term care. This document is designed to provide a vehicle for sharing podiatric knowledge and skills with long-term care personnel. By increasing the awareness of long term care facility personnel to pedal health needs, it is our hope that residents will benefit by receiving appropriate preventive measures, as well as remedial intervention in pedal health problems.

We are pleased to have supported the development of these materials through our program funds and anticipate that they will contribute to the well-being of long-term care residents.

Bernice Catherine Harper

PREFACE

The purpose of this training program is to help long-term care (LTC) personnel present training programs which will improve the level of podiatric care rendered to the aged and chronically ill in LTC facilities. It has been designed for use by medical directors, doctors of podiatric medicine, registered nurses, and in-service education personnel. Additionally, this material may serve as a self-teaching tool for all levels of personnel.

This program consists of three main parts. The first consists of a recommended example of a foot health presentation designed for use by the practical nurse and nurse's aide, including a printed text of the presentation and a 2 × 2 inch color slide accompaniment to enhance information presented.[a]

The second is a series of five lectures for the use of medical directors, podiatrists, directors of nursing, and LTC in-service educators as in-depth training resources. Materials include recommended pre- and postlecture discussions for trainees, lecture outlines, lecture text, glossary, and a recommended reading list.

The third is a listing of additional resource materials available to the LTC in-service educator. It includes additional printed resource articles, a listing of State podiatry societies (for obtaining speakers, etc.), a listing of audio-visual training aids available to the educator, and information related to financing foot-health care.

METHOD OF PRESENTATION

This guide has been designed so that the following methods of presentation are available to the instructor.

---

[a] The LTC slide series is available for loan or purchase upon request from the American Podiatry Association, 20 Chevy Chase Circle, N.W., Washington, DC 20015 (Attn: Audio-visual Department).

The instructor can show the slides along with his or her own version of the sample narrative. This may range from slight modification in the wording of the prepared material to a highly altered narrative. A blank page has been provided after the text of each lecture so the instructor can add his or her own prepared text or notes.

Slides can be extracted from the package or requested from the American Podiatry Association as per the attached catalogue and used as adjuncts to a presentation substantially different from the text in this guide. Each slide is numbered on the mounting frame.

In some settings, the instructor may wish to use the slide-text combination as a self-teaching tool for individual trainees or small groups of trainees.

SECTION A
EXAMPLE OF A SLIDE-TEXT PRESENTATION

This section contains a recommended example of a foot-health presentation designed for the nurse and nurse's aide. It includes a printed text of the presentation, and a visual 2 × 2 inch color slide accompaniment is availabe upon request to enhance the presentation.

Improving Foot Care in the Long-Term Care Facility

Slide
No.

1. This presentation is designed for use by nurse's aides and licensed nurses in learning basic concepts related to improving foot health care given LTC residents. It has been designed with the knowledge that each facility operates under its own guidelines and may differ in its approach to personal responsibility and direction. Therefore, the following information is general and basic and should be considered in the context of the procedures of your facility.

2. Foot health for our aged and chronically ill population has become of increasing importance to our society. We now have a better understanding of the importance of ambulation and independent activity to individual dignity and well-being.
The foot problem of this person has caused disability and pain which commonly lead to inactivity, listlessness, and worsening mental, as well as physical, health.

3. Because many of the aged and chronically ill consider their feet unattractive they are reluctant to talk about their foot problems. Rather than seek help, even from you, a nurse or nurse's aide, whom they see everyday, they may resort to using canes and cut-out shoes, and endure tremendous pain.

4. One serious problem which is very common among the elderly is the ulcer or open sore. This condition, if unattended by a professional, may become increasingly infected and ultimately necessitate amputation to save the resident's life.

5. Equally as dangerous is the ulcerated lesion which may have been caused by a trauma or injury, diabetes, circulatory complications, or a combination of these disorders.

6. The foot is a specialized appendage. A medical specialist, the podiatrist, has been trained to care for it.

7. The podiatrist, seen here doing a foot examination, is establishing the nature of the resident's foot problem. He evaluates the pulse, reflexes, muscle strength, color, skin temperature, skin texture, swelling, and also detects points of discomfort.

8. The role of the podiatrist, like that of the nurse, is threefold. In prevention, they together provide routine patient evaluation, screening, and education. The nurse and the podiatrist can detect problems early through knowledge of the history of the patient, careful examination, and sometimes x-rays and laboratory tests. The podiatrist treats foot problems through general foot care, foot prothesis, surgery, and medication.

9. The foot is a very complex structure. Its 26 bones make up one-fourth of the body's total number of bones. With the ligaments, muscles, nerves, and blood vessels, the foot makes up an appendage that is rivaled in lifetime work only by the heart and lung. The typical individual will walk some 250,000 miles in a lifetime.

10. Aging produces many changes that will affect the feet. Bones become brittle, the skin becomes dry and discolored, ligaments lose elasticity, and the muscles waste and lose strength.

11. Specifically, because of these changes, the elderly commonly suffer soreness, stiffness and fatigue associated with muscle strain, arthritic conditions, and everyday wear and tear or stress on the feet.

12. Poor blood flow to the extremities produces shiny, dry, parchment-like skin with hair loss that is susceptible to ulceration and infection.

13. The aging process changes the foot's shape as the arch becomes enlarged and inflamed. The bony joints enlarge and

become inflamed; the ligaments and muscles stretch and weaken. Thus, the foot becomes distorted and painful.

14. Lastly, aging causes slower healing. For example, the dark skin pigment around this diabetic ulcer is associated with poor circulation and repeated injury to the site will take a long time and special care to heal.

15. Some common foot problems of the LTC
16. resident are influenced by hereditary fac-
17. tors. For example, bunions, hammer toes and flat feet are frequently seen in succeeding generations.

18. Foot imbalance, stress, friction, and obesity are some factors influencing local foot problems. The foot strain during our everyday activities is accentuated by the hard surfaces we walk on.

19. Prompt professional attention will provide a diagnosis and effective treatment of these foot problems and will result in restored patient comfort and activity.

20. Communication between the podiatrist and nurse will help in prevention, early detection and treatment of existing foot problems. Early recognition is important in such detection. Remember, the doctor sees the patient only on routine visits. The nurse sees the individual every day.

21. Here are some examples of conditions that a nurse must be aware of and recognize.

22. This ram's horn nail has a thickened, malformed appearance. The nail itself is softened and yellowish or brown in color. The ram's horn nail commonly results from injury, nail infection or ringworm. The nurse plays a vital role in prevention of the condition by her early detection and referral.

23. This untreated ram's horn nail has produced an ulcer of the nail bed due to prolonged or continued pressure from the nail itself and the shoe.

24. Swelling and inflammation of this bunion has resulted from irritation. A bursitis is often present, contributing to the pain and swelling.

25. Infection of this bunion joint has developed, producing disability and increased pain.

26. This local foot problem is a simple corn. It has been affected by friction and pressure.

27. The patient's abuse and neglect of this foot problem has led to ulceration and infection of this corn.

28. General disease of the body can often be spotted first in the foot. Frequently these general (systemic) ailments can be detected and diagnosed at an early stage by the podiatrist.

29. General diseases such as gout may tend to affect certain areas of the foot. The first joint (bunion) area is usually involved, and the symptoms commonly produced are redness, edema and sudden excruciating pain. Heart and kidney diseases may produce swelling and discomfort affecting the foot, ankle or leg.

30. Diabetes—diabetic neuropathy (a lack of nerve sensation due to nerve degeneration), obesity and foot imbalance combined to produce this ulcer.

31. Osteoarthritis—Swelling and inflammation over the great toe joints produce the soreness and stiffness commonly seen in this disease.

32. Rheumatoid arthritis—This deforming disease of bones and joints has produced dislocations, hammer toes and limited mobility.

33. Peripheral vascular disease—This ailment produces a shiny, parchment-like appearance of skin and nails and loss of hair growth. Complications of this disease can produce gangrene and may require amputation.

34. Cardiac produced edema—This disease is pitting in nature. The distention of the tissue causes discomfort and pain.

35. The heal spur is an extension or shelf of
36. bone projecting out on the bottom surface of the heal. This is usually associated with painful bursitis and arch strain.

37. We have now discussed the following areas in our basic review of LTC foot health:
    1. Importance of foot health
    2. The podiatrist's role in health care
    3. Effects of aging upon feet
    4. Local and general foot conditions
    Now, let us direct our attention to the nurse's role in promoting good foot health.

38. As stated earlier, the nurse has three key functions in foot health:
    1. Observing and detecting

2. Administering basic foot health care

3. Advising patients on foot health

39. Early detection of foot problems can often be accomplished during the bathing period, thus not adding to the work schedule. The nurse can observe the nails, skin texture, temperature, color and swelling.

40. Following bathing, check between the

41. toes and inspect for soft corns, fungus (athletes foot), fissures (cracks), or infection.

42. Observe the nails for thickness, discolor-

43. ation, irritation and infection. These nail problems can be easily detected and referred to the podiatrist or facility doctor.

44. Another duty of the nurse is administering basic foot health care.

45. After bathing, proper drying of the foot is essential to prevent oversoft skin; feet should be blotted dry. Tender loving care is important. Inspection at this time reveals any irritation, infection or injury.

46. Massage is helpful in maintaining basic

47. foot health. In dry skin conditions and foot dermatitis, specific medications may be prescribed by the doctor. Massage stimulates circulation and is therapeutic. It must be done gently.

48. Applying a foot powder helps keep the

49. skin dry and avoids skin cracks and infection. The foot powder may be antiseptic, antifungal or both.

50. After skin care, the nurse can often help handle simple nail conditions under the direction of the podiatrist or medical director.

51. The podiatrist uses many instruments in basis LTC. Seen here on the podiatry tray are podiatry nail drill (maintained only for the podiatrist on his patient visits), scissors, nail spatula, curette, nail nippers and tissue nippers.
The nail nipper is probably the only instrument the nurse will use after instructions from the podiatrist for simple nail care.

52. Observe how the nurse holds and posi-

53. tions the large nail nipper. The nurse should cut the nail straight across and avoid probing in the corners.

54. The nurse or nurse's aide may also advise the patient about helpful drugs that have been prescribed, and explain about daily foot care using skin creams, antiseptics, foot powders, and soaps.

55. Daily exercises are important in maintaining health. Walking helps maintain muscle strength and tone. This leads to a sense of well-being and should be encouraged. Other exercises can be recommended by the podiatrist to enhance ambulation.

56. Unfortunately, the elderly are not always

57. careful in treating their feet. Each year,

58. home treatments and remedies are used improperly and lead to many serious foot complications. The use of certain drugs and instruments has resulted in acid burns, infections, ulcers and even gangrene. Too often, these problems are not reported promptly and treated professionally. Consult with the podiatrist when residents are using over-the-counter foot remedies.

59. Extreme temperature changes can be

60. harmful to the feet. Avoid excessive heat in foot soaks, heating pads, compresses, etc. Encourage bathing in warm water. Remember that vascular deficiencies in the elderly may cause loss of sensation and make the individual unaware of dangerous heat, pain, etc.

61. Foot and leg bindings can restrict blood flow. Panty girdles can be binding to a person with varicose veins. Rubber bands or garters should be discarded as a means of holding up stockings. Crossing the legs for long periods can cut of blood flow and limit sensation to the legs.

62. Bed socks may provide warmth and comfort to an individual with poor circulation or arthritis. Cotton or wool will absorb perspiration and provide comfort; nylon and other synthetic materials should not be used.

63. Fractures and sprains often result from

64. accidental bumping into obstacles, particularly when barefoot. If an injury occurs, repeated use of cold compresses or ice are indicated over a 24-hour period. Injuries should be promptly inspected and treated. Call the doctor—don't wait!

65. Well-fitted, sturdy shoes should be worn.

66. They help provide support and protection to the feet. Sturdy shoes should also be worn following a lengthy period of bedrest and/or inactivity. Avoid plastic or rubber shoes; leather will conform to

the shape of the foot and allow the foot to breathe.

67. Again, a team effort helps promote better foot health for LTC residents. The nurse plays an essential role in detecting foot problems early and in assisting in daily foot care. Early recognition by the nurse and the nurse's aide leads to prompt referral and treatment by the podiatrist, helping to avoid serious complications.

68. An example of this team effort: note the nurse and the doctor examining a patient with a decubitus ulcer (bed sore) on her heel.

69. The nurse is loosening bed linen to pre-
70. vent any binding pressures on this foot. This helps prevent sores.

71. The nurse, or aide, may also enhance

72. prevention of foot problems by using the
73. (1) air mattress (relieves undue pressures); (2) bed cradle (removes pressures); and (3) block elevation (assists in blood flow to our feet).

74. In this brief outlined presentation, we
75. have emphasized that cooperation between the podiatrist and the nurse leads to a program of beneficial foot care. Detecting disease early, spotting infections, referring the patient promptly, providing basic daily foot-health care techniques with massages, foot powder, lotions, nail trimming, and warm soaks and advising the patient about proper shoes and rules for better foot health all help in resolving foot problems.

SECTION B
FOOT HEALTH LECTURES

The following lectures have been prepared to provide the medical director, the director of nursing, the doctor of podiatric medicine, and other inservice educators with more specific resource information related to foot health. Accompanying each lecture text are questions to consider as one reads the material. An outline of the material has been added to provide additional assistance.

LECTURE 1
PEDAL HEALTH AND THE LONG-TERM CARE RESIDENT:
AN INTRODUCTION

Purpose

This lecture is designed to:

Inform trainees of the basic objectives of foot health in the LTC program.

Impress upon trainees the importance of the lower extremities as functioning parts of the total body.

Sensitize trainees to the complications that inadequate foot care can bring.

Enable trainees to readily understand and recognize the normal foot through review of basic foot anatomy.

Familiarize trainees with the many potential roles of the podiatrist in LTC foot-health programs and how those roles complement the roles of the LTC personnel.

Acquaint the trainee with important concepts concerning resources available to the LTC resident to help improve foot health.

Outline

I. Need for foot health
  A. The lower extremities as cause of morbidity, disease change, disability and limitation of activity
  B. Objectives of good podiatric care
  C. Complications of inadequate foot care
  D. Incidence and prevalence of foot disease in TLC residents
II. Nature of the lower extremities and their properties
  A. Definition of normal foot
  B. The skeletal system and changes occurring in the aged and chronically ill
  C. The ligament and joint systems and changes occurring in the aged and chronically ill
  D. The muscular system and changes occurring in the aged and chronically ill

  E. The nervous system and changes occurring in the aged and chronically ill
  F. The arterial system and changes occurring in the aged and chronically ill
  G. The skin and nails and changes occurring in the aged and chronically ill
III. Administrative information related to financing podiatric services
  A. Foot health and the Medicare program
  B. Foot health and the Medicaid program
  C. Foot health and other third party insurers
IV. Summary

Pre- and Postlecture Discussion Questions

1. What would you consider some basic objectives of good foot-health care programs in a LTC facility?
2. What do you feel the role of the LTC personnel should be in providing quality foot-health care? Administrators? Nurses? Aides?
3. What are some possible complications which can result from inadequate foot care?
4. What are some examples of the social, psychological and economic implications of the inability of LTC residents to walk?
5. How would you define the role of the podiatrist in health care delivery? Include in your definition what you feel a podiatrist can and cannot do.
6. What do you consider the most important functions of the foot?
7. What percent of the body's total bones are in the feet?

8. What are some detrimental effects of modern civilization on the lower extremities?
9. What common changes occur in the anatomy of the feet in aging?
   a. skeletal system   b. ligaments—joints

c. muscles, fascia   d. innervation
e. blood vessels   f. skin

10. What are some common types of programs which provide financial reimbursement for foot-health care given in the LTC resident?

LECTURE 1
PEDAL HEALTH AND THE LONG-TERM CARE RESIDENT: AN INTRODUCTION

Have you ever stopped to think how important your feet are in your daily activities? Imagine just for a moment how limited you would be if they were in such condition that you couldn't stand or walk without chronic, unbearable pain, or if you couldn't stand or walk at all. Not a pleasant thought is it? It has been estimated that by the time we reach 65 years of age, 95% of us will have developed some chronic foot disorder which will require continued management if we are to stay active and productive. Yes, our feet are important to us, and they need more attention as we grow older. This presentation, the first in a series of five, will attempt to provide you with an overall look at the importance of the foot of the LTC resident. This information may prove useful as you care for the residents in your daily routine.

This presentation will address three basic issues. First, the need for foot-health; second, the nature of the lower extremities and their properties; and third, administrative responsibilities relating to financing podiatric services in the LTC care facility.

Before the LTC resident's need for foot care can be evaluated, long term care must be viewed in its entirety. It once related only to geriatric institutions or facilities for the mentally retarded, but the term has come to mean much more. Today, long term care might be broadly defined as the management of any disease process, whether it be physical, functional or mental, that requires extended care.

People involved in LTC management, in or out of institutions, must have special understanding, special knowledge about many unusual problems, and the ability to adapt treatment methods to various circumstances.

The foot generally has received less attention than other parts of the human anatomy. It is seldom the cause of mortality. It is,

however, many times the cause of morbidity, disease change, disability and limited activity. Many initial signs of systemic disease may be seen first in the foot.

If the institutionalized patient is to function to the best of his ability, he must be able to walk. This permits that patient to act for himself, to obtain his own food, to maintain an exercise program, to adjust his own television set, to take care of his personal needs, and, most importantly, to maintain his self-dignity.

Good podiatric care and good foot health have three main objectives in the LTC program: to relieve pain, to limit disability and to restore the independent activity of the patient.

Many complications can result from inadequate foot care. Loss of mobility has already been mentioned. A second complication is increased discomfort. Third is the increase in complications accompanying chronic disease. Fourth is the likelihood of prolonged institutional care or bed confinement. Fifth is an increase in the likelihood of hospitalization as a result of foot infection.

Several surveys in LTC facilities have shown foot problems of residents to be widespread. The most extensive study was conducted for a period of 7 years at the South Mountain Restoration Center, a LTC facility for the elderly and mentally ill operated by the Commonwealth of Pennsylvania. A final report concluded that foot problems were prevalent. Of 1,366 patients evaluated, each averaged more than three foot complaints—75% complaining of pain. It also concluded that patients entering LTC facilities usually have had a recent history of foot problems and that, unless appropriately treated, even simple foot problems can become serious and require more intensive care than might be available at the institution. Such problems can require so much care by nursing personnel that they might detract from the care provided to other patients.

This study also showed that when foot health was emphasized at that institution, the patient's foot health improved or stablized. Even as a patient grew older and the chronic disease grew worse with potential for complication greater, adequate foot care helped prevent the development of new foot problems.

So the foot does deserve attention. What about this familiar appendage? What about the foot itself? What is it? How does it function? Why is it so special? The foot is an efficient structure of propulsion and locomotion. Through the years, it must carry a physical work load exceeded only by organs such as the heart and lungs. In addition to its workload, we must add that the human foot is a flexible structure not designed to walk on modern civilization's hard surfaces.

The human foot is complex. Each foot has 26 bones (together constituting one-fourth of the body's total), ossicles, ligaments, muscles, tendons, arteries, veins, nerves and, of course, its covering of skin. It normally bears weight on a triangular base with the long sides being the inner and outer borders of the foot, or longitudinal arches, and the short side being the basis along the five metatarsal bone heads at the toes. Weight is transferred from the heel bone to the first and fifth metatarsals at the base of the toes where the angles of this triangle can be found and where the basic anatomical arches of the foot can be demonstrated easily.

A normal foot in an aged person cannot be defined anatomically. By the time a person is classified as aged, some deformity has taken place. The skin has undergone changes, the bones have deviated or shifted, the muscles have wasted and a limitation of motion has occurred. Significant changes occur in toenails of elderly patients; they become thickened, brittle and do not resemble the nails of people in other age groups. They are misshapen or diseased, but as long as they do not limit function and may be easily managed, they may be broadly defined as normal. So, it might be better to consider the foot of the elderly person as normal if it permits the individual to perform independent tasks. Keep in mind that the normal foot of an aged individual will differ from the normal foot of a 20-year-old athlete.

But let's get back to what the foot is. The basic structures are bone. The talus, which with the lower portions of the leg bones (tibia and fibula) makes up part of the ankle joint, is an interesting bone. It has no muscular attachment, and thus its activity is controlled by the tendons and muscles which parallel it.

Beneath the talus is the heel bone, or calcaneus. It is a much longer bone attached to the Achilles tendon or heel cord. It is a major contributor to foot function. In front of the calcaneus is the cuboid, a rectangular shaped bone, which adds structural support to the foot. In front of the talus is the navicular, a coin-like bone which also provides muscular attachments. In front of the navicular and adjacent to the cuboid are three wedge-shaped bones called the first, second and third cuniforms. These help provide stability to the foot. These bones make up the rear foot.

In front of these bones are the five metatarsals. Each consists of a base, a shaft and a head. They are anatomically classed as long bones. Their general makeup is similar to that of the thigh bones or bones in the arm.

In front of the metatarsals are the phalanges. Each of the smaller toes contains three phalanges. The great toe contains two.

Each bone attaching to another forms a joint. Bones are attached to each other by a series of ligaments or fibrous bands which hold them together. Their functional role is to maintain proximity. Their properties are strength and rigidity with limited elasticity.

The ligament attachments of all of the joints are numerous. They generally include ligaments on the top, bottom and to the sides, depending upon the joint. There are stronger joints and weaker joints, but one fact should be mentioned in understanding foot anatomy. Each toe joint has what are called membranous expansions, so that the attachments of muscles and ligaments truly bind all of the joints of each toe together in a firm manner. These expansions permit all of the muscles in the foot to aid in its propulsive activity.

Bone changes that occur in aging might be defined as a loss of mineral substance and, therefore, an actual weakening of the bone itself. A common fracture that occurs as a result of this weakening, coupled with a twisting or bending of tissue without evidence of injury, is called a pathologic fracture.

The basic change in foot ligaments as a

result of aging is from elasticity to rigidity. A ligament which binds one bone to another is strong. It takes force to sever it. When a ligament is pulled away from bone, it generally pulls some bone cells with it, causing a sprain, which, if severe, can be worse than a fracture. There is less chance of healing once this occurs.

The most predominant and significant membranous covering in the foot is known as the plantar fascia. It attaches to the back of the heel bone and fans out forward into the metatarsal area just under the skin. It covers all the foot muscles, all the ligaments and all the bones on the bottom of the foot. It acts as a spring to aid in function and protects all of the structures on the bottom of the foot. It is a very elastic mass in youth which becomes wasted and rigid with age.

The upper part of the foot, the top or dorsum, does not have such a strong fascial attachment. In fact, most of the structures there are just beneath the skin. Therefore, any severe trauma on the dorsum tends to be more of a problem than an injury on the plantar or bottom.

The muscles of the foot are guided by muscles from the leg. On the upper surface they include the tendon which controls the great toe (extensor hallicus longus) and four tendons which control the lesser toes (extensor digitorum longus). In addition, a shorter ligament (tibialus anterior) coming from the inner portion of the leg functions to turn the foot inward. The ligaments on the outside of the foot (perioneus longus and brevis) together permit the foot to be pulled outward. One muscle rises from the top of the foot. Its function is to pull the foot toward the leg.

A decrease in muscle strength can be seen in the aged and chronically ill. This can result in foot drop, a condition where stronger extending muscles overpower those on top of the foot.

The nerves of the foot come from the spinal cord by way of the sciatic nerve in the leg. Through branches, it supplies both the upper and lower portions of the foot. The nerves on the bottom of the foot include the lateral plantar nerve and the medial planter nerve. They subdivide into branches and supply all the toes with both sensation and function. On the upper portion of the foot, the superficial plantar nerve does the same. The sapenous nerve supplies the outer portion of the great toe area, and the sural nerve supplies the outer portion of the fifth toe area.

The blood vessels of the foot also come from the leg, each branching off from a larger blood vessel. The main arterial vessels in the foot are near the bones. They include the major artery to the upper portion of the foot (dorsalis pedis). This can be palpated just beside the tendon leading to the great toe. This major vessel then subdivides into metatarsal arteries, digital arteries and then into capillaries.

The major artery on the bottom of the foot (posterior tibialis) is also close to bone, thus affording foot protection to the vital blood supply. It can be palpated just behind the inner portion of the ankle. It provides more blood to the foot than does the artery on top of the foot (dorsalis pedis). This also subdivides into metatarsal arteries and provides blood supply to the toes.

The function of the blood vessels is to bring blood to the foot. The changes they undergo during the aging process are especially important. Because of the accumulation of fatty material inside the arteries (arteriosclerosis), blood flow to the foot decreases. When blood flow is sufficiently blocked, the development of gangrene or death of a part of the foot can follow.

The skin of the foot is made up of fitted, flexible, elastic inner dermis covered by an insensitive outer epidermis or cuticle. It varies in thickness from .05 mm. (as in the eyelid) to 4 to 5 mm. in the sole. The skin of the foot undergoes many changes in aging. It becomes thinner, even parchment-like, loses its elasticity, may atrophy and may lose hair. It loses its hydration or water content because there is generally less perspiration and lubrication. It loses its suppleness. It becomes brittle and injures easily. This condition, accompanied by a diminished blood supply, can be quite serious. These are the important properties making up the foot. Knowing them will help you to understand common foot problems and principles of foot care.

Since the foot is such a specialized structure, a medical discipline—podiatry—has arisen to provide specialized foot care. There are more than 8,000 doctors of podiatric medicine in the United States. With colleagues in medicine, osteopathic medicine, and dentistry, the podiatrist is a member of one of the four professions permitted by law to prescribe and treat, medically and surgically, a part of the human anatomy. The podiatrist's scope of practice is defined in each state by law. He is licensed to diagnose and treat foot problems, to correct or revise deformities, to manage the foot complications of chronic disease in cooperation with an attending physician, to treat injuries and deformities of the foot, including the surgical correction of bones, muscles, and tendons. But general podiatric care includes more. It includes the concept of prevention, the key to good foot health.

The podiatrist is a graduate of an accredited college of podiatric medicine. He or she enters podiatry college with 3 or 4 years of undergraduate study and completes a four-academic-year medical curriculum. During the last 2 years, much time is spent in clinical and hospital rotations. Upon completion of podiatry school, a graduate must pass either national or state board examinations for a license. Additionally, the podiatrist may complete a hospital residency program.

The podiatrist's responsibility to the LTC patient begins only when the LTC institution decides to provide comprehensive care which includes adequate foot care. This decision may result in hiring a consultant who meets with the administrator, the nurses, and the nurse's aides to determine the foot-health problems within the facility. This consultant may not be the podiatrist ultimately responsible for patient care; he may obtain others to provide care and to maintain quality for a foot-health program.

The consulting podiatrist may function as a health educator in informal and practical inservice educational programs for staff. He may also provide or supplement patient education when the patient is able to comprehend his problems and what is to be done for him. When patient involvement is possible, the duties of the practitioner, the nurse, the aide, and the administrator become lighter and, perhaps, less costly.

Upon request, state podiatry associations will recommend qualified consultants to administrators of LTC facilites. They will also usually recommend an individual who will be able to assist the institution or program in establishing a needed level of foot care. They will recommend a podiatrist who understands the financial problems of foot care and the mechanics of delivery within the current payment system.

As for financing problems, podiatry services can be paid for by Medicare, by Medicaid, by other third party carriers, and, finally, by the patient himself. The law does state that a podiatrist is a physician for purposes of payment under Medicare. The Medicare program will pay for the treatment of foot conditions with few exceptions. These exceptions are the routine foot care procedures. Exceptions are waived when the patient has an overlying cardiovascular systemic disease or a condition such as diabetes mellitus. Medicare will not cover the treatment of nonsurgical correction of deformities of the foot, such as orthosis, or specialized footwear or modification of footwear.

Foot services covered by Medicaid programs vary from state to state. Generally, when Medicaid pays for podiatric care, reimbursement may not be reasonable. There are no categorical exclusions in Medicaid regulations. Determinations on specific procedures are made at the state level, and many states provide for a full range of foot health services through Medicaid.

Other sources of outside payment for podiatric care are third party carriers. Carrier programs must be studied on an individual basis to determine the limits of coverage, what exclusions exist, and what the exceptions are to such exclusions. It is essential in a foot care program that, even if coverage is not available and even if the patient or his family cannot pay, the podiatrist be willing to provide necessary services.

This presentation has attempted to briefly describe the importance of foot-health care programs, to take a new look at the dynamic structure of the foot, to introduce the foot care professional—the doctor of podiatric medicine—and to outline current financial plans for foot care.

Remember, foot health is accomplished by a team effort. Everyone can play an important role, as foot health and foot care are extremely important to the patient's total health. It is an important link in maintaining the LTC patient's mobility and dignity.

LECTURE 2
IMPROVING THE ABILITY FOR EARLY RECOGNITION OF FOOT PROBLEMS IN THE LONG-TERM CARE RESIDENT

Purpose

This lecture is designed to enable trainees to better recognize the early symptoms of foot problems in the elderly through an understanding of basic foot examination techniques and procedures.

Outline

I. Foot problem recognition and LTC personnel
   A. Importance of LTC staff in early detection and reporting
   B. Use of patient histories to indicate problems
      1. Patient medical history
      2. Environmental influences
      3. Racial-hereditary factors
      4. Age of patient
      5. Nutritional habits
      6. Family history
      7. Social habits
II. Use of examination and observation as foot problem indicators
   A. What to look for as indicators of problems
   B. Checking temperatures of extremities
   C. Checking pulses of extremities
   D. Checking blood pressures of the extremities
   E. Podiatric uses of reflex tests
   F. Use of manual muscle testing

III. Pain as the most important indicator of foot problems
   A. Types of pain and their possible meanings
   B. Complications arising from painful conditions
   C. Lack of pain and possible meanings
IV. Summary

Pre- and Postlecture Discussion Questions

1. List some specific ways in which a patient history can indicate the potential of foot problems occurring in a resident.
2. What are some basic observable abnormalities in the foot indicating the need for further examination by an M.D. or a podiatrist?
3. Why is the temperature of the feet an important indicator of problems in the LTC resident?
4. What are some common types of pain that occur in the feet indicating the need for further examination by an M.D. or a podiatrist?
5. What are some common reasons many elderly individuals do not complain of existing foot problems?
6. Why is taking the foot pulse an important procedure in foot health?
7. What are some important reflex tests used on the foot?

LECTURE 2
IMPROVING THE ABILITY FOR EARLY RECOGNITION OF FOOT PROBLEMS IN THE LONG-TERM CARE RESIDENT

Early detection and treatment of health problems are of paramount importance in preventive health care practice. But how do many of us practice this concept when it concerns the feet?

This presentation is designed to educate nurses and nurses' aides in LTC facilities about the specifics of early detection of common foot disorders among elderly and chronically ill patients. These key people must use their experience, knowledge and observations to detect problems and report them to the podiatrist and physician.

We will review the use of patient histories, physical examination of the foot, interpretation of various foot complaints, and the difference between a normal foot and abnormal one, as basic tools in your everyday contact with the resident.

As has been previously stated, the role of the LTC staff in detecting and preventing foot disorders is important. One important tool available to them in accomplishing this is the resident patient's medical and family history. A history should contain information on the patient's present and past diseases and physical condition, as well as a comprehensive review of medical problems prevalent in his family.

It should include his former address, which may help determine whether new environmental influences are affecting his medical condition. Knowing whether a patient lived in a tenement building or next to a polluted river, or in an area with a healthier environment, can help interpret a patient's symptoms, even those in his feet.

Racial background and hereditary factors should also be noted in the history and can help to associate environment with the patient's condition.

A patient's age is another aid to proper diagnosis. We know that changes occur in the aging foot and have an idea what is normal and what is not. Yet, while age can be a determining factor in disease, it cannot be used alone. For example, a child may have a condition that is completely ignored by medical personnel simply because he is young. Or a middle-aged woman may have a real medical problem missed simply because she is nearing menopause. The ages of parents, if they are still living, and the ages of all brothers and sisters are also important. If any members of the family are deceased, their ages at death and causes of death are facts doctors should know when diagnosing a patient's condition.

Finally, the history should contain a record of social habits, such as smoking, drinking and drug use. Smoking directly affects the circulatory system by constricting the blood vessels, thus reducing blood flow. Alcoholism, or alcohol consumption, can lead to numbness in the feet, liver problems and retarded mental function.

We have established that knowledge of the patient's background, medical history, family history, age, sex and social habits can be a great aid to the nursing staff in detecting a potential problem in a resident. These items will be important to us later when we discuss certain diseases and conditions caused by heredity, environment, nutrition or social habits.

Perhaps more important to the nursing staff than the family and personal history is the constant observation and examination of the feet of the patient. Each time a patient is bathed, dressed, fed, walked or exercised, the staff person should be observing the patient for rashes, sores, painful joints and other problems, particularly in the feet and legs.

One of the first things to notice is the color of the skin. In the elderly patient, the skin color usually varies from red to red-blue. Skin that is marble white is associated with pain or numbness. This may indicate an acute vascular insufficiency, which is a medical emergency. Color changes which affect only one foot are also very important. Areas of dark pigmentation over major arteries can mean circulation deficits or stagnation of blood. Red spots in areas of pressure on the bottom of the foot can be a precursor to ulceration which may be connected with diabetes. Black or blue moles that change color, enlarge, or bleed may become malignant.

Variations in texture (smooth, rough, glossy, dull, pigmented, scaly, clear) are helpful, if recognized, in determining the potential presence of circulatory and dermatological problems and other systemic conditions.

Checking the temperature of the foot is a good diagnostic procedure. The normal foot temperature varies anywhere between 92 and 98 degrees Farenheit and may be determined by a skin thermometer. Touching both feet at the same time provides an indication of the relative temperature of the feet. Disparity is what is important to notice. Excessive warmth in one foot may mean an inflammation or infection. Coldness in one foot may mean poor circulation or a neurological deficit affecting the vascular system. Perspiring feet may indicate nervous conditions, faulty foot mechanics, or pain. Temperature of individual toes can also be determined. If one toe is colder than the others, this could signify a local vascular deficit which could lead to gangrene and possible amputation if not found and treated.

Checking pulses in the foot and leg can be very important. The foot has two pulses, one located on top of the foot, the other located behind the innermost part of the ankle. Occasionally, the pulse on the top of the foot (dorsalis pedis pulse) may be impalpable, but this is normal in some people. The pulse behind the ankle, the posterior tibial pulse, is usually palpable, except in cases of decreased circulation. The staff person must not confuse his own pulse, which is best felt in the thumb, with the patient's. For this reason the middle three fingers are used to feel the pulsations. There is also a pulse behind the knee, the popliteal pulse, which can be felt by holding the knee from the front with thumbs placed on the knee cap and fingers exerting mild pressure behind the knee. With practice you will be able to find these pulses and differentiate normal from abnormal. The rate of the pulse is not as important as the strength and fullness of that pulse for both feet. Are they equally strong? If not, there should be further investigation.

Other means of examination include checking blood pressures in both the leg and the arm which can be valuable in diagnosing problems such as vascular insufficiency, aortic insufficiency, and coarctation of the aorta. Like the pulse, blood pressure readings should be observed for equal strength. If a wide disparity occurs, further investigation should be initiated.

Determining the presence or absence of tendon reflexes can also be helpful. The knee jerk or knee reflex test, in which a rubber hammer is used to strike the area below the knee cap, is well known. The same procedure can be performed at the ankle and on the side of the foot by the podiatrist. The lack of reflexes or the increased force of a reflex can lead the podiatrist to uncovering neurological conditions which may not be evident by observing the patient.

Manual testing of muscles is another important procedure used by physicians in diagnosing foot problems. This can be done simply by applying pressure to each of the four sides of the foot and having the patient exert an opposite force. This provides a relative indication of the strength of the patient's individual leg muscles.

The previous portion of this presentation has dealt with six physical indicators of foot problems: color and texture of skin, temperature, pulses, blood pressures, reflexes, and muscle strength. However, the most important intangible indicator is pain. When a patient complains of pain or burning or itching, it should always be investigated. The fact that a patient is old and sometimes incoherent or senile should not prevent staff persons from listening to and acting on any complaint.

Foot pain is a common complaint, especially in elderly patients. As age increases, joints become arthritic, circulation decreases, muscles become wasted, and the chances of injury and damage to the foot and leg increase. Even simple problems can become complicated. For example, a corn on a toe or a callous on the bottom of the foot may cause the patient to limp and favor that foot, thus shifting weight abnormally and causing other problems to develop. Pain may be reported as cramping, burning, dull aching, tingling, or sharp shooting pains.

Cramping is a common complaint usually caused by an unnatural position of or impaired circulation in the foot. Cramps in the foot and leg while sleeping or while walking can signify arterial insufficiency. This condition is known as intermittent claudication. Deformities and nutritional deficiencies can also cause cramping.

A complaint of tingling or numbness and burning can be due to many disorders. A nerve tumor between two toes can cause tingling in those toes and burning between the toes. Compression of the sciatic nerve in the back can cause tingling in the heel and the back of the leg. Numbness can be due to nerve irritation or vascular insufficiency, or such systemic diseases as diabetes or chronic alcoholism. Vitamin deficiencies, anemia, and dietary problems are also common causes of tingling and burning.

Soreness can be due to overworked muscles, stretched ligaments and joints, and inflammation of veins (phlebitis) in the leg. A common complaint in the elderly is soreness on the top and inside of the big toe. This is one of the early signs of arteriosclerosis of the foot.

Sharp shooting pains may be due to a nerve that is entrapped or a fracture of a bone in the foot. If it occurs on arising, and stepping out of bed in the morning, it is probably due to arthritic changes.

Just as important as the complaint of pain is the situation in which an obvious problem or condition exists, but elicits no complaint. Ulcers on the foot or leg that are not painful should be suspect. These may be caused by diabetes or other systemic diseases and should be reported and thoroughly investigated. Many elderly patients, because of embarrassment or modesty, will not complain of problems. Most patients feel their feet are ugly and do not like to show them. Additionally, it is likely that often a problem will be present, but the patient will not feel pain or be aware of sensation changes. Circulatory deficiencies in the elderly can cause a gradual loss of sensation that precludes pain. This is an especially dangerous situation and further adds to the importance of the staff using all examination techniques.

We have briefly explored methods that can be used to recognize foot problems common in the elderly and chronically ill patient. The difference between the normal and abnormal foot and the functions of nurses and nursing assistants in observing and identifying foot problems have also been defined. The various methods of determining the general state of the health or disease of a foot have been explained. These have included observing skin color, temperature and texture, looking for rashes, and the testing of muscles, tendon reflexes, and blood pressure of the extremities. When performed by either the podiatrist or the nurse, these tests take only a few minutes and give a good indication not only of the patient's foot health, but of his overall health, as well. Nurses and nurses' aides are in constant contact with patients in LTC facilities, and they carry the primary responsibility for observing, discovering, and reporting foot problems for necessary care.

LECTURE 3
IDENTIFYING AND CARING FOR COMMON SKIN AND NAIL PROBLEMS OF THE LONG-TERM CARE RESIDENT

Purpose

This lecture is designed to:

Enable trainees to recognize the most common skin and nail foot problems found in the LTC resident and understand the various causes.

Acquaint trainees with recommended principles and techniques used by podiatrists in caring for such problems.

Teach trainees to contribute to the prevention and management of these conditions through early recognition, and the use of foot hygiene as a deterrent to complications.

Outline

I. Normal skin and the aged
   A. Normal signs of aging skin
   B. Appearance of aging skin
   C. Causes of signs of aging
   D. Anatomical structure of the skin
II. Common dermatological foot problems of LTC residents
   A. Hyperkeratotic lesions (corns and callouses)
   B. Verrucae (warts)
   C. Mycotic infections (fungus infections, etc.)
   D. Contact dermatitis
   E. Ulcers
   F. Neoplasms—tumors
III. Management as classified by cause
   A. Congenitally caused
   B. Trauma-induced
   C. Allergies
   D. Nutritional changes
   E. Other infections
   F. Nail conditions associated with other pathology
IV. Summary

Pre- and Postlecture Discussion Questions

The Skin

1. What are some common observable signs of aging in the skin of the elderly?
2. List some common dermatological problems incurred by LTC residents.

3. What are some causes of determatological problems in LTC residents?
4. What are some common principles and techniques of preventive care for dermatological problems?

The Nails

1. What are some common signs of nail problems of the LTC resident?

2. List some common nail problems incurred by LTC residents.
3. What are some common causes of nail problems in LTC residents?
4. What are some common principles and techniques of preventive care for nail problems?

LECTURE 3
IDENTIFYING AND CARING FOR COMMON SKIN AND NAIL PROBLEMS OF THE LONG-TERM CARE RESIDENT

During the course of a lifetime, the human foot endures much use, misuse, trauma and neglect. The stresses of daily activity, the fact that the foot is constantly enclosed, and the degenerative changes of aging require special attention for the individual to remain ambulant.

Given this information, it is easy to understand that the most common local, chronic foot problems are those of the skin and the nail. This presentation will review some of the common foot complaints associated with these areas.

The skin of the elderly patient's foot is noticeably different from that of a younger person. It is less supple than youthful skin because of diminished elasticity of the fibers beneath the epidermis and dermis. There may be a loss of hair on the outer side of the leg and on the foot, distinctive brownish pigmentation changes, some dryness, scaling, and atrophy. This dryness comes from naturally diminishing oily secretions. Other changes are due to metabolic and nutritional factors.

Common dermatological problems in feet of the aged or chronically ill are varied and because of the delicate nature of the individual's normal condition, treatment must be approached conservatively. An individual often comes to an LTC facility with chronic foot conditions. The problems in treating these patients are multiple. Future problems as well as complications in the existing condition must be prevented.

Let's quickly review the structure and composition of the foot's skin. The skin consists of the epidermis (outer layer), which varies in thickness, and the dermis (inner layer). The outermost layer of the epidermis (stratum corneum) consists of cells containing keratin, a fibrous protein. It is thickest where external trauma is greatest, such as on the soles. This stratum corneum actually increases in thickness with trauma. The outer layers peel off as new cells are formed continuously to maintain this thickness. The deeper layer of the stratum corneum serves as a barrier to absorption of substances through the skin. The dermis (corium) is the inner section of the skin, containing blood vessels, nerves, and such tissues as sweat glands, ducts and hair follicles and their sebaceous glands.

The nerve supply of the skin conducts both sensory and motor impulses. Sensory nerves transmit perception of touch, temperature and pain. Motor nerves control sweat glands, arterioles and smooth muscle of the skin.

Six types of skin problems of the foot are often encountered in LTC facilities. The first are hyperkeratotic lesions; these result from many minimal traumas, initiative frictions, and pressures on the skin which cause an abnormally thickened mass of keratin. The term "hyperkeratotic" means overactive production of keratinic tissue. The most common hyperkeratotic lesions are forms of callouses (tyloma) and corns (heloma). Callouses often occur over a bony enlargement or at a site of abnormal weight distribution. Corns are usually found about the toes and are commonly caused by pressure from ill-fitting footwear or by bony prominences.

Two common corns are the hard corn (heloma durum) and the soft corn (heloma molle). The soft corn differs from the hard corn in that it absorbs perspiration and moisture as it is commonly found between the toes. Another common corn is the heloma neurofibrosum, which contains a core of fibrous tissue. It is especially painful with a throbbing, burning, and stabbing pain found in an area of extreme friction and pressure or at a site of direct trauma. It can be recognized by its irregular outline and white and grey color.

Heloma vascularis is like heloma durum, but the abnormally thickened tissue also bleeds. Its orange and red to yellow linear discolorations are separated by a callous and covered with dry or moist tissue.

Miliary helomas consist of multiple localized spotty areas of hyperkeratosis, measuring about 1 to 3 mm. in diameter. They are multiple, deeply imbedded, and appear nearly white to yellow in color.

Callouses look different depending upon which part of the foot (including heel and toes) they occur. They can be extremely painful.

Corns and callouses can be treated both palliatively and surgically. Treatment of both depends upon etiology, size, location, and the patient's health and age. Both must be treated judiciously as they are capable of causing further difficulty.

Even though corns and callouses can be removed surgically, the more common treatment is to soften the involved area and thus reduce keratosis. Next, removal of pressure in the involved area is necessary. This can be accomplished by a change in footwear and by the prescription of an orthotic. An orthotic is a device made of plastic, rubber, felt and other materials that is used to shield painful areas. Additionally, the patient should be instructed how to use emollients and skin-softening foot soaps.

A second common foot complaint is warts (verrucae); there are many types. Warts are seldom found in the elderly, but they often occur in the younger chronically ill patient. The causes of these benign growths, which cause excruciating pain when weight is put on them, are not known. Some possible causes may be viruses, irritations, psychosomatic factors, endocrine changes, and metabolic disorders.

Many foot warts are extremely difficult to remove. Common methods are surgical excision and chemosurgery. In the elderly, management of warts is best accomplished with simple relief of pressure and the use of emollients.

A third common type of foot complaint may be classified as disorders of the sweat glands and fungus (or mycotic) infections. Because of glandular and metabolic changes, the elderly can suffer from two basic disorders involving the sweat glands. Hyperidrosis, an abnormal increase in perspiration, and anidrosis, an abnormal decrease in perspiration. Hyperidrosis, or excessive perspiration, and bromidrosis, accompanied by a fetid odor, both specifically result from ill-fitting footwear or unbalanced diets. Treatment of these conditions depends on normalizing the functions of the sweat glands and the general physical status of the patient.

The patient should wear hosiery that can absorb perspiration but that has a weave wide enough to allow for evaporation. Lightweight woolen hose or good quality absorbent cotton are recommended. Synthetic substances—nylon or orlon—do not permit adequate evaporation of excessive perspiration and may cause the skin to become soggy, irritated, macerated and painful. Poorly constructed and ill-fitting footwear contribute to excessive perspiration. Shoes made of plastic or rubber compounds prevent evaporation and cause maceration and discomfort.

The following regimen has been used successfully to combat hyperidrosis and many of its complicating factors. The patient should bathe feet daily in lukewarm water and tetramethylthiuram disulfide or hexachlorophene—a bacteriostatic product. The skin should be patted dry, not rubbed. A suitable astringent should be applied between the toes and over areas that perspire more than others. Prescribed solutions may be swabbed daily over the perspiring feet and toes to decrease the excessive perspiration.

Hyperidrosis and bromidrosis may also be helped by using a dusting powder, which the doctor will be able to prescribe.

Anidrosis is the abnormally low output of perspiration. It may be caused either by sluggish sweat glands or by mechanical obstruction of the sweat ducts and pores, limiting normal excretion of perspiration and thereby causing the skin to be dry, scaly and sometimes parchment-like. Though foot soaking is important, one should avoid excessive use of strong soap and hot salt water. In addition to local and systemic medical treatment of the problem, the use of emollient creams and moisturizing agents is suggested.

One possible complication of anidrosis is fissured heels, in which the skin cracks into fissures and ulcerations. Fissured heels can be serious when there is an associated poor blood supply to the heel. The broken skin is susceptible to infection. Therapy is aimed at closing the fissures and at future prevention.

Next, we will explore fungus (mycotic) infections. One of the most common is athlete's foot or tinea pedis. Symptoms in the younger individual are itching or maceration between the toes. However, in the elderly individual with diminishing sensation, there may be no complaint. There will be scaling and redness, particularly between the toes. Treatment is usually topical with drugs. Using topical foot powders helps prevent recurrences.

Contact dermatitis is a fourth dermatological problem which the LTC patient may suffer. Its causes are normally shoe dyes and various foot-covering materials. It is characterized by a limited and circumscribed area of inflammation and a previous history of allergy. The primary irritant must be isolated and removed. Therapy is then aimed at the various skin manifestations and would usually include mild soaks, such as Burrows solution or saline solutions, and topical application of steroids and related drugs.

A fifth skin problem—ulcers—may result from external problems or systemic disease. Ulcers resulting from external causes include trauma, decubitus ulceration (bed sores), trophic ulceration, scratches from excessive itching, and burns, either thermal, electrical or chemical, or burns from use of corn cure medications. The internal or systemic diseases that can cause ulcers include arterial or venous insufficiencies, diabetes mellitus, gout and residuals of syphilis.

Treatment of any ulcerated area in the LTC patient should be approached conservatively by the doctor. Further infection and even gangrene due to vascular insufficiency is a possibility.

A sixth type of common foot problem is various forms of neoplasms, or tumors, such as small fibromas and other cysts. These may require surgical excision. However, when they are benign and pose no immediate problem, they may be left alone.

The second part of this presentation will review common nail problems found in LTC patients. Chief nail complaints usually relate to thickness, hardness, and the inability to cut one's own nails. These simple problems can be magnified by poor eyesight and the inability to bend. The normal nail is somewhat thin, translucent, and has a fresh pinkish color beneath the nail. However, it is generally hard and thickened in the elderly individual. This is largely the result of a decreasing vascular supply to the nail bed.

Among the causes of geriatric nail pathology are trauma, infectious dermatoses, and degenerative diseases, such as arteriosclerosis and arthritis.

LTC staff should be aware that the geriatric patient may commonly demonstrate anonychia (absence of a nail), macronychia (enlarged nails), and micronychia (a small nail). These conditions are asymptomatic.

What are some of the more common nail problems of the elderly? Congenital thickening of the nail may be common, and treatment may include periodic reduction by sandpaper, electric drill, and burrs accompanied by home care measures.

A thickening of the nail plate is also associated with aging, nutritional disturbances, repeated trauma, inflammation, local infection, various infectious diseases, such as syphilis, and various degenerative diseases, such as arteriosclerosis. The nail appears thickened and discolored, and onychophosis (callous nail groove), subungual hyperkeratosis, debris, and fungus infection usually accompanies this condition. Pain may be present due to the pressure of the nail plate against the upper part of the shoe. Again, periodic reduction of the nail plate is the customary treatment.

A sudden traumatic blow to the nail can result in a subungual hematoma, which is quite painful. Bleeding can usually be seen through the translucent nail plate. A small hole may be drilled through the nail plate to permit blood to escape, immediately relieving the the pain. X-rays should be taken to rule out a fracture of bone. Thickening may follow any acute injury to the nail root (matrix). A severe injury to the matrix may also cause loss of the nail, starting at the base. Beau's lines (transverse striations) may be present when nail growth is interrupted, but the injury is not severe enough to cause shedding.

Onychophosis (callous nail groove) is usually the result of trauma to the nail plate or some external pressure. Treatment consists of excision, the use of emollients to moisten and lubricate the hyperkeratosis, thinning of the nail plate to permit flexibility, and the removal of any external pressures.

Onychocryptosis (ingrown toenail) may occur when a fragment of a nail pierces the skin of the nail lip (ungualabia). It may be the result of improper self-treatment or external pressure. It may be accompanied by secondary infection and granulation tissue.

Conservative treatment consists of excising the offending portion of the nail, followed by saline soaks, and packing until the corner of the nail reaches the free edge. When secondary infection is present, antibiotics are used. Total treatment can be complicated by a thickened nail. An ingrown toenail can be quite serious when systemic disease, such as arteriosclerosis or diabetes, is present. Neglect by the patient in these circumstances can result in gangrene. When this condition becomes chronic, surgical excision or cautery of a portion of the nail matrix must be considered to prevent further infection.

Pinpoint pressure on any nail bed may result in a corn (subungual heloma). A bony tumor (subungual exostosis) or chondroma (tumor formed from cartilage cells) must be ruled out by use of x-rays. The corn usually appears as a dark spot beneath the nail plate. Treatment consists of excising the lesion and removing pressure. A cancerous tumor (subungual melanoma) may present a similar dark appearance through the nail plate and must be ruled out before treatment begins.

Allergic reactions in the nails may be due to primary irritants, such as bacteria and fungi, or to repeated exposures to secondary irritants, such as nail polish and shoe dyes. Inflammation (onychia) is usually present and is followed by separation of the nail from the bed starting at the free edge (onycholysis). Treatment should try to eliminate the cause, following up with medication for both infection and inflammation. Topical steroids are useful in chronic cases.

Remember that diet plays an important role in all body structures. In poor nutritional states, the nails usually become thin and brittle and lose their luster. Onychomadesis, which is the shedding of nails, may occur for this reason.

Onychomycosis is a fungus infection of the nail which usually causes a severe disturbance of nail growth accompanied by local nail plate destruction. Onychomycosis can be incapacitating and always remains as a focal point for reinfection. These nails may appear opaque, scaly, and hypertrophic. The areas of destruction may be granular and may separate. Inflammation may be a complicating factor. Treatment includes culture, mechanical debridement, chemical debridement, and the use of antifungal agents. Antibiotics can be utilized but results are dependent upon the arterial supply to the nail bed. Topical preparations require meticulous care by both the patient and the podiatrist. This problem is notably resistant to treatment.

Varieties of bacteria and other organisms can cause nail infections. The cardinal signs of inflammation are always present. Therapy consists of warm saline soaks and antibiotics. Inflammation is common in diabetes.

Various neoplasms or tumors may affect the nail area. Therapy depends upon the cause.

Psoriatic nails are usually opaque and lose their luster. Loosening of the nails, debris, retarded growth, and Beau's lines are common. Inflammation is the classical diagnostic sign that a problem exists. Chronic eczema usually produces a disturbed growth pattern and a marked nail distortion. Chronic long-standing endocrine disturbances usually produce atrophy of the nail plate and surrounding tissues.

Restrictions of the blood supply may produce atrophy and widening of the cuticle. The organic vascular diseases, such as arteriosclerosis and Beurger's disease, usually produce local ischemia and retarded linear growth. Splitting, brittleness and overgrowth are usually also present. When there is an associated diabetic problem, minor nail pathology can require hospitalization.

The nails of the arthritic patient are usually dry and brittle. These nails usually become inflamed and separated in the early stages and demonstrate hypertrophy in the latter stages.

As you can see, the skin and the nails are the easiest parts of the foot to observe. Aged patients will have a variety of common skin and nail problems. These are but a few. Many of these can be managed easily with basic care, cleanliness, common foot medications and relief from pressure or allergic substances. Others will require professional care and can be serious if not detected early.

In addition to being important for the comfort of the patient, many of the skin and nail conditions are significant because they are symptomatic of serious health problems. Those involving constriction of blood supply can lead, in extreme cases, to gangrene and a need for amputation of the affected parts.

Observation and treatment of foot problems are important for foot health and for the overall health of the patient. You, as a responsible member of the LTC staff, must assist in the early detection of these dangerous foot problems.

LECTURE 4
IDENTIFYING AND CARING FOR MUSCULAR AND SKELETAL PROBLEMS OF THE LONG-TERM CARE RESIDENT

Purpose

This lecture is designed to:

Enable trainees to recognize the most common muscular and skeletal problems found in the LTC resident, and their various causes.

Acquaint trainees with recommended principles and techniques used by podiatrists for the care of the muscular and skeletal problems of the LTC resident.

Teach trainees to contribute to the prevention and management of muscular and skeletal problems.

Outline

I. Muscular and skeletal changes that occur in the feet of the LTC resident.
II. Muscular and skeletal problems suffered by LTC residents
  A. Definition of conditions
    1. Corns and callouses
    2. Hammer toes
    3. Osteoarthritis or degenerative joint disease
    4. Rheumatoid arthritis
    5. Flat feet (pes planus)
    6. Bunions
    7. Matatarsalgia (painful ball of foot)
    8. Bunionette or tailors bunion
    9. Stiffened big toe joint (hallux rigidus)
    10. Nerve impairments
    11. Heel spurs
  B. Causes and contributing factors to conditions
  C. Techniques and principles of treatment and management
    1. Palliative care
    2. Surgical applications by physicians
    3. Recommended exercises and other physical measures
III. Summary

Pre- and Postlecture Discussion Questions

1. Why is ambulation so important to LTC resident foot health?
2. What are common muscular-skeletal changes that occur in the lower extremities of the aged and chronically ill?
3. What are some common specific mechanical problems that occur in the feet of LTC residents?
4. What are some principles and techniques of podiatric care for muscular-skeletal problems?
5. What are the most basic types of exercises to strengthen muscles of the feet?

LECTURE 4
IDENTIFYING AND CARING FOR MUSCULAR AND SKELETAL PROBLEMS OF THE LONG-TERM RESIDENT

"When your feet hurt, you hurt all over." This often quoted adage probably originated because an elderly gentleman's feet hurt so badly that when he walked, he shifted his weight, walked abnormally, and thus caused other joints to hurt. While this may not be a true story, it is true that painful feet can cause pains elsewhere. These foot problems are often due to arthritic joints, partial dislocations, and other mechanical disorders that affect the feet of elderly patients.

Movement is accomplished by the force of muscles acting on bones of the body. Mechanical disorders occur when either the muscles or the bones are impaired. Thus, they are called musculoskeletal disorders. The following discussion will examine the most common musculoskeletal problems, the techniques and principles in caring for them, and how each of us might contribute to their prevention.

As most things grow older, they tend to wear out and break down. This is true of automobiles and other machines with moving parts. It is also true of the human body. Years of use and abuse take their toll. Probably no area is affected more than the foot. It has been estimated that a 65-year-old person has walked a distance of over 250,000 miles during his lifetime, a figure that the most well-constructed car, with interchangeable parts, cannot match. During the course of a lifetime many changes occur, including wearing out of joints and loss of soft tissue. These changes affect not only the local area where they occur, but also other joints and areas that have to function with the affected joints. These cause changes in posture, balance, and gait and may contribute to musculoskeletal problems.

Musculoskeletal problems reveal themselves in many ways, by forming bumps, painful spurs, thick skin, and crooked toes. Probably the most common of these are the corn and the callous. People still consider these two problems as primarily skin problems and, consequently, apply corn plasters and medicines to remove them. Actually a corn's thick skin is caused by an underlying bony prominence pushing the skin from the inside and the shoe exerting pressure from the outside. When intermittent friction occurs, the skin toughens to protect itself and a corn begins. Medication for corns, which in most cases is merely acid, will remove the thick skin and good skin as well, but does nothing to solve the real problem, which is the bony prominence beneath the corn.

A corn can be treated surgically by removing the piece of bone causing it or by releasing the tendon (which is pulling the toe upward) to allow the toe, if it is flexible, to flatten.

Padding and flexible shielding can be used for patients for whom surgical treatment is not recommended. Shoes can be altered by removing the top portion so that the toe has no pressure; this will cure the symptom and relieve pain, but will not cure the real problem.

Callouses are also a common occurrence in LTC patients. They can be caused by the misalignment of metatarsals, or bones behind the toes, by a bone that is too rigid and does not move or one that is too loose and moves constantly, or by a mechanical fault in which the bone is pushed downward by a toe out of line.

Again, treatment can be surgical removal of the bony part, or surgical correction of the tendon pull that causes the bone to be depressed. More often in LTC patients, the areas will be padded or a shoe or orthosis built to relieve pressure from this area. Relief of pressure is essential in the care of diabetics and patients with circulatory problems, to prevent ulceration, infection, and need for possible amputation.

In the elderly, the type of bony prominence seen most often is a condition called hammer toes. In a hammer toe, a toe joint hammers or curves upward in the middle subjecting the toe to shoe pressure and causing the formation of a corn. At one time, hammer toes were thought to be caused by tight shoes. However, doctors came to realize that shoes tight enough to cause hammer toes would be too painful to wear. Actually, hammer toes can be caused by problems in mechanics of the foot or diseases such as rheumatoid arthritis.

One mechanical cause of hammer toes is the tendon on the top of the foot, which exerts a pull on the toe. If the toe is not in proper alignment, the tendon will pull the toe abnormally and cause it to curve upward. Pressure from the shoe pushing downward on this dislocated toe causes a corn, which can become ulcerated, infected, and occasionally requires amputation. Nursing personnel must watch the toes daily, especially in patients with vascular diseases and diabetes.

Other musculoskeletal problems often seen in the elderly are caused by osteoarthritis or degenerative joint disease. It affects almost all elderly prsons because, in this form of arthritis, the joints begin to wear out. The cartilage between the bones begins to erode, causing bone to rub against bone, which causes pain. These patients can usually forecast the weather mainly by the pain they experience before a change in humidity or barometric pressure. X-rays show areas of bone spur formation around the joints and a narrowing of the spaces between the joints. There might also be some observable thickening in the joints of the fingers and toes. Most people with degenerative joint disease experience stiffness in the morning, which decreases as the day progresses and the joints are exercised.

Treatment of degenerative joint disease may consist of physical therapy, such as whirlpool and ultrasound treatments, paraffin baths, or other means by which heat surrounds the part. This seems to relax the muscles, relieve some of the joint pressure and allow smoother and less painful motion. Aspirin or other mild analgesics will control moderate discomfort. If deterioration is severe, surgical replacement or fusion of painful joints may be indicated.

Another type of arthritis seen in LTC facilities, which may strike at any age, is rheumatoid arthritis, a disease affecting connective tissue. It differs from degenerative joint disease in that the joints do not merely wear out from long use, but instead are eventually destroyed completely. The causes of rheumatoid arthritis are still unknown, but some feel that it may be an autoimmune disease. In other words, the patient may be allergic to something within his own body.

Rheumatoid arthritis causes dislocations of joints, usually laterally, joint fusions and bunion formation. Many musculoskeletal disorders can be caused by rheumatoid arthritis, including hammer toes, bowstringing of tendons, complete disappearance of toe bones and other dramatic changes. X-rays of rheumatoid arthritic patients show joints destroyed, bones losing calcium, brittleness, and toes dislocated and misaligned.

Because there is no known cure for rheumatoid arthritis, the treatment is concerned with the symptoms, that is, stopping the pain; trying to slow down the deformities with braces, shoes and orthoses; and physical therapy methods, such as whirlpool, ultrasound, and daily exercises. The surgical replacement of joints has been a great help to patients with rheumatoid arthritis. With today's advanced medical technology, almost every joint in the body can be replaced surgically. When successful, these operations bring pain relief and comfort to the patient.

Another musculoskeletal condition seen in LTC patients is flat feet (pes planus) in which the arch is broken down and the entire sole touches the ground. Detecting whether or not a foot is truly flat can be difficult, because the foot may be flat when it is bearing weight and completely normal when at rest. A podiatrist can detect flat feet and provide treatment if the problem is painful. Usually flat feet will have associated problems, including corns, callouses, and bunions.

The bunion is a term used to describe the inside of the joint of the big toe when it becomes enlarged, inflamed, or painful. In most cases this area is actually normal bone that has been forced outward when the big toe moves laterally toward the second toe. Bunions are not caused by shoes, but by a mechanical problem in the foot that causes the foot to be flat and most often hypermobile.

Bunions, if detected in the early stages, can be arrested by using orthoses to stop excessive motion and stabilize the foot. In healthy patients, surgery may be indicated to remove the bunion and straighten the big toe. When all else fails, padding and the use of orthodigital devices to protect the area and cutting out of shoes may be the final answer. This area must be observed by LTC personnel and the signs of inflammation, excessive pressure, etc. must be seen and reported to the podiatrist. X-rays can be taken to determine the extent of damage and the choice of a therapeutic method.

In the high arched foot or cavus foot, it is not uncommon to see callouses, corns, bunions and hammer toes all at the same time. The reasons are the same as in the condition of flat footedness; only the mechanics are different.

Again, this condition can be handled surgically if the patient can tolerate surgery. However, it is more common to use orthotic devices or shoe therapy to make the patient as comfortable as possible, and mobile.

Another musculoskeletal disorder involves a painful ball of the foot, called metatarsalgia. Patients who are ambulatory will compain of a dull ache or burning sensation in this area. In elderly patients, the fatty tissue formerly on the ball of the foot to absorb shock and disperse pressure has disappeared, and the bones can be felt readily just beneath the skin. The area now has only fascia and tendons left to absorb the pressure. When they become irritated and inflamed they cause pain. Physical therapy will help this condition, along with padding or shifting the pressure to another area. Shoe therapy and orthoses may also be used to give more lasting relief.

On the outside of the foot, behind the little toe, a lump may sometimes form what is known as a bunionette or tailor's bunion. It is so named because of the way tailors used to sit crosslegged for hours of work. Pressure is exerted on the little toe forcing it to the middle of the foot and pushing the bones behind it outward. Constant pressure on those bones causes a callous to form, so there is an enlarged bump much like the bunion formed behind the big toe. This condition can also be controlled surgically or with orthoses and padding.

Another mechanical disorder, which stiffens the big toe joint, is called hallux limitus or hallux rigidus. Hallux limitus allows little motion, and hallux rigidus allows no motion. Pain may be stopped by restricting the motion in the joint, utilizing a steel insole and a steel shank in the shoe to prevent it from bending, by physical therapy, and by regional injections or cortisone type drugs. Pressure around the joint can be relieved by padding, by using a low vamp shoe, and by skipping an eyelet at the site if shoes which tie are worn.

Occasionally a patient will complain of sharp burning pain between two toes that occurs while walking and stops when no weight is on the foot. This is usually due to an enlarged nerve and is directly associated with musculoskeletal problems. It usually occurs between the third and fourth toes where two metatarsal heads compress the nerve between them. Relief can be obtained by cortisone injection, by padding, and by vitamin B-12. If symptoms persist, surgical removal is indicated.

Heel spurs causing heel pain are another manifestation of musculoskeletal problems. The aged heel, just as other areas once covered by a shock-absorbing fatty pad, has only skin to protect it. Also, the ligaments are relaxed and weakened, and they stretch, allowing the foot to become more flattened. This places a stretch and pull on the plantar fascia which is attached to the heel bone. The pain symptoms are usually due either to plantar fascitis, or to a bruise on the heel bone itself.

In the case of fascitis, simply relieving the pressure in the heel bone from the pull of the fascia will often control the pain. This can be done with padding and eventually an orthotic device to control pronation of the foot and prevent fascial stretch.

In the cases where periostitis or a stone bruise occurs on the bone, padding may be used with a cut-out beneath the spot of tenderness, or appliances can be made to do the same thing. Physical therapy is very helpful here to give penetrating heat and increased circulation.

This lecture has explained some of the musculoskeletal problems that plague LTC residents. We have established that as the muscles age, they begin to get smaller and weaken or atrophy. These muscle weaknesses affect not only the immediate local area but every associated bone, joint and muscle. Painful deformities can result.

Subjects covered have included simple musculoskeletal problems, such as hammer toes and corns, as well as more complex disorders such as cavus feet and flat feet. They all have one thing in common: they force the patient to live and walk in pain and distress. Elderly patients seem to lose all enthusiasm when they become bedridden or helpless because of foot problems. Pressure and pain can be relieved or lessened through physical therapy, surgery, padding and appliance therapy.

Walking, next to swimming, is the best exercise for joints and muscles and should be encouraged daily in LTC facilities. Other exercises that are beneficial include merely wiggling the toes, extending and flexing the knee, and pushing against the wall or floor with the foot. Anything that encourages muscle use is helpful. Muscle contraction is an aid to circulation, and when muscles are not used, patients with peripheral vascular disease may find themselves in trouble. Their failure to exercise could lead to inadequate blood supply, lack of oxygen in the tissue, ulceration, gangrene and eventual need for amputation.

Proper care of the musculoskeletal system by nursing personnel is vital to the survival and overall health and well-being of the LTC patient. Mechanical disorders can be a deterrent to good health maintenance. Deformities that cause pain, inhibit ambulation, and encourage patients to stay seated or remain in bed, are devastating if left unattended. If a patient limps, shifts weight abnormally, winces when walking, favors one side over the other, or just refuses to walk, the nursing staff's responsibility is to find out why and to report these findings immediately. As emphasized before, observation is the most important way to detect problems and prevent complications.

Podiatrists have for many years used the old adage, "Keep them walking" as a sort of motto. LTC facilities would do well to adopt it for their residents, too.

LECTURE 5
IDENTIFYING AND CARING FOR
PERIPHERAL VASCULAR PROBLEMS
OF THE LONG-TERM RESIDENT

Purpose

This lecture is designed to:

Enable trainees to recognize the most common peripheral vascular problems found in the LTC resident and their various causes.

Acquaint trainees with recommended principles and techniques of caring for the LTC resident with peripheral vascular problems. enable trainees to better understand, recognize and treat the special needs of this group of individuals.

Outline

I. Defining systemic vascular problems manifested in lower extremities
   A. Characteristics and appearances of peripheral vascular problems
   B. Causes of peripheral vascular diseases manifested in the lower extremities
II. Four common peripheral vascular diseases found in the LTC resident
   A. Arteriosclerosis
      1. Characteristics
      2. Symptoms and signs
      3. Treatment-management in the LTC facility
   B. Atherosclerosis
      1. Characteristics
      2. Symptoms and signs

3. Treatment-management in the LTC facility
   C. Varicose veins
      1. Characteristics
      2. Symptoms and signs
      3. Treatment-management in the LTC facility
   D. Vascular complications of diabetes
      1. Characteristics
      2. Symptoms and signs
      3. Treatment-management in the LTC facility
III. Summary

Pre- and Postlecture Discussion Questions

1. Why are peripheral vascular problems in the LTC resident a critical aspect of the foot health program?
2. What are some common peripheral vascular diseases which can be observed initially in the foot?
3. What are some observable characteristics of peripheral vascular diseases manifested in the foot?
4. Can you explain the difference between arteriosclerosis and atherosclerosis?
5. What are some important facets of the prevention and management of systemic vascular problems in the LTC resident?
6. What are some of the areas of special need for this group of people?

LECTURE 5
IDENTIFYING AND CARING FOR
PERIPHERAL VASCULAR PROBLEMS
OF THE LONG-TERM CARE RESIDENT

The most dangerous condition that can affect the foot of the LTC resident is peripheral vascular disease. It is of paramount importance that in their daily activities of observation and inspection, the nursing staff be aware of its presence and understand its initial signs of complications.

Vascular diseases are ailments that affect

blood vessels. In this discussion, emphasis will be placed on vascular diseases that affect the blood supply to the legs and feet. There are many peripheral vascular diseases. We will attempt to cover the most common ones, to acquaint personnel with techniques used by podiatrists for their management, and to create a better understanding of the special needs of patients afflicted with these disorders. We will also relate the types of disease, their symptoms, signs, and treatments.

The symptoms of peripheral vascular diseases include pain, changes in skin color, texture and temperature, tingling, burning and numbness, ulcerations, hair loss, nail changes and edema.

Vascular diseases to be covered are arteriosclerosis (including arteriosclerosis obliterans), artherosclerosis, varicose veins, and the vascular complications of diabetes. Arteriosclerosis is a disease characterized by a thickening of the middle layer of muscles in the artery and a loss of its elasticity. It is commonly called hardening of the arteries and eventually affects nearly all elderly patients.

Atherosclerosis is very similar to arteriosclerosis in that the vessels get thicker and lose elasticity, but in atherosclerosis, the narrowing of the artery is due to fatty deposits within the vessel. These diseases have similar symptoms, since they both cause a decrease in blood flow.

Pain is the most common symptom in arteriosclerosis and atherosclerosis. When any muscle is exercised, it requires oxygen. If its blood supply is diminished, the muscle starves for oxygen and a cramp occurs. Upon cessation of exercise, the pain stops. It usually occurs in the calf muscles and will be described by the patient as a tightness or cramp. In the foot, the pain is manifested by a feeling that the patient is walking on gravel or cobblestones. The pain is usually exhibited at or below the area where the vessel is narrowed. The skin is usually thin and atrophic and its temperature is cool. Patients also complain of numbness, edema and weakness of muscles. The toenails usually demonstrate thickening and, occasionally, fungus infections. Patients must care for their feet to prevent cuts and infections. With the circulation decreased, the body's ability to fight infection may be reduced. Thus infection may spread and lead to gangrene and the need for amputation. These patients need constant observation by nursing personnel for skin changes, ulcers, and cuts. These symptoms must be reported immediately to the podiatrist or physician.

The treatment of these sclerotic conditions is mainly symptomatic. No way has yet been found to dissolve the fatty plaques within the vessel or to increase the size of the artery. Exercise to tolerance can help to expand the vessels slightly. Warm soaks and heating elements will also cause some dilation of the vessels and increase circulation.

The most devastating form of atherosclerosis occurs in diabetes mellitus. Diabetes is usually associated with high blood sugar. Diabetics rarely associate circulatory problems with their disease. Diabetes mainly affects the small arteries in the eye, kidneys and feet. Diabetics complain of paresthesias, motor weakness, atrophic skin, tingling, numbness and burning of the feet and toes, cramping, and nearly all the other symptoms of vascular insufficiency.

Diabetics exhibit nail changes that include thickening and occasional fungus infections. Nails should be cut by a podiatrist to prevent the possibility of creating an ingrown toenail. Diabetics lose feeling in their feet due to the vascular insufficiency and must be aware of that. Feet should be inspected daily for cuts, bruises, and ulcers, and should be washed daily to ensure cleanliness. This responsibility belongs solely to nursing personnel in LTC facilities. Their attention to the diabetic patient can insure the patient's reaching the highest potential of health and well-being.

The chief diabetic complication in the foot is ulceration. It can become infected, gangrenous, and eventually require amputation. If ulceration appears, it should be treated immediately by a podiatrist. Proper care by the patient and nursing personnel can help eliminate diabetic complications.

The usual treatment involves several steps. The first is to cleanse the area to prevent infection. Ulcers usually appear on weight-bearing surfaces of the foot or on areas that undergo constant or intermittent friction. This friction and pressure must be relieved either by padding the area or prohibiting the patient from putting weight on the foot.

Next, the devitalized tissue must be removed so that good tissue is able to heal. Since diabetes causes a decrease in sensation debriding ulcerated areas is usually painless. Following this, a tissue stimulant is applied to form a granulation tissue and speed up the healing process. During healing, adequate blood flow to the area must be maintained and encouraged by keeping the area warm and very still, if possible. Treatment can include the use of plaster casting to immobilize the ulcerated area completely. This not only prevents weight bearing and friction, but restricts the edema that often causes an ulcer to remain open. Once an ulcer heals, the podiatrist should fabricate either an orthosis or a special shoe to prevent recurrences. Occasionally, if the cause of the ulcer was a bony prominence, surgical excision of the prominence may be indicated.

Another type of arterial disease that affects the lower extremities is arteriosclerosis obliterans. It is similar to arteriosclerosis and atherosclerosis in symptoms, but is more severe and more acutely painful. The deposits on the inner wall of a major artery cause an occlusion or blockage which reduces blood supply to the lower legs and feet. It is found predominantly in males between the ages of 50 and 70 years.

Intermittent claudication (mentioned earlier as pain and cramping of a calf muscle with exercise) is a major diagnostic sign in arteriosclerosis obliterans. In severe cases, there is also pain when resting or sleeping. The pain worsens as the occlusion grows larger. Pulses of the foot and leg are diminished or absent. Skin color may change to a dark red, especially in the toes. If the occlusion is acute and large, the affected foot may be very pale and appear smaller than the other. Severity of the disease can also be judged by changes in color when the foot is elevated. Abnormal loss of color on elevation and redness on lowering, with delayed return of color, are characteristic of occlusive arterial disease. The decreased blood flow to the foot often causes foot temperature to be abnormally low.

Small infections, such as ingrown toenails, which appear in patients with arteriosclerosis obliterans may develop into large ulcers, become gangrenous and require amputation. Advanced cases will also show osteoporosis, or bone demineralization, on x-ray.

Treatment of the disease is usually aimed toward increasing circulation to the affected limb by using heating elements, exercise to tolerance, and vasodilating drugs. In severe cases, surgery may be indicated. Surgery involves constructing a bypass graft which will circumvent the area of the blockage and restore adequate blood flow to the foot. This can be done, however, only if the arteries above and below the occlusion are open and have not been affected by the disease.

In arteriosclerosis obliterans, as in the other arterial diseases already described, the nursing staff must be aware of the potential complications and keep the patient as free as possible from adverse factors which might endanger him. The affected extremity must be protected at all times. It is essential that the leg and foot be observed daily for any signs of edema, redness, breakdown, infection, etc. The patient must be advised of the inherent dangers of his condition and instructed in the care of his problem.

In arteriosclerosis obliterans, long term survival of both the limb and the patient depends on the extent and rapidity of the occlusion. In a slow occlusive process, the vessels around the occlusion may have time to establish and continue uninterrupted blood flow. At the other extreme, a massive, rapid occlusion is a surgical emergency.

So far, this discussion has concentrated on arterial diseases characterized by a thickening of the inner vessel wall that reduces adequate blood flow. Another important vascular disorder that affects the lower leg and foot is varicose veins. Varicose veins are dilated, enlarged, and tortuous veins with defective valves that cause the vessels to swell and blood to pool within them.

The most common symptom is aching legs; this occurs in approximately 70 percent of all patients. When the veins become swollen and engorged with blood, they cause pain and a full feeling in the legs. Frequently, these veins will break, causing leakage of blood beneath the skin, more swelling, and more pain.

Varicosities in the elderly are especially harmful. If the veins are allowed to continue to expand, complications may arise. Among these are increased pigmentation, dermatitis, cellulitis, skin erosion and ulceration. Darkened skin is an indication of rupture of capillaries. Varicosities can cause dermatitis (skin eruptions) and, occasionally, ulcers on the lower leg and ankle. An inflammation of a vein with formation of a thrombus or clot may also occur. This is very dangerous. This clot may break away from the vein wall, work its way up the veins into a lung, and cause a pulmonary embolism, which could eventually lead to death.

The treatment of severe varicose veins consists of surgical removal. In some elderly debilitated patients, treatment may have to be more conservative. The vein may be injected with a sclerosing agent if the patient is able to tolerate it. Therapy in debilitated patients and in patients with less severe varicose veins may involve the use of elastic support stockings, which compress the engorged vein and allow muscle action to aid in moving the blood back up to the heart. Or, it may include elevating the leg above the level of the heart by placing it on pillows. Gravity then forces blood out of the engorged vessels and back toward the heart. Elevation can be periodic, but it is especially helpful in the afternoon or evening after the patient has had a lot of swelling. Walking is also therapeutic because it helps to force this blood up to the heart.

In LTC facilities, nursing staff must observe the patient with varicose veins and see that the legs are kept elevated, warpped in elastic stockings and ace bandages. The patient should also have frequent exercising walks. Again, the staff should be aware of possible dangerous complications and be on the lookout for them.

This lecture has contained an explanation of several common peripheral vascular diseases, their symptoms and their treatments. While much of the presentation has focused on the various diseases, the most important point to remember is that personnel in the LTC facility, because of their everyday contact with patients, are responsible for noting these conditions and preventing their complications.

In closing, several points should be reemphasized. Peripheral vascular disease can be one of the most devastating conditions affecting elderly patients. Those with vascular problems must be observed constantly for skin lesions, rashes, ulcerations, increases in pain or swelling, and changes in skin color or temperature. Those patients with arterial insufficiency, such as arteriosclerosis, atherosclerosis, or arteriosclerosis obliterans, must be watched for signs of ulceration and infection. Diabetics, too, require special care and attention. In all patients, complications may lead to gangrene and a possible need for amputation. The ultimate responsibility for observing the patient, identifying problems, and notifying the doctor of these problems is in the hands of the nursing staff and nursing aides.

GLOSSARY

Terms Used to Denote Location

Dorsum	The top surface of the foot	
Plantar	Pertaining to the sole of the foot	**Superior**
Medial	Middle, closer to the mid-line of the body	
Lateral	Side, a position away from the mid-line of the body	**Inferior**
Distal	Farthest from any point of reference (as opposed to proximal)	**Anterior**
Proximal	Nearest or closest to any	**Posterior**

point of reference (as opposed to distal)

Superior Situated above, a structure occupying a higher position

Inferior Situated below, a structure occupying the lowest position

Anterior Situated in front of or forward part of the body

Posterior Situated in back of or back part of the body

Anatomic Definitions

Bone	Substance that makes up the skeletal framework; gives the body form and rigidity
Ligament	Fibrous band of tissue that connects bones
Muscle	Organ attached to the

bones which, by contracting, provides movement of the body

Tendon Fibrous band of tissue that connects the muscles to the bones

Artery Tubular vessel that car-

ries the blood from the
heart to other parts of
the body

Vein   Tubular vessel that carries the blood from other
parts of the body back

Nerve   Cord-like structure that
conveys impulses be-
tween the brain and cen-
tral nervous system to
other parts of the body

to the heart

Other Terms

Abduction   To move away from a
center line (as if it is
drawn between the feet)

Abscess   Localized collection of
pus in a cavity

Achilles tendon   A tendon attached to the
posterior of the calca-
neus that flexes the foot

Adduction   To move toward a center
line (as if it is drawn be-
tween the feet)

Adhesion   Fibrous connection between two structures,
whether soft tissue or
hard, that may be a re-
sult of surgery, trauma
or infection

Amputation   Partial or total removal
of an extremity

Anatomy   Science of the structure
of the body and relation
of its parts

Anesthesia   Induced loss of feeling
or sensation to permit
surgery or other painful
procedures

Antibiotic   Chemical   substance
with the ability to inhibit
the growth of, or to de-
stroy, bacteria and other
microorganisms

Antiseptic   Substance that will inhibit the growth and de-
velopment of microor-
ganisms without neces-
sarily destroying them

Appliance   Mechanical device used
to support or align parts
of the body to facilitate
a particular function

Areolar tissue   Loose connective tissue

Arteriosclerosis   Hardening of the arteries

Arthrectomy   Excision of a joint by
surgical means

Arthritis   Inflammation of a joint;
there are many different
types due to different
causes

Atherosclerosis   Fatty   tissues   in   the
blood vessels

Arthrodesis   Surgical fixation of a
joint by fusion of the
joint surfaces

Arthrography   X-ray visualization and
recording of a joint by
introduction of contrast
media into the joint for
purposes of visualizing
the joint structures

Arthroplasty   Reconstruction or plastic repair of a joint with
the formation of a mov-
able joint

Articulation   Place of union or junc-
tion between two or
more bones of the skel-
eton

Aspiration   Withdrawal of fluid or
gas from a cavity or joint
space

Athlete's foot   Layman's term for fungus infection of the foot

Atrophy   Defect or wasting away
or diminution in size of
cells, tissues or organs

Avulsion   Forceable removal of
some part or all of a
toenail

Balanced inlay   Flexible support worn in
a shoe to balance weight
and structure of the foot

Bar   Build-up on the exterior
of the sole of a shoe to
control distribution of
weight of the foot

Bunion   Swelling of the outer
side of the ball of the
great toe, with a thick-
ening of the overlaying

skin and forcing of the toe inward toward the lesser toes

Bunionectomy Excision of a bunion by arthroplasty of the metatarsophalangeal joint

Bunionette Bunion-like enlargement of the joint of the little toe due to pressure over the lateral surface of the foot

Bursa Sac or sac-like cavity filled with a fluid and situated at places in the area at which friction would otherwise develop

Callosity Circumscribed thickening of the skin; hypertrophy of the horny layer, from friction, pressure or other irritations

Callous (callus) Same as callosity; also used to describe the healing following the fracture of a bone

Calvus molle Soft corn found between the toes, also referred to as heloma molle

Cautery Application of burning agent (chemical or electrical), cold (as produced by carbon dioxide), actual cautery (as fire or actual burning), potential cautery (as by escharotic agent without applying heat)

Chemosurgery Surgical removal of diseased or unwanted tissue by application of caustic chemicals

Clubfoot Congenital deformity of the foot with multiple abnormalities

Collateral ligament Ligament connecting one bone to another across joint spaces

Contracted toe Also called hammer toes, toe bent upward at the middle joint

Corn Horny induration and thickening of the skin, produced by friction and pressure, producing pain and irritation

Cryocautery Destruction of tissue by application of extreme cold

Cyst Pouch or sac, normal or abnormal, especially one that contains liquid or semi-solid material

Debridement Surgical removal of foreign material or devitalized tissue from an area

Dermatological Having to do with skin

Dermatomycosis A superficial infection of the skin or its appendages by a fungi

Dermatophytosis (Tinea pedis) Same as dermatomycosis, but more often used to specifically designate infection of the skin of the feet

Diabetes Deficiency condition marked by excessive quantity of discharge of urine; diabetes mellitus, the most common form, is a metabolic disorder usually due to faulty pancreas, thus producing high blood sugar with resulting sugar in the urine. Condition usually manifested in lower extremities in addition to elsewhere in body.

Dorsalis pedis pulse Pulse on top of the foot

Dorsiflexion Backward bending or flexation, as of the hand or foot

Eczema An inflammatory condition of the skin

Edema Swelling, the presence of an abnormally large amount of fluid in body tissues

Erythema Redness of the skin produced by congestion of the capillaries

Exostoses Bony growth projecting outward from the bone surface

Extensor Muscle or tendon on the

Fascia — dorsum of the foot that bends the foot, or part of the foot, up toward the leg

Fascia — A sheet or band of fibrous tissue

Fibroma — Tumor composed mainly of fibrous or fully developed connective tissues

Fissure — Any crack, cleft or groove, normal or otherwise, in skin of the foot—usually the heel

Flatfoot — Flattening of the arch

Flexor — Muscle that bends a limb or part (as opposed to an extensor)

Footstrain — Strain or stretching of muscles and ligaments of the foot

Functional insole — Lightweight thin appliance to accommodate minor foot problems

Ganglion — Cyst of a joint capsule, tendon sheath or aponeurosis

Gangrene — An eating sore which ends in mortification

Granulation tissue — Abnormal growth of tissue associated with inflammation and healing

Hallux — Great toe or first digit of the foot

Heloma — Corn of the foot

Hematoma — Localized collection of blood

Hydrotherapy — Use of water for therapeutic purposes

Inflammation — Condition into which tissues enter as a reaction to injury or disease

Ingrown nail — Nail that breaks through the skin or tissue causing pain

Metatarsal — One of the long bones of the foot

Metatarsalgia — Pain in metatarsal area

Mycotic — Infection caused by a fungus

Neoplasm — A new growth of tissue (tumor) serving no physiological function

Neuralgia — Condition of pain along the course of a nerve

Neuritis — Inflammation of a nerve

Neuroma — A nerve tumor

Onychectomy — Surgical removal of a nail

Onychia — Inflammation or infection of nail matrix resulting in loss of the nail

Onycho — Combining word form denoting relationship to the nails

Onychocryptosis — Ingrown nail

Orthodigita — Correcting deformities of the toes and fingers

Orthomechano-therapy — Treatment of foot and ankle problems with mechanical devices

Orthosis — An orthopedic appliance or apparatus used to support, align, prevent or correct deformities

Os — Bone

Ossification — Formation of bone, conversion of fibrous tissue or cartilage into bone

Osteoarthritis — Chronic multiple degenerative joint disease

Osteochronditis — Inflammation of both bone and cartilage

Osteoma — Tumor of bone

Osteomyelitis — Infection and inflammation of the bone marrow

Osteotomy — Surgical cutting of a bone

Palliative — Affording relief, but not a cure

Pes cavus — Exaggerated height of long arch of the foot

Pes planus — Deformed foot structure in which the bones of long arch have been altered to lower position

Phalangeal — Phalanx bones

Plates — Foot orthoses, rigid types used for correction, stabilization and gait training of the foot

Posterior tibial pulse — Pulse in the foot located at the inside of ankle

Pronation — Result of a combination of factors in the tarsal and metatarsal areas of the foot that lowers the arch and allows the forefoot to splay or turn

	outward from the mid-line of the body
Sesamoid	Small bone usually located beneath the head of the first metatarsal bone
Sprain	Joint injury where the supporting ligaments are stretched or ruptured, but the continuity of the ligaments remains intact
Spur	Projecting body, as from a bone
Strain	Overstretching of the muscles due to excessive effort or undue exercise
Subluxation	Partial dislocation of a bone
Subungual	Beneath the nail
Syndactylism	Condition in which two or more digits are fused together; also referred to as web toes
Tarsal bone	Of or pertaining to a bone in the tarsal region of the foot
Tarsal joint	Of or pertaining to the articulation between tarsal bones
Tarsus	Bone of the rear and midfoot, comprised of seven bones called tarsal bones
Tendo-Achilles	Tendon that connects the posterior calf muscles to the heel bone, the thickest and strongest tendon in the body
Tenotomy	Surgical incision of a tendon
Tibialis anterior	Leg muscle attached to the foot which pulls the foot inward
Tyloma	Callous of the foot

Ulcer	Open sore on the skin or mucous surface of a body organ, characterized by gradual disintegration and necrosis of tissues
Ungual	Pertaining to nails
Valgus	Eversion or turning out of the plantar aspect of the toes or foot
Varicose	Unnaturally swollen or enlarged and tortuous, as a vein, artery or lymphatic vessel
Varus	Inversion or turning up of the plantar aspect of toes or foot
Verruca	Wart, tumorous growth of the skin caused by a virus

Selected Readings

American Podiatry Association, Audio-visual informational and educational materials, Catalogue, 1976.

American Podiatry Association, Foot Health and Aging, pamphlet. Washington, D. C., 1976.

American Podiatry Association, Foot Health Literature and Material, catalogue. Washington, D. C., 1976.

American Podiatry Association, Podiatrist Services Under Medicare, pamphlet, Washington, D. C., February, 1977.

American Podiatry Association, Podiatry in Today's Hospital. Washington, D. C., October 1973.

Department of Health, Education and Welfare, Medicaid Regulation Summary Chart Pertaining to Individual States, Washington, D. C., June 1, 1976.

LeBendig, M., Diamond, E., A Podiatric Resource Guide for Preventive and Rehabilitation Foot and Leg Care. Futura Publishing Co., Mt. Kisco, New York, 1976.

Loche, R., Minnell, J., Sgarlato, T., Foot Complaints—Doctor My Feet Are Killing Me. Patient Care, Vol. IX, No. 6, March 15, 1975.

O'Brien, D., This Team Keeps Patients on Their Feet. Modern Nursing Home Administrator, Vol. 21, July/August 1967.

Working With Older People, A Guide to Practice, Volume IV, Clinical Aspects of Aging, Section C., part XX, Podiatry. U.S. Department of Health, Education and Welfare, Public Health Service.

Index